Color Atlas of Pharmacology

2nd edition, revised and expanded

Heinz Lüllmann, M. D.
Professor Emeritus
Department of Pharmacology
University of Kiel
Germany

Albrecht Ziegler, Ph. D.
Professor
Department of Pharmacology
University of Kiel
Germany

Klaus Mohr, M. D.
Professor
Department of Pharmacology
and Toxicology
Institute of Pharmacy
University of Bonn
Germany

Detlef Bieger, M. D.
Professor
Division of Basic Medical Sciences
Faculty of Medicine
Memorial University of
Newfoundland
St. John's, Newfoundland
Canada

164 color plates by Jürgen Wirth

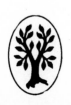

Thieme
Stuttgart · New York · 2000

Library of Congress Cataloging-in-Publication Data

Taschenatlas der Pharmakologie. English.
    Color atlas of pharmacology / Heinz Lullmann ... [et al.] ; color plates by Jurgen Wirth. — 2nd ed., rev. and expanded.
    p. cm.
    Rev. and expanded translation of: Taschenatlas der Pharmakologie. 3rd ed. 1996.
    Includes bibliographical references and indexes.
    ISBN 3-13-781702-1 (GTV). — ISBN 0-86577-843-4 (TNY)
    1. Pharmacology Atlases.   2. Pharmacology Handbooks, manuals, etc.
I. Lullmann, Heinz.   II. Title.
    [DNLM: 1. Pharmacology Atlases.   2. Pharmacology Handbooks.   QV
17 T197c 1999a]
    RM301.12.T3813   1999
    615'.1—dc21
    DNLM/DLC
for Library of Congress   99-33662
                                                                 CIP

Illustrated by Jürgen Wirth, Darmstadt, Germany

This book is an authorized revised and expanded translation of the 3rd German edition published and copyrighted 1996 by Georg Thieme Verlag, Stuttgart, Germany. Title of the German edition:
Taschenatlas der Pharmakologie

©2000 Georg Thieme Verlag, Rüdigerstrasse 14, D-70469 Stuttgart, Germany
Thieme New York, 333 Seventh Avenue, New York, NY 10001, USA

Typesetting by Gulde Druck, Tübingen
Printed in Germany by Staudigl, Donauwörth

ISBN 3-13-781702-1 (GTV)
ISBN 0-86577-843-4 (TNY)   1 2 3 4 5 6

Important Note: Medicine is an ever-changing science undergoing continual development. Research and clinical experience are continually expanding our knowledge, in particular our knowledge of proper treatment and drug therapy. Insofar as this book mentions any dosage or application, readers may rest assured that the authors, editors and publishers have made every effort to ensure that such references are in accordance **with the state of knowledge at the time of production of the book.**

Nevertheless this does not involve, imply, or express any guarantee or responsibility on the part of the publishers in respect of any dosage instructions and forms of application stated in the book. **Every user is requested to** examine carefully the manufacturers' leaflets accompanying each drug and to check, if necessary in consultation with a physician or specialist, whether the dosage schedules mentioned therein or the contraindications stated by the manufacturers differ from the statements made in the present book. Such examination is particularly important with drugs that are either rarely used or have been newly released on the market. **Every dosage schedule or every form of application used is entirely at the user's own risk and responsibility.** The authors and publishers request every user to report to the publishers any discrepancies or inaccuracies noticed.

Preface

The present second edition of the Color Atlas of Pharmacology goes to print six years after the first edition. Numerous revisions were needed, highlighting the dramatic continuing progress in the drug sciences. In particular, it appeared necessary to include novel therapeutic principles, such as the inhibitors of platelet aggregation from the group of integrin GPIIB/IIIA antagonists, the inhibitors of viral protease, or the non-nucleoside inhibitors of reverse transcriptase. Moreover, the re-evaluation and expanded use of conventional drugs, e.g., in congestive heart failure, bronchial asthma, or rheumatoid arthritis, had to be addressed. In each instance, the primary emphasis was placed on essential sites of action and basic pharmacological principles. Details and individual drug properties were deliberately omitted in the interest of making drug action more transparent and affording an overview of the pharmacological basis of drug therapy.

The authors wish to reiterate that the Color Atlas of Pharmacology cannot replace a textbook of pharmacology, nor does it aim to do so. Rather, this little book is designed to arouse the curiosity of the pharmacological novice; to help students of medicine and pharmacy gain an overview of the discipline and to review certain bits of information in a concise format; and, finally, to enable the experienced therapist to recall certain factual data, with perhaps some occasional amusement.

Our cordial thanks go to the many readers of the multilingual editions of the Color Atlas for their suggestions. We are indebted to Prof. Ulrike Holzgrabe, Würzburg, Doc. Achim Meißner, Kiel, Prof. Gert-Hinrich Reil, Oldenburg, Prof. Reza Tabrizchi, St. John's, Mr Christian Klein, Bonn, and Mr Christian Riedel, Kiel, for providing stimulating and helpful discussions and technical support, as well as to Dr. Liane Platt-Rohloff, Stuttgart, and Dr. David Frost, New York, for their editorial and stylistic guidance.

Heinz Lüllmann
Klaus Mohr
Albrecht Ziegler
Detlef Bieger
Jürgen Wirth

Fall 1999

Contents

VIII Contents

General Pharmacology

History of Pharmacology

Since time immemorial, medicaments have been used for treating disease in humans and animals. The herbals of antiquity describe the therapeutic powers of certain plants and minerals. Belief in the curative powers of plants and certain substances rested exclusively upon traditional knowledge, that is, empirical information not subjected to critical examination.

The Idea

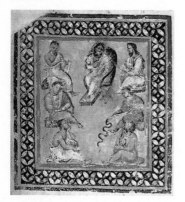

Claudius Galen (129–200 A.D.) first attempted to consider the theoretical background of pharmacology. Both theory and practical experience were to contribute equally to the rational use of medicines through interpretation of observed and experienced results.
"The empiricists say that all is found by experience. We, however, maintain that it is found in part by experience, in part by theory. Neither experience nor theory alone is apt to discover all."

The Impetus

Theophrastus von Hohenheim (1493–1541 A.D.), called Paracelsus, began to quesiton doctrines handed down from antiquity, demanding knowledge of the active ingredient(s) in prescribed remedies, while rejecting the irrational concoctions and mixtures of medieval med-

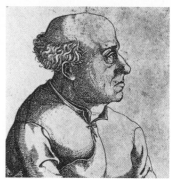

icine. He prescribed chemically defined substances with such success that professional enemies had him prosecuted as a poisoner. Against such accusations, he defended himself with the thesis that has become an axiom of pharmacology:
"If you want to explain any poison properly, what then isn't a poison? All things are poison, nothing is without poison; the dose alone causes a thing not to be poison."

Early Beginnings

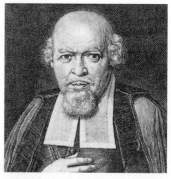

Johann Jakob Wepfer (1620–1695) was the first to verify by animal experimentation assertions about pharmacological or toxicological actions.
"I pondered at length. Finally I resolved to clarify the matter by experiments."

Foundation

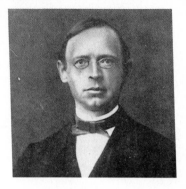

Rudolf Buchheim (1820–1879) founded the first institute of pharmacology at the University of Dorpat (Tartu, Estonia) in 1847, ushering in pharmacology as an independent scientific discipline. In addition to a description of effects, he strove to explain the chemical properties of drugs.

"The science of medicines is a theoretical, i.e., explanatory, one. It is to provide us with knowledge by which our judgement about the utility of medicines can be validated at the bedside."

Consolidation – General Recognition

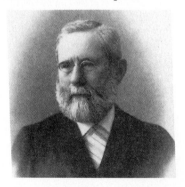

Oswald Schmiedeberg (1838–1921), together with his many disciples (12 of whom were appointed to chairs of pharmacology), helped to establish the high reputation of pharmacology. Fundamental concepts such as structure-activity relationship, drug receptor, and selective toxicity emerged from the work of, respectively, T. Frazer (1841–1921) in Scotland, J. Langley (1852–1925) in England, and P. Ehrlich (1854–1915) in Germany. Alexander J. Clark (1885–1941) in England first formalized receptor theory in the early 1920s by applying the Law of Mass Action to drug-receptor interactions. Together with the internist, Bernhard Naunyn (1839–1925), Schmiedeberg founded the first journal of pharmacology, which has since been published without interruption. The "Father of American Pharmacology", John J. Abel (1857–1938) was among the first Americans to train in Schmiedeberg's laboratory and was founder of the *Journal of Pharmacology and Experimental Therapeutics* (published from 1909 until the present).

Status Quo

After 1920, pharmacological laboratories sprang up in the pharmaceutical industry, outside established university institutes. After 1960, departments of clinical pharmacology were set up at many universities and in industry.

Drug and Active Principle

Until the end of the 19th century, medicines were natural organic or inorganic products, mostly dried, but also fresh, plants or plant parts. These might contain substances possessing healing (therapeutic) properties or substances exerting a toxic effect.

In order to secure a supply of medically useful products not merely at the time of harvest but year-round, plants were preserved by drying or soaking them in vegetable oils or alcohol. Drying the plant or a vegetable or animal product yielded a **drug** (from French "drogue" – dried herb). Colloquially, this term nowadays often refers to chemical substances with high potential for physical dependence and abuse. Used scientifically, this term implies nothing about the quality of action, if any. In its original, wider sense, drug could refer equally well to the dried leaves of peppermint, dried lime blossoms, dried flowers and leaves of the female cannabis plant (hashish, marijuana), or the dried milky exudate obtained by slashing the unripe seed capsules of *Papaver somniferum* (**raw opium**). Nowadays, the term is applied quite generally to a chemical substance that is used for pharmacotherapy.

Soaking plants parts in alcohol (ethanol) creates a **tincture**. In this process, pharmacologically active constituents of the plant are extracted by the alcohol. Tinctures do not contain the complete spectrum of substances that exist in the plant or crude drug, only those that are soluble in alcohol. In the case of opium tincture, these ingredients are **alkaloids** (i.e., basic substances of plant origin) including: morphine, codeine, narcotine = noscapine, papaverine, narceine, and others.

Using a natural product or extract to treat a disease thus usually entails the administration of a number of substances possibly possessing very different activities. Moreover, the dose of an individual constituent contained within a given amount of the natural product is subject to large variations, depending upon the product's geographical origin (biotope), time of harvesting, or conditions and length of storage. For the same reasons, the relative proportion of individual constituents may vary considerably. Starting with the extraction of morphine from opium in 1804 by F. W. Sertürner (1783–1841), the active principles of many other natural products were subsequently isolated in chemically pure form by pharmaceutical laboratories.

The aims of isolating active principles are:

1. Identification of the active ingredient(s).
2. Analysis of the biological effects (pharmacodynamics) of individual ingredients and of their fate in the body (pharmacokinetics).
3. Ensuring a precise and constant dosage in the therapeutic use of chemically pure constituents.
4. The possibility of chemical synthesis, which would afford independence from limited natural supplies and create conditions for the analysis of structure-activity relationships.

Finally, derivatives of the original constituent may be synthesized in an effort to optimize pharmacological properties. Thus, derivatives of the original constituent with improved therapeutic usefulness may be developed.

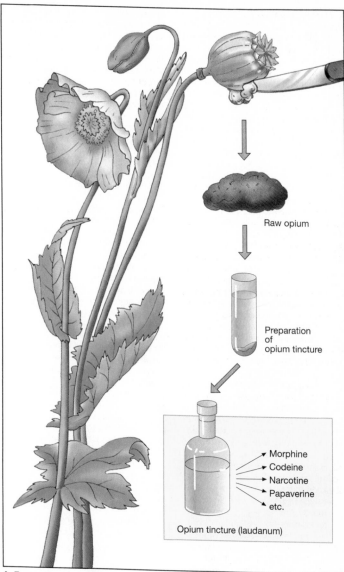

Raw opium

Preparation
of
opium tincture

Morphine
Codeine
Narcotine
Papaverine
etc.

Opium tincture (laudanum)

A. From poppy to morphine

Drug Development

This process starts with the **synthesis** of novel chemical compounds. Substances with complex structures may be obtained from various sources, e.g., plants (cardiac glycosides), animal tissues (heparin), microbial cultures (penicillin G), or human cells (urokinase), or by means of gene technology (human insulin). As more insight is gained into structure-activity relationships, the search for new agents becomes more clearly focused.

Preclinical testing yields information on the biological effects of new substances. Initial screening may employ *biochemical-pharmacological investigations* (e.g., receptor-binding assays p. 56) or experiments on cell cultures, isolated cells, and isolated organs. Since these models invariably fall short of replicating complex biological processes in the intact organism, any potential drug must be tested in the whole animal. Only animal experiments can reveal whether the desired effects will actually occur at dosages that produce little or no toxicity. *Toxicological investigations* serve to evaluate the potential for: (1) toxicity associated with acute or chronic administration; (2) genetic damage (genotoxicity, mutagenicity); (3) production of tumors (onco- or carcinogenicity); and (4) causation of birth defects (teratogenicity). In animals, compounds under investigation also have to be studied with respect to their absorption, distribution, metabolism, and elimination *(pharmacokinetics)*. Even at the level of preclinical testing, only a very small fraction of new compounds will prove potentially fit for use in humans.

Pharmaceutical technology provides the methods for drug formulation.

Clinical testing starts with **Phase I** studies on healthy subjects and seeks to determine whether effects observed in animal experiments also occur in humans. Dose-response relationships are determined. In **Phase II**, potential drugs re first tested on selected patients for therapeutic efficacy in those disease states for which they are intended. Should a beneficial action be evident and the incidence of adverse effects be acceptably small, **Phase III** is entered, involving a larger group of patients in whom the new drug will be compared with standard treatments in terms of therapeutic outcome. As a form of human experimentation, these clinical trials are subject to review and approval by institutional ethics committees according to international codes of conduct (Declarations of Helsinki, Tokyo, and Venice). During clinical testing, many drugs are revealed to be unusable. Ultimately, only one new drug remains from approximately 10,000 newly synthesized substances.

The decision to **approve a new drug** is made by a national regulatory body (Food & Drug Administration in the U.S.A., the Health Protection Branch Drugs Directorate in Canada, UK, Europe, Australia) to which manufacturers are required to submit their applications. Applicants must document by means of appropriate test data (from preclinical and clinical trials) that the criteria of efficacy and safety have been met and that product forms (tablet, capsule, etc.) satisfy general standards of quality control.

Following approval, the new drug may be marketed under a trade name (p. 333) and thus become available for prescription by physicians and dispensing by pharmacists. As the drug gains more widespread use, regulatory surveillance continues in the form of post-licensing studies (**Phase IV** of clinical trials). Only on the basis of long-term experience will the risk: benefit ratio be properly assessed and, thus, the therapeutic value of the new drug be determined.

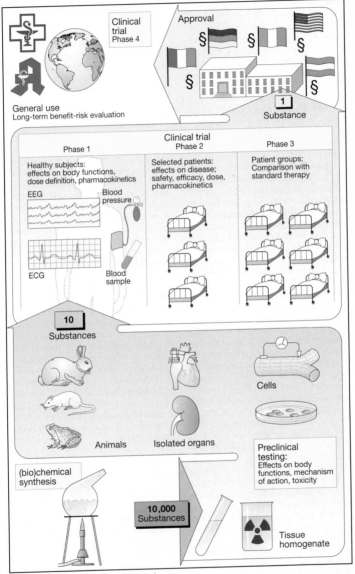

A. From drug synthesis to approval

Dosage Forms for Oral, Ocular, and Nasal Applications

A medicinal agent becomes a medication only after formulation suitable for therapeutic use (i.e., in an appropriate **dosage form**). The dosage form takes into account the intended mode of use and also ensures ease of handling (e.g., stability, precision of dosing) by patients and physicians. *Pharmaceutical technology* is concerned with the design of suitable product formulations and quality control.

Liquid preparations (A) may take the form of **solutions, suspensions** (a sol or mixture consisting of small water-insoluble solid drug particles dispersed in water), or **emulsions** (dispersion of minute droplets of a liquid agent or a drug solution in another fluid, e.g., oil in water). Since storage will cause sedimentation of suspensions and separation of emulsions, solutions are generally preferred. In the case of poorly watersoluble substances, solution is often accomplished by adding ethanol (or other solvents); thus, there are both *aqueous* and *alcoholic solutions*. These solutions are made available to patients in specially designed drop bottles, enabling single doses to be measured exactly in terms of a defined number of drops, the size of which depends on the area of the drip opening at the bottle mouth and on the viscosity and surface tension of the solution. The advantage of a drop solution is that the dose, that is, the number of drops, can be precisely adjusted to the patient's need. Its disadvantage lies in the difficulty that some patients, disabled by disease or age, will experience in measuring a prescribed number of drops.

When the drugs are dissolved in a larger volume — as in the case of *syrups or mixtures* — the single dose is measured with a measuring spoon. Dosing may also be done with the aid of a tablespoon or teaspoon (approx. 15 and 5 ml, respectively). However, due to the wide variation in the size of commercially available spoons, dosing will not be very precise. (Standardized medicinal teaspoons and tablespoons are available.)

Eye drops and **nose drops** (A) are designed for application to the mucosal surfaces of the eye (conjunctival sac) and nasal cavity, respectively. In order to prolong contact time, nasal drops are formulated as solutions of increased viscosity.

Solid dosage forms include **tablets**, **coated tablets**, and **capsules** (B). **Tablets** have a disk-like shape, produced by mechanical compression of active substance, filler (e.g., lactose, calcium sulfate), binder, and auxiliary material (excipients). The filler provides bulk enough to make the tablet easy to handle and swallow. It is important to consider that the individual dose of many drugs lies in the range of a few milligrams or less. In order to convey the idea of a 10-mg weight, two squares are marked below, the paper mass of each weighing 10 mg. Disintegration of the tablet can be hastened by the use of dried starch, which swells on contact with water, or of $NaHCO_3$, which releases CO_2 gas on contact with gastric acid. Auxiliary materials are important with regard to tablet production, shelf life, palatability, and identifiability (color).

Effervescent tablets (compressed effervescent powders) do not represent a solid dosage form, because they are dissolved in water immediately prior to ingestion and are, thus, actually liquid preparations.

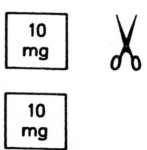

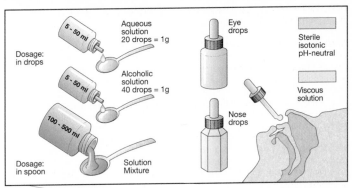

A. Liquid preparations

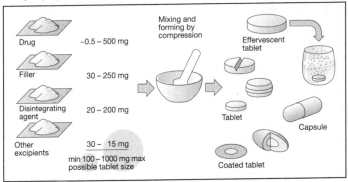

B. Solid preparations for oral application

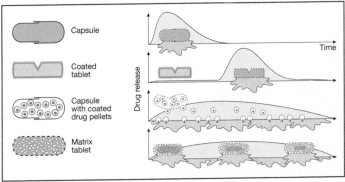

C. Dosage forms controlling rate of drug dissolution

The **coated tablet** contains a drug within a core that is covered by a shell, e.g., a wax coating, that serves to: (1) protect perishable drugs from decomposing; (2) mask a disagreeable taste or odor; (3) facilitate passage on swallowing; or (4) permit color coding.

Capsules usually consist of an oblong casing — generally made of gelatin — that contains the drug in powder or granulated form (See. p. 9, C).

In the case of the **matrix-type** tablet, the drug is embedded in an inert meshwork from which it is released by diffusion upon being moistened. In contrast to *solutions,* which permit direct absorption of drug (**A**, track 3), the use of solid dosage forms initially requires *tablets* to break up and *capsules* to open (**disintegration**) before the drug can be dissolved (**dissolution**) and pass through the gastrointestinal mucosal lining (**absorption**). Because disintegration of the tablet and dissolution of the drug take time, absorption will occur mainly in the intestine (**A**, track 2). In the case of a solution, absorption starts in the stomach (**A**, track 3).

For acid-labile drugs, a coating of wax or of a cellulose acetate polymer is used to prevent disintegration of solid dosage forms in the stomach. Accordingly, disintegration and dissolution will take place in the duodenum at normal speed (**A**, track 1) and drug liberation *per se* is not retarded.

The **liberation of drug**, hence the site and time-course of absorption, are subject to modification by appropriate production methods for matrix-type tablets, coated tablets, and capsules. In the case of the matrix tablet, the drug is incorporated into a lattice from which it can be slowly leached out by gastrointestinal fluids. As the matrix tablet undergoes enteral transit, drug liberation and absorption proceed en route (**A**, track 4). In the case of coated tablets, coat thickness can be designed such that release and absorption of drug occur either in the proximal (**A**, track 1) or distal (**A**, track 5) bowel. Thus, by matching dissolution time with small-bowel transit time, drug release can be timed to occur in the colon.

Drug liberation and, hence, absorption can also be spread out when the drug is presented in the form of a granulate consisting of pellets coated with a waxy film of graded thickness. Depending on film thickness, gradual dissolution occurs during enteral transit, releasing drug at variable rates for absorption. The principle illustrated for a *capsule* can also be applied to tablets. In this case, either drug pellets coated with films of various thicknesses are compressed into a tablet or the drug is incorporated into a *matrix-type tablet.* Contrary to timed-release capsules (Spansules®), *slow-release tablets* have the advantage of being dividable *ad libitum;* thus, fractions of the dose contained within the entire tablet may be administered.

This kind of **retarded drug release** is employed when a rapid rise in blood level of drug is undesirable, or when absorption is being slowed in order to prolong the action of drugs that have a short sojourn in the body.

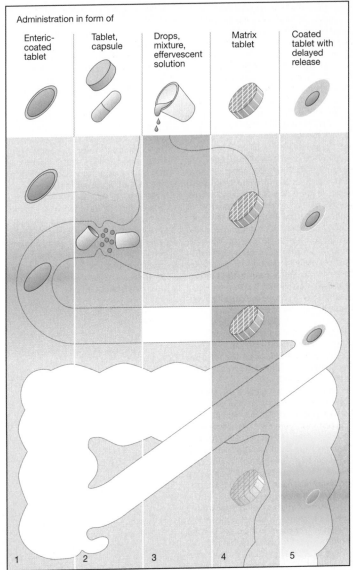

Administration in form of

| Enteric-coated tablet | Tablet, capsule | Drops, mixture, effervescent solution | Matrix tablet | Coated tablet with delayed release |

1   2   3   4   5

A. Oral administration: drug release and absorption

Dosage Forms for Parenteral (1), Pulmonary (2), Rectal or Vaginal (3), and Cutaneous Application

Drugs need not always be administered **orally** (i.e., by swallowing), but may also be given **parenterally**. This route usually refers to an injection, although enteral absorption is also bypassed when drugs are inhaled or applied to the skin.

For intravenous, intramuscular, or subcutaneous injections, drugs are often given as solutions and, less frequently, in crystalline suspension for intramuscular, subcutaneous, or intraarticular injection. An **injectable solution** must be free of infectious agents, pyrogens, or suspended matter. It should have the same osmotic pressure and pH as body fluids in order to avoid tissue damage at the site of injection. Solutions for injection are preserved in airtight glass or plastic sealed containers. From **ampules for multiple or single use**, the solution is aspirated via a needle into a syringe. The **cartridge ampule** is fitted into a special injector that enables its contents to be emptied via a needle. An infusion refers to a solution being administered over an extended period of time. **Solutions for infusion** must meet the same standards as solutions for injection.

Drugs can be sprayed in **aerosol** form onto mucosal surfaces of body cavities accessible from the outside (e.g., the respiratory tract [p. 14]). An aerosol is a dispersion of liquid or solid particles in a gas, such as air. An aerosol results when a drug solution or micronized powder is reduced to a spray on being driven through the nozzle of a pressurized container.

Mucosal application of drug via the rectal or vaginal route is achieved by means of **suppositories** and **vaginal tablets,** respectively. On rectal application, absorption into the systemic circulation may be intended. With vaginal tablets, the effect is generally confined to the site of application. Usually the drug is incorporated into a fat that solidifies at room temperature, but melts in the rectum or vagina. The resulting oily film spreads over the mucosa and enables the drug to pass into the mucosa.

Powders, ointments, and **pastes** (p. 16) are applied to the skin surface. In many cases, these do not contain drugs but are used for skin protection or care. However, drugs may be added if a topical action on the outer skin or, more rarely, a systemic effect is intended.

Transdermal drug delivery systems are pasted to the epidermis. They contain a reservoir from which drugs may diffuse and be absorbed through the skin. They offer the advantage that a drug depot is attached noninvasively to the body, enabling the drug to be administered in a manner similar to an infusion. Drugs amenable to this type of delivery must: (1) be capable of penetrating the cutaneous barrier; (2) be effective in very small doses (restricted capacity of reservoir); and (3) possess a wide therapeutic margin (dosage not adjustable).

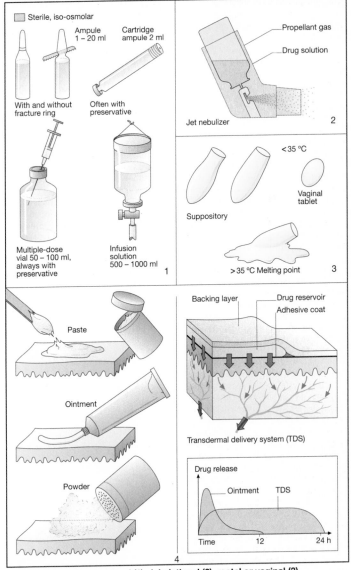

☐ Sterile, iso-osmolar

Ampule 1 – 20 ml

Cartridge ampule 2 ml

With and without fracture ring

Often with preservative

Multiple-dose vial 50 – 100 ml, always with preservative

Infusion solution 500 – 1000 ml

1

Propellant gas

Drug solution

Jet nebulizer

2

< 35 °C

Vaginal tablet

Suppository

> 35 °C Melting point

3

Paste

Ointment

Powder

Backing layer

Drug reservoir

Adhesive coat

Transdermal delivery system (TDS)

Drug release

Ointment TDS

Time 12 24 h

4

A. Preparations for parenteral (1), inhalational (2), rectal or vaginal (3), and percutaneous (4) application

Drug Administration by Inhalation

Inhalation in the form of an aerosol (p. 12), a gas, or a mist permits drugs to be applied to the bronchial mucosa and, to a lesser extent, to the alveolar membranes. This route is chosen for drugs intended to affect bronchial smooth muscle or the consistency of bronchial mucus. Furthermore, gaseous or volatile agents can be administered by inhalation with the goal of alveolar absorption and systemic effects (e.g., inhalational anesthetics, p. 218). **Aerosols** are formed when a drug solution or micronized powder is converted into a mist or dust, respectively.

In conventional sprays (e.g., nebulizer), the air blast required for aerosol formation is generated by the stroke of a pump. Alternatively, the drug is delivered from a solution or powder packaged in a pressurized canister equipped with a valve through which a metered dose is discharged. During use, the inhaler (spray dispenser) is held directly in front of the mouth and actuated at the start of inspiration. The effectiveness of delivery depends on the position of the device in front of the mouth, the size of aerosol particles, and the coordination between opening of the spray valve and inspiration. The size of aerosol particles determines the speed at which they are swept along by inhaled air, hence the **depth of penetration into the respiratory tract.** Particles > 100 μm in diameter are trapped in the oropharyngeal cavity; those having diameters between 10 and 60 μm will be deposited on the epithelium of the bronchial tract. Particles < 2 μm in diameter can reach the alveoli, but they will be largely exhaled because of their low tendency to impact on the alveolar epithelium.

Drug deposited on the mucous lining of the bronchial epithelium is partly absorbed and partly transported with bronchial mucus towards the larynx. Bronchial mucus travels upwards due to the orally directed undulatory beat of the epithelial cilia. Physiologically, this mucociliary transport functions to remove inspired dust particles. Thus, only a portion of the drug aerosol (~ 10%) gains access to the respiratory tract and just a fraction of this amount penetrates the mucosa, whereas the remainder of the aerosol undergoes mucociliary transport to the laryngopharynx and is swallowed. The advantage of inhalation (i.e., localized application) is fully exploited by using drugs that are poorly absorbed from the intestine (isoproterenol, ipratropium, cromolyn) or are subject to first-pass elimination (p. 42; beclomethasone dipropionate, budesonide, flunisolide, fluticasone dipropionate).

Even when the swallowed portion of an inhaled drug is absorbed in unchanged form, administration by this route has the advantage that drug concentrations at the bronchi will be higher than in other organs.

The efficiency of mucociliary transport depends on the force of kinociliary motion and the viscosity of bronchial mucus. Both factors can be altered pathologically (e.g., in smoker's cough, bronchitis) or can be adversely affected by drugs (atropine, antihistamines).

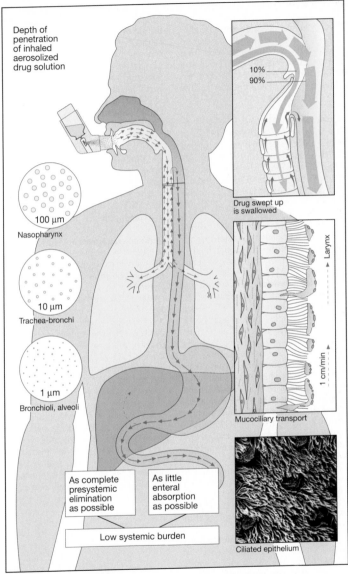

Depth of penetration of inhaled aerosolized drug solution

10%
90%

Drug swept up is swallowed

100 µm
Nasopharynx

10 µm
Trachea-bronchi

1 µm
Bronchioli, alveoli

Larynx

1 cm/min

Mucociliary transport

As complete presystemic elimination as possible

As little enteral absorption as possible

Low systemic burden

Ciliated epithelium

A. Application by inhalation

Dermatologic Agents

Pharmaceutical preparations applied to the outer skin are intended either to provide skin care and protection from noxious influences (A), or to serve as a vehicle for drugs that are to be absorbed into the skin or, if appropriate, into the general circulation (B).

Skin Protection (A)

Protective agents are of several kinds to meet different requirements according to skin condition (dry, low in oil, chapped vs moist, oily, elastic), and the type of noxious stimuli (prolonged exposure to water, regular use of alcohol-containing disinfectants [p. 290], intense solar irradiation).

Distinctions among protective agents are based upon consistency, physicochemical properties (lipophilic, hydrophilic), and the presence of additives.

Dusting Powders are sprinkled onto the intact skin and consist of talc, magnesium stearate, silicon dioxide (silica), or starch. They adhere to the skin, forming a low-friction film that attenuates mechanical irritation. Powders exert a drying (evaporative) effect.

Lipophilic ointment (oil ointment) consists of a lipophilic base (paraffin oil, petroleum jelly, wool fat [lanolin]) and may contain up to 10% powder materials, such as zinc oxide, titanium oxide, starch, or a mixture of these. Emulsifying ointments are made of paraffins and an emulsifying wax, and are miscible with water.

Paste (oil paste) is an ointment containing more than 10% pulverized constituents.

Lipophilic (oily) cream is an emulsion of water in oil, easier to spread than oil paste or oil ointments.

Hydrogel and water-soluble ointment achieve their consistency by means of different gel-forming agents (gelatin, methylcellulose, polyethylene glycol). **Lotions** are aqueous suspensions of water-insoluble and solid constituents.

Hydrophilic (aqueous) cream is an emulsion of an oil in water formed with the aid of an emulsifier; it may also be considered an oil-in-water emulsion of an emulsifying ointment.

All dermatologic agents having a lipophilic base adhere to the skin as a water-repellent coating. They do not wash off and they also prevent (**occlude**) outward passage of water from the skin. The skin is protected from drying, and its hydration and elasticity increase.

Diminished evaporation of water results in warming of the occluded skin area. Hydrophilic agents wash off easily and do not impede transcutaneous output of water. Evaporation of water is felt as a cooling effect.

Dermatologic Agents as Vehicles (B)

In order to reach its site of action, a drug (D) must leave its pharmaceutical preparation and enter the skin, if a local effect is desired (e.g., glucocorticoid ointment), or be able to penetrate it, if a systemic action is intended (transdermal delivery system, e.g., nitroglycerin patch, p. 120). The tendency for the drug to leave the drug vehicle (V) is higher the more the drug and vehicle differ in lipophilicity (high tendency: hydrophilic D and lipophilic V, and vice versa). Because the skin represents a closed lipophilic barrier (p. 22), only lipophilic drugs are absorbed. Hydrophilic drugs fail even to penetrate the outer skin when applied in a lipophilic vehicle. This formulation can be meaningful when high drug concentrations are required at the skin surface (e.g., neomycin ointment for bacterial skin infections).

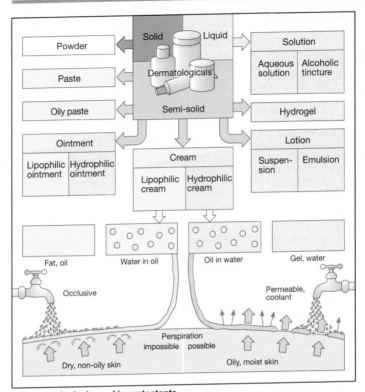

A. Dermatologicals as skin protectants

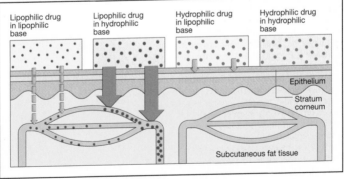

B. Dermatologicals as drug vehicles

From Application to Distribution in the Body

As a rule, drugs reach their target organs via the blood. Therefore, they must first enter the blood, usually the venous limb of the circulation. There are several possible sites of entry.

The drug may be injected or infused **intravenously,** in which case the drug is introduced directly into the bloodstream. In **subcutaneous** or **intramuscular** injection, the drug has to diffuse from its site of application into the blood. Because these procedures entail injury to the outer skin, strict requirements must be met concerning technique. For that reason, the **oral** route (i.e., simple application by mouth) involving subsequent uptake of drug across the gastrointestinal mucosa into the blood is chosen much more frequently. The disadvantage of this route is that the drug must pass through the liver on its way into the general circulation. This fact assumes practical significance with any drug that may be rapidly transformed or possibly inactivated in the liver (first-pass hepatic elimination; p. 42). Even with **rectal** administration, at least a fraction of the drug enters the general circulation via the portal vein, because only veins draining the short terminal segment of the rectum communicate directly with the inferior vena cava. Hepatic passage is circumvented when absorption occurs buccally or sublingually, because venous blood from the oral cavity drains directly into the superior vena cava. The same would apply to administration by **inhalation** (p. 14). However, with this route, a local effect is usually intended; a systemic action is intended only in exceptional cases. Under certain conditions, drug can also be applied percutaneously in the form of a **transdermal** delivery system (p. 12). In this case, drug is slowly released from the reservoir, and then penetrates the epidermis and subepidermal connective tissue where it enters blood capillaries. Only a very few drugs can be applied transdermally. The feasibility of this route is determined by both the physicochemical properties of the drug and the therapeutic requirements (acute vs. long-term effect).

Speed of absorption is determined by the route and method of application. It is fastest with **intravenous** injection, less fast with **intramuscular** injection, and slowest with **subcutaneous** injection. When the drug is applied to the oral mucosa (**buccal, sublingual** route), plasma levels rise faster than with conventional oral administration because the drug preparation is deposited at its actual site of absorption and very high concentrations in saliva occur upon the dissolution of a single dose. Thus, uptake across the oral epithelium is accelerated. The same does not hold true for poorly water-soluble or poorly absorbable drugs. Such agents should be given orally, because both the volume of fluid for dissolution and the absorbing surface are much larger in the small intestine than in the oral cavity.

Bioavailability is defined as the fraction of a given drug dose that reaches the circulation in unchanged form and becomes available for systemic distribution. The larger the presystemic elimination, the smaller is the bioavailability of an orally administered drug.

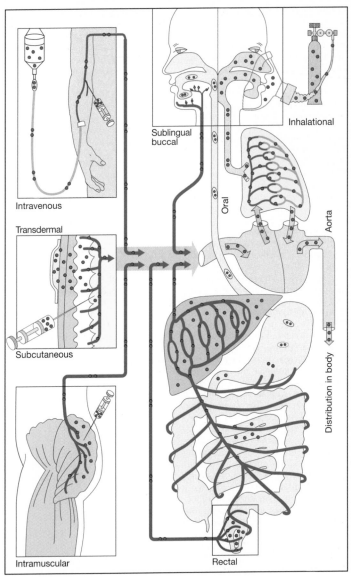

Intravenous

Transdermal

Subcutaneous

Intramuscular

Sublingual buccal

Inhalational

Oral

Aorta

Rectal

Distribution in body

A. From application to distribution

Potential Targets of Drug Action

Drugs are designed to exert a selective influence on vital processes in order to alleviate or eliminate symptoms of disease. The smallest basic unit of an organism is the **cell**. The outer cell membrane, or plasmalemma, effectively demarcates the cell from its surroundings, thus permitting a large degree of internal autonomy. Embedded in the plasmalemma are **transport proteins** that serve to mediate *controlled metabolic exchange with the cellular environment.* These include energy-consuming pumps (e.g., Na, K-ATPase, p. 130), carriers (e.g., for Na/glucose-cotransport, p. 178), and ion channels e.g., for sodium (p. 136) or calcium (p. 122) (**1**).

Functional coordination between single cells is a prerequisite for viability of the organism, hence also for the survival of individual cells. Cell functions are regulated by means of messenger substances for the transfer of information. Included among these are "transmitters" released from nerves, which the cell is able to recognize with the help of specialized membrane binding sites or **receptors.** Hormones secreted by endocrine glands into the blood, then into the extracellular fluid, represent another class of chemical signals. Finally, signalling substances can originate from neighboring cells, e.g., prostaglandins (p. 196) and cytokines.

The **effect of a drug** frequently results from interference with cellular function. Receptors for the recognition of endogenous transmitters are obvious sites of drug action (receptor agonists and antagonists, p. 60). Altered activity of transport systems affects cell function (e.g., cardiac glycosides, p. 130; loop diuretics, p. 162; calcium-antagonists, p. 122). Drugs may also directly interfere with intracellular metabolic processes, for instance by inhibiting (phosphodiesterase inhibitors, p. 132) or activating (organic nitrates, p. 120) an enzyme (**2**).

In contrast to drugs acting from the outside on cell membrane constituents, agents acting in the cell's interior need to penetrate the cell membrane.

The **cell membrane** basically consists of a **phospholipid bilayer** (80Å = 8 nm in thickness) in which are embedded proteins (integral membrane proteins, such as receptors and transport molecules). **Phospholipid** molecules contain two long-chain *fatty acids* in ester linkage with two of the three hydroxyl groups of *glycerol.* Bound to the third hydroxyl group is *phosphoric acid,* which, in turn, carries a further *residue,* e.g., choline, (phosphatidylcholine = lecithin), the amino acid serine (phosphatidylserine) or the cyclic polyhydric alcohol inositol (phosphatidylinositol). In terms of solubility, phospholipids are amphiphilic: the tail region containing the apolar fatty acid chains is lipophilic, the remainder – the polar head – is hydrophilic. By virtue of these properties, phospholipids aggregate spontaneously into a bilayer in an aqueous medium, their polar heads directed outwards into the aqueous medium, the fatty acid chains facing each other and projecting into the inside of the membrane (**3**).

The **hydrophobic interior** of the phospholipid membrane constitutes a **diffusion barrier** virtually impermeable for charged particles. Apolar particles, however, penetrate the membrane easily. This is of major importance with respect to the absorption, distribution, and elimination of drugs.

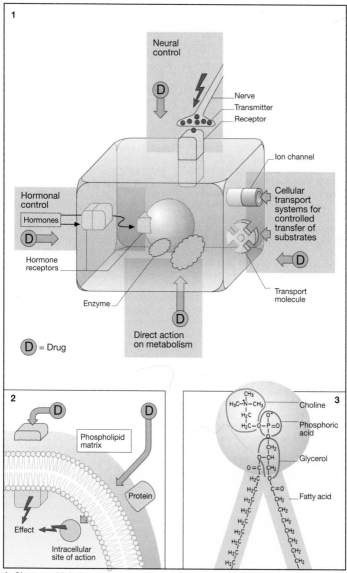

A. Sites at which drugs act to modify cell function

External Barriers of the Body

Prior to its uptake into the blood (i.e., during absorption), a drug has to overcome barriers that demarcate the body from its surroundings, i.e., separate the internal milieu from the external milieu. These boundaries are formed by the skin and mucous membranes.

When absorption takes place in the **gut** (enteral absorption), the intestinal epithelium is the barrier. This single-layered epithelium is made up of enterocytes and mucus-producing goblet cells. On their luminal side, these cells are joined together by *zonulae occludentes* (indicated by black dots in the inset, bottom left). A *zonula occludens* or tight junction is a region in which the phospholipid membranes of two cells establish close contact and become joined via integral membrane proteins (semicircular inset, left center). The region of fusion surrounds each cell like a ring, so that neighboring cells are welded together in a continuous belt. In this manner, an unbroken phospholipid layer is formed (yellow area in the schematic drawing, bottom left) and acts as a continuous barrier between the two spaces separated by the cell layer – in the case of the gut, the intestinal lumen (dark blue) and the interstitial space (light blue). The efficiency with which such a barrier restricts exchange of substances can be increased by arranging these occluding junctions in multiple arrays, as for instance in the endothelium of cerebral blood vessels. The connecting proteins (connexins) furthermore serve to restrict mixing of other functional membrane proteins (ion pumps, ion channels) that occupy specific areas of the cell membrane.

This phospholipid bilayer represents the intestinal mucosa-blood barrier that a drug must cross during its enteral absorption. Eligible drugs are those whose physicochemical properties allow permeation through the lipophilic membrane interior (yellow) or that are subject to a special carrier transport mechanism. Absorption of such drugs proceeds rapidly, because the absorbing surface is greatly enlarged due to the formation of the epithelial brush border (submicroscopic foldings of the plasmalemma). The absorbability of a drug is characterized by the *absorption quotient*, that is, the amount absorbed divided by the amount in the gut available for absorption.

In the **respiratory tract**, cilia-bearing epithelial cells are also joined on the luminal side by *zonulae occludentes,* so that the bronchial space and the interstitium are separated by a continuous phospholipid barrier.

With sublingual or buccal application, a drug encounters the non-keratinized, multilayered squamous epithelium of the **oral mucosa**. Here, the cells establish punctate contacts with each other in the form of desmosomes (not shown); however, these do not seal the intercellular clefts. Instead, the cells have the property of sequestering phospholipid-containing membrane fragments that assemble into layers within the extracellular space (semicircular inset, center right). In this manner, a continuous phospholipid barrier arises also inside squamous epithelia, although at an extracellular location, unlike that of intestinal epithelia. A similar barrier principle operates in the multilayered keratinized squamous epithelium of the outer **skin**. The presence of a continuous phospholipid layer means that squamous epithelia will permit passage of lipophilic drugs only, i.e., agents capable of diffusing through phospholipid membranes, with the epithelial thickness determining the extent and speed of absorption. In addition, cutaneous absorption is impeded by the keratin layer, the stratum corneum, which is very unevenly developed in various areas of the skin.

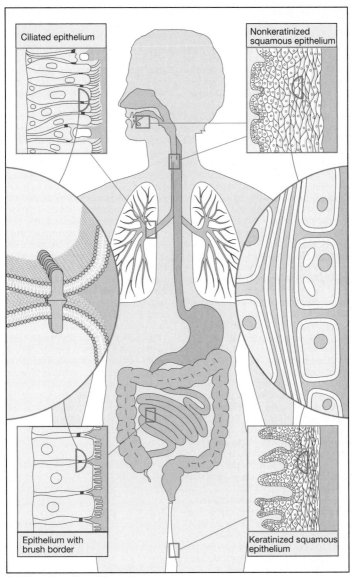

Ciliated epithelium

Nonkeratinized squamous epithelium

Epithelium with brush border

Keratinized squamous epithelium

A. External barriers of the body

Blood-Tissue Barriers

Drugs are transported in the blood to different tissues of the body. In order to reach their sites of action, they must leave the bloodstream. Drug permeation occurs largely in the capillary bed, where both surface area and time available for exchange are maximal (extensive vascular branching, low velocity of flow). The capillary wall forms the **blood-tissue barrier**. Basically, this consists of an endothelial cell layer and a basement membrane enveloping the latter (solid black line in the schematic drawings). The endothelial cells are "riveted" to each other by tight junctions or occluding zonulae (labelled Z in the electron micrograph, top left) such that no clefts, gaps, or pores remain that would permit drugs to pass unimpeded from the blood into the interstitial fluid.

The blood-tissue barrier is developed differently in the various capillary beds. Permeability to drugs of the capillary wall is determined by the structural and functional characteristics of the endothelial cells. In many capillary beds, e.g., those of **cardiac muscle**, endothelial cells are characterized by pronounced **endo-** and **transcytotic activity**, as evidenced by numerous invaginations and vesicles (arrows in the EM micrograph, top right). Transcytotic activity entails transport of fluid or macromolecules from the blood into the interstitium and vice versa. Any solutes trapped in the fluid, including drugs, may traverse the blood-tissue barrier. In this form of transport, the physicochemical properties of drugs are of little importance.

In some capillary beds (e.g., in the **pancreas**), endothelial cells exhibit **fenestrations**. Although the cells are tightly connected by continuous junctions, they possess **pores** (arrows in EM micrograph, bottom right) that are closed only by diaphragms. Both the diaphragm and basement membrane can be readily penetrated by substances of low molecular weight — the majority of drugs — but less so by macromolecules,

e.g., proteins such as insulin (G: insulin storage granules). Penetrability of macromolecules is determined by molecular size and electrical charge. Fenestrated endothelia are found in the capillaries of the *gut* and *endocrine glands*.

In the central nervous system (**brain and spinal cord**), capillary endothelia lack pores and there is little transcytotic activity. In order to cross the **blood-brain barrier**, drugs must diffuse transcellularly, i.e., penetrate the luminal and basal membrane of endothelial cells. Drug movement along this path requires specific physicochemical properties (p. 26) or the presence of a transport mechanism (e.g., L-dopa, p. 188). Thus, the blood-brain barrier is permeable only to certain types of drugs.

Drugs exchange freely between blood and interstitium in the **liver**, where endothelial cells exhibit large fenestrations (100 nm in diameter) facing Disse's spaces (D) and where neither diaphragms nor basement membranes impede drug movement. Diffusion barriers are also present beyond the capillary wall: e.g., *placental barrier* of fused syncytiotrophoblast cells; blood: testicle barrier — junctions interconnecting Sertoli cells; *brain choroid plexus: blood barrier* — occluding junctions between ependymal cells.

(Vertical bars in the EM micrographs represent 1 μm; E: cross-sectioned erythrocyte; AM: actomyosin; G: insulin-containing granules.)

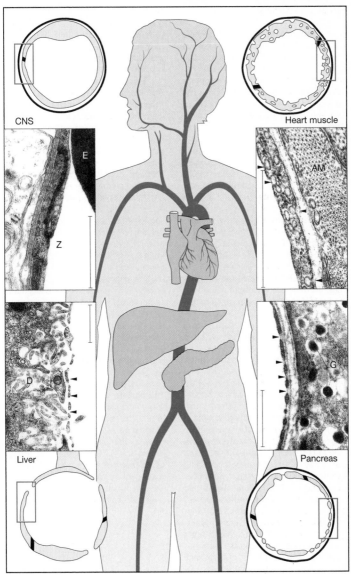

A. Blood-tissue barriers

Membrane Permeation

An ability to penetrate lipid bilayers is a prerequisite for the absorption of drugs, their entry into cells or cellular organelles, and passage across the blood-brain barrier. Due to their amphiphilic nature, phospholipids form bilayers possessing a hydrophilic surface and a hydrophobic interior (p. 20). Substances may traverse this membrane in three different ways.

Diffusion (A). Lipophilic substances (red dots) may enter the membrane from the extracellular space (area shown in ochre), accumulate in the membrane, and exit into the cytosol (blue area). Direction and speed of permeation depend on the relative concentrations in the fluid phases and the membrane. The steeper the gradient (concentration difference), the more drug will be diffusing per unit of time (Fick's Law). The lipid membrane represents an almost insurmountable obstacle for hydrophilic substances (blue triangles).

Transport (B). Some drugs may penetrate membrane barriers with the help of transport systems (carriers), irrespective of their physicochemical properties, especially lipophilicity. As a prerequisite, the drug must have affinity for the carrier (blue triangle matching recess on "transport system") and, when bound to the latter, be capable of being ferried across the membrane. Membrane passage via transport mechanisms is subject to competitive inhibition by another substance possessing similar affinity for the carrier. Substances lacking in affinity (blue circles) are not transported. Drugs utilize carriers for physiological substances, e.g., L-dopa uptake by L-amino acid carrier across the blood-intestine and blood-brain barriers (p. 188), and uptake of aminoglycosides by the carrier transporting basic polypeptides through the luminal membrane of kidney tubular cells (p. 278). Only drugs bearing sufficient resemblance to the physiological substrate of a carrier will exhibit affinity for it.

Finally, membrane penetration may occur in the form of small membrane-covered vesicles. Two different systems are considered.

Transcytosis (vesicular transport, C). When new vesicles are pinched off, substances dissolved in the extracellular fluid are engulfed, and then ferried through the cytoplasm, vesicles (phagosomes) undergo fusion with lysosomes to form phagolysosomes, and the transported substance is metabolized. Alternatively, the vesicle may fuse with the opposite cell membrane (cytopempsis).

Receptor-mediated endocytosis (C). The drug first binds to membrane surface receptors (1, 2) whose cytosolic domains contact special proteins (adaptins, 3). Drug-receptor complexes migrate laterally in the membrane and aggregate with other complexes by a clathrin-dependent process (4). The affected membrane region invaginates and eventually pinches off to form a detached vesicle (5). The clathrin coat is shed immediately (6), followed by the adaptins (7). The remaining vesicle then fuses with an "early" endosome (8), whereupon proton concentration rises inside the vesicle. The drug-receptor complex dissociates and the receptor returns into the cell membrane. The "early" endosome delivers its contents to predetermined destinations, e.g., the Golgi complex, the cell nucleus, lysosomes, or the opposite cell membrane (transcytosis). Unlike simple endocytosis, receptor-mediated endocytosis is contingent on affinity for specific receptors and operates independently of concentration gradients.

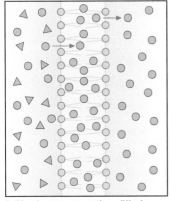

A. Membrane permeation: diffusion

B. Membrane permeation: transport

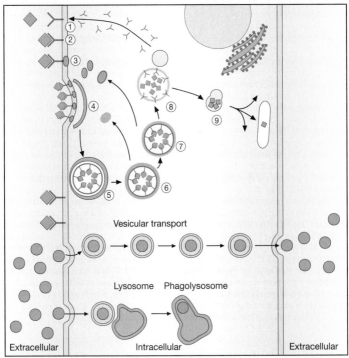

Vesicular transport

Lysosome   Phagolysosome

Extracellular   Intracellular   Extracellular

C. Membrane permeation: receptor-mediated endocytosis, vesicular uptake, and transport

Possible Modes of Drug Distribution

Following its uptake into the body, the drug is distributed in the blood (**1**) and through it to the various tissues of the body. Distribution may be restricted to the extracellular space (plasma volume plus interstitial space) (**2**) or may also extend into the intracellular space (**3**). Certain drugs may bind strongly to tissue structures, so that plasma concentrations fall significantly even before elimination has begun (**4**).

After being distributed in blood, macromolecular substances remain largely confined to the vascular space, because their permeation through the blood-tissue barrier, or endothelium, is impeded, even where capillaries are fenestrated. This property is exploited therapeutically when loss of blood necessitates refilling of the vascular bed, e.g., by infusion of dextran solutions (p. 152). The vascular space is, moreover, predominantly occupied by substances bound with high affinity to plasma proteins (p. 30; determination of the plasma volume with protein-bound dyes). Unbound, free drug may leave the bloodstream, albeit with varying ease, because the blood-tissue barrier (p. 24) is differently developed in different segments of the vascular tree. These regional differences are not illustrated in the accompanying figures.

Distribution in the body is determined by the ability to penetrate membranous barriers (p. 20). Hydrophilic substances (e.g., inulin) are neither taken up into cells nor bound to cell surface structures and can, thus, be used to determine the extracellular fluid volume (**2**). Some lipophilic substances diffuse through the cell membrane and, as a result, achieve a uniform distribution (**3**).

Body weight may be broken down as follows:

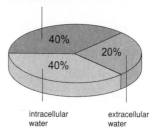

Solid substance and structurally bound water

40%

20%

40%

intracellular water

extracellular water

Potential aqueous solvent spaces for drugs

Further subdivisions are shown in the table.

The volume ratio interstitial: intracellular water varies with age and body weight. On a percentage basis, interstitial fluid volume is large in premature or normal neonates (up to 50% of body water), and smaller in the obese and the aged.

The concentration (c) of a solution corresponds to the amount (D) of substance dissolved in a volume (V); thus, c = D/V. If the dose of drug (D) and its plasma concentration (c) are known, a volume of distribution (V) can be calculated from V = D/c. However, this represents an *apparent* volume of distribution (V_{app}), because an even distribution in the body is assumed in its calculation. Homogeneous distribution will not occur if drugs are bound to cell membranes (**5**) or to membranes of intracellular organelles (**6**) or are stored within the latter (**7**). In these cases, V_{app} can exceed the actual size of the available fluid volume. The significance of V_{app} as a pharmacokinetic parameter is discussed on p. 44.

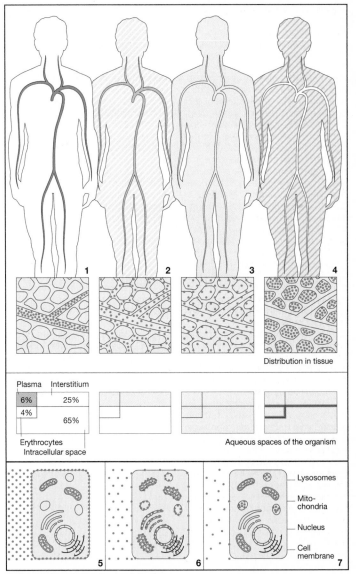

Distribution in tissue

Plasma	Interstitium
6%	25%
4%	65%

Erythrocytes
Intracellular space

Aqueous spaces of the organism

Lysosomes

Mito-
chondria

Nucleus

Cell
membrane

A. Compartments for drug distribution

Binding to Plasma Proteins

Having entered the blood, drugs may bind to the protein molecules that are present in abundance, resulting in the formation of drug-protein complexes.

Protein binding involves primarily albumin and, to a lesser extent, β-globulins and acidic glycoproteins. Other plasma proteins (e.g., transcortin, transferrin, thyroxin-binding globulin) serve specialized functions in connection with specific substances. The degree of binding is governed by the concentration of the reactants and the affinity of a drug for a given protein. Albumin concentration in plasma amounts to 4.6 g/100 mL or 0.6 mM, and thus provides a very high binding capacity (two sites per molecule). As a rule, drugs exhibit much lower affinity (K_D approx. 10^{-5}–10^{-3} M) for plasma proteins than for their specific binding sites (receptors). In the range of therapeutically relevant concentrations, protein binding of most drugs increases linearly with concentration (exceptions: salicylate and certain sulfonamides).

The albumin molecule has different binding sites for anionic and cationic ligands, but *van der Waals'* forces also contribute (p. 58). The extent of binding correlates with drug hydrophobicity (repulsion of drug by water).

Binding to plasma proteins is instantaneous and reversible, i.e., any change in the concentration of unbound drug is immediately followed by a corresponding change in the concentration of bound drug. Protein binding is of great importance, because it is the concentration of free drug that determines the intensity of the effect. At an identical total plasma concentration (say, 100 ng/mL) the *effective* concentration will be 90 ng/mL for a drug 10 % bound to protein, but 1 ng/mL for a drug 99 % bound to protein. The reduction in concentration of free drug resulting from protein binding affects not only the intensity of the effect but also biotransformation (e.g., in the liver) and elimination in the kidney, because only free drug will enter hepatic sites of metabolism or undergo glomerular filtration. When concentrations of free drug fall, drug is resupplied from binding sites on plasma proteins. Binding to plasma protein is equivalent to a depot in prolonging the duration of the effect by retarding elimination, whereas the intensity of the effect is reduced. If two substances have affinity for the same binding site on the albumin molecule, they may compete for that site. One drug may displace another from its binding site and thereby elevate the free (effective) concentration of the displaced drug (a form of **drug interaction**). Elevation of the free concentration of the displaced drug means increased effectiveness and accelerated elimination.

A decrease in the concentration of albumin (liver disease, nephrotic syndrome, poor general condition) leads to altered pharmacokinetics of drugs that are highly bound to albumin.

Plasma protein-bound drugs that are substrates for transport carriers can be cleared from blood at great velocity, e.g., *p*-aminohippurate by the renal tubule and sulfobromophthalein by the liver. Clearance rates of these substances can be used to determine renal or hepatic blood flow.

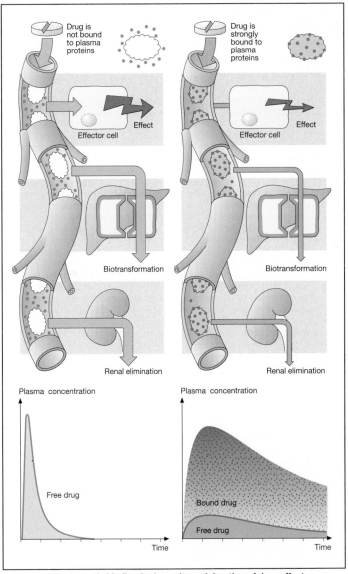

A. Importance of protein binding for intensity and duration of drug effect

The Liver as an Excretory Organ

As the chief organ of drug biotransformation, the liver is richly supplied with blood, of which 1100 mL is received each minute from the intestines through the portal vein and 350 mL through the hepatic artery, comprising nearly $1/3$ of cardiac output. The blood content of hepatic vessels and sinusoids amounts to 500 mL. Due to the widening of the portal lumen, intrahepatic blood flow decelerates (**A**). Moreover, the endothelial lining of hepatic sinusoids (p. 24) contains pores large enough to permit rapid exit of plasma proteins. Thus, blood and hepatic parenchyma are able to maintain intimate contact and intensive exchange of substances, which is further facilitated by microvilli covering the hepatocyte surfaces abutting Disse's spaces.

The hepatocyte secretes biliary fluid into the bile canaliculi (dark green), tubular intercellular clefts that are sealed off from the blood spaces by tight junctions. Secretory activity in the hepatocytes results in movement of fluid towards the canalicular space (**A**). The hepatocyte has an abundance of enzymes carrying out metabolic functions. These are localized in part in mitochondria, in part on the membranes of the rough (rER) or smooth (sER) endoplasmic reticulum.

Enzymes of the sER play a most important role in drug biotransformation. At this site, molecular oxygen is used in oxidative reactions. Because these enzymes can catalyze either hydroxylation or oxidative cleavage of -N-C- or -O-C-bonds, they are referred to as "mixed-function" oxidases or hydroxylases. The essential component of this enzyme system is cytochrome P450, which in its oxidized state binds drug substrates (R-H). The Fe^{III}-P450-RH binary complex is first reduced by NADPH, then forms the ternary complex, O_2-Fe^{II}-P450-RH, which accepts a second electron and finally disintegrates into Fe^{III}-P450, one equivalent of H_2O, and hydroxylated drug (R-OH).

Compared with hydrophilic drugs not undergoing transport, lipophilic drugs are more rapidly taken up from the blood into hepatocytes and more readily gain access to mixed-function oxidases embedded in sER membranes. For instance, a drug having lipophilicity by virtue of an aromatic substituent (phenyl ring) (**B**) can be hydroxylated and, thus, become more hydrophilic (Phase I reaction, p. 34). Besides oxidases, sER also contains reductases and glucuronyl transferases. The latter conjugate glucuronic acid with hydroxyl, carboxyl, amine, and amide groups (p. 38); hence, also phenolic products of phase I metabolism (Phase II conjugation). Phase I and Phase II metabolites can be transported back into the blood — probably via a gradient-dependent carrier — or actively secreted into bile.

Prolonged exposure to certain substrates, such as phenobarbital, carbamazepine, rifampicin results in a proliferation of sER membranes (cf. **C** and **D**). This **enzyme induction**, a load-dependent hypertrophy, affects equally all enzymes localized on **sER** membranes. Enzyme induction leads to accelerated biotransformation, not only of the inducing agent but also of other drugs (a form of **drug interaction**). With continued exposure, induction develops in a few days, resulting in an increase in reaction velocity, maximally 2–3 fold, that disappears after removal of the inducing agent.

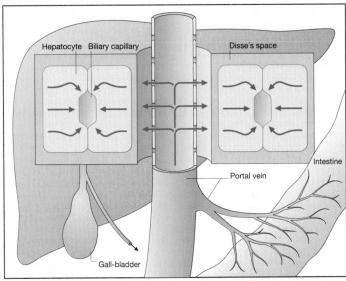

A. Flow patterns in portal vein, Disse's space, and hepatocyte

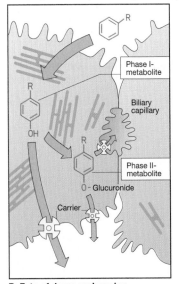

B. Fate of drugs undergoing hepatic hydroxylation

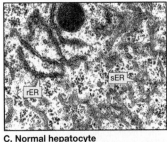

C. Normal hepatocyte

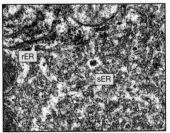

D. Hepatocyte after phenobarbital administration

Biotransformation of Drugs

Many drugs undergo chemical modification in the body (**biotransformation**). Most frequently, this process entails a loss of biological activity and an increase in hydrophilicity (water solubility), thereby promoting elimination via the renal route (p. 40). Since rapid drug elimination improves accuracy in titrating the therapeutic concentration, drugs are often designed with built-in weak links. Ester bonds are such links, being subject to hydrolysis by the ubiquitous esterases. *Hydrolytic cleavages,* along with *oxidations, reductions, alkylations,* and *dealkylations,* constitute **Phase I reactions** of drug metabolism. These reactions subsume all metabolic processes apt to alter drug molecules chemically and take place chiefly in the liver. In **Phase II (synthetic) reactions, conjugation products** of either the drug itself or its Phase I metabolites are formed, for instance, with glucuronic or sulfuric acid (p. 38).

The special case of the endogenous transmitter acetylcholine illustrates well the high velocity of ester hydrolysis. Acetylcholine is broken down at its sites of release and action by acetylcholinesterase (pp. 100, 102) so rapidly as to negate its therapeutic use. Hydrolysis of other esters catalyzed by various esterases is slower, though relatively fast in comparison with other biotransformations. The local anesthetic, procaine, is a case in point; it exerts its action at the site of application while being largely devoid of undesirable effects at other locations because it is inactivated by hydrolysis during absorption from its site of application.

Ester hydrolysis does not invariably lead to inactive metabolites, as exemplified by acetylsalicylic acid. The cleavage product, salicylic acid, retains pharmacological activity. In certain cases, drugs are administered in the form of esters in order to facilitate absorption (enalapril → enalaprilate; testosterone undecanoate → testosterone) or to reduce irritation of the gastrointestinal mucosa (erythromycin succinate → erythromycin). In these cases, the ester itself is not active, but the cleavage product is. Thus, an inactive precursor or **prodrug** is applied, formation of the active molecule occurring only after hydrolysis in the blood.

Some drugs possessing amide bonds, such as prilocaine, and of course, peptides, can be hydrolyzed by peptidases and inactivated in this manner. Peptidases are also of pharmacological interest because they are responsible for the formation of highly reactive cleavage products (fibrin, p. 146) and potent mediators (angiotensin II, p. 124; bradykinin, enkephalin, p. 210) from biologically inactive peptides.

Peptidases exhibit some substrate selectivity and can be selectively inhibited, as exemplified by the formation of angiotensin II, whose actions inter alia include vasoconstriction. Angiotensin II is formed from angiotensin I by cleavage of the C-terminal dipeptide histidylleucine. Hydrolysis is catalyzed by "angiotensin-converting enzyme" (ACE). Peptide analogues such as captopril (p. 124) block this enzyme. Angiotensin II is degraded by angiotensinase A, which clips off the N-terminal asparagine residue. The product, angiotensin III, lacks vasoconstrictor activity.

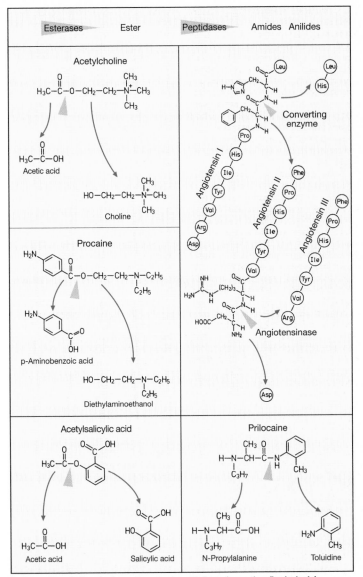

A. Examples of chemical reactions in drug biotransformation (hydrolysis)

Oxidation reactions can be divided into two kinds: those in which oxygen is incorporated into the drug molecule, and those in which primary oxidation causes part of the molecule to be lost. The former include **hydroxylations, epoxidations,** and **sulfoxidations.** Hydroxylations may involve alkyl substituents (e.g., pentobarbital) or aromatic ring systems (e.g., propranolol). In both cases, products are formed that are conjugated to an organic acid residue, e.g., glucuronic acid, in a subsequent Phase II reaction.

Hydroxylation may also take place at nitrogen atoms, resulting in hydroxylamines (e.g., acetaminophen). Benzene, polycyclic aromatic compounds (e.g., benzopyrene), and unsaturated cyclic carbohydrates can be converted by mono-oxygenases to **epoxides,** highly reactive electrophiles that are hepatotoxic and possibly carcinogenic.

The second type of oxidative biotransformation comprises **dealkylations.** In the case of primary or secondary amines, dealkylation of an alkyl group starts at the carbon adjacent to the nitrogen; in the case of tertiary amines, with hydroxylation of the nitrogen (e.g., lidocaine). The intermediary products are labile and break up into the dealkylated amine and aldehyde of the alkyl group removed. O-dealkylation and S-dearylation proceed via an analogous mechanism (e.g., phenacetin and azathioprine, respectively).

Oxidative **deamination** basically resembles the dealkylation of tertiary amines, beginning with the formation of a hydroxylamine that then decomposes into ammonia and the corresponding aldehyde. The latter is partly reduced to an alcohol and partly oxidized to a carboxylic acid.

Reduction reactions may occur at oxygen or nitrogen atoms. Keto-oxygens are converted into a hydroxyl group, as in the reduction of the prodrugs cortisone and prednisone to the active glucocorticoids cortisol and prednisolone, respectively. N-reductions occur in azo- or nitro-compounds (e.g., nitrazepam). Nitro groups can be reduced to amine groups via nitroso and hydroxylamino intermediates. Likewise, dehalogenation is a reductive process involving a carbon atom (e.g., halothane, p. 218).

Methylations are catalyzed by a family of relatively specific methyltransferases involving the transfer of methyl groups to hydroxyl groups (O-methylation as in norepinephrine [noradrenaline]) or to amino groups (N-methylation of norepinephrine, histamine, or serotonin).

In thio compounds, **desulfuration** results from substitution of sulfur by oxygen (e.g., parathion). This example again illustrates that biotransformation is not always to be equated with bioinactivation. Thus, paraoxon (E600) formed in the organism from parathion (E605) is the actual active agent (p. 102).

Desalkylierung

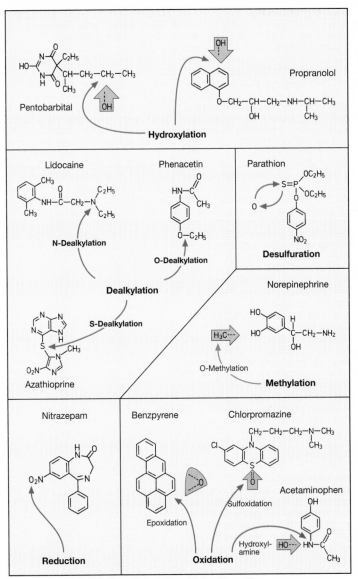

A. Examples of chemical reactions in drug biotransformation

Enterohepatic Cycle (A)

After an orally ingested drug has been absorbed from the gut, it is transported via the portal blood to the liver, where it can be conjugated to glucuronic or sulfuric acid (shown in **B** for salicylic acid and deacetylated bisacodyl, respectively) or to other organic acids. At the pH of body fluids, these acids are predominantly ionized; the negative charge confers high polarity upon the conjugated drug molecule and, hence, low membrane penetrability. The conjugated products may pass from hepatocyte into biliary fluid and from there back into the intestine. O-glucuronides can be cleaved by bacterial β-glucuronidases in the colon, enabling the liberated drug molecule to be **reabsorbed**. The **enterohepatic cycle** acts to trap drugs in the body. However, conjugated products enter not only the bile but also the blood. Glucuronides with a molecular weight (MW) > 300 preferentially pass into the blood, while those with MW > 300 enter the bile to a larger extent. Glucuronides circulating in the blood undergo glomerular filtration in the kidney and are excreted in urine because their decreased lipophilicity prevents tubular reabsorption.

Drugs that are subject to enterohepatic cycling are, therefore, excreted slowly. Pertinent examples include digitoxin and acidic nonsteroidal anti-inflammatory agents (p. 200).

Conjugations (B)

The most important of phase II conjugation reactions is *glucuronidation.* This reaction does not proceed spontaneously, but requires the activated form of glucuronic acid, namely glucuronic acid uridine diphosphate. Microsomal glucuronyl transferases link the activated glucuronic acid with an acceptor molecule. When the latter is a phenol or alcohol, an ether glucuronide will be formed. In the case of carboxyl-bearing molecules, an ester glucuronide is the result. All of these are O-glucuronides.

Amines may form N-glucuronides that, unlike O-glucuronides, are resistant to bacterial β-glucuronidases.

Soluble cytoplasmic sulfotransferases conjugate *activated sulfate* (3'-phosphoadenine-5'-phosphosulfate) with alcohols and phenols. The conjugates are acids, as in the case of glucuronides. In this respect, they differ from conjugates formed by acetyltransferases from *activated acetate* (acetylcoenzyme A) and an alcohol or a phenol.

Acyltransferases are involved in the conjugation of the amino acids *glycine* or *glutamine* with carboxylic acids. In these cases, an amide bond is formed between the carboxyl groups of the acceptor and the amino group of the donor molecule (e.g., formation of salicyluric acid from salicylic acid and glycine). The acidic group of glycine or glutamine remains free.

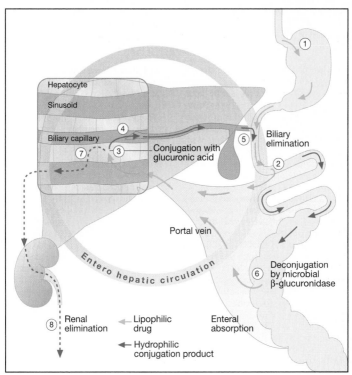

A. Enterohepatic cycle

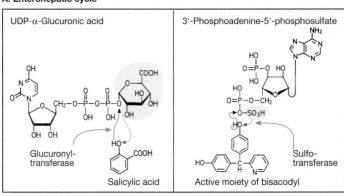

B. Conjugation reactions

The Kidney as Excretory Organ

Most drugs are eliminated in urine either chemically unchanged or as metabolites. The kidney permits elimination because the vascular wall structure in the region of the glomerular capillaries (**B**) allows unimpeded passage of blood solutes having molecular weights (MW) < 5000. Filtration diminishes progressively as MW increases from 5000 to 70000 and ceases at MW > 70000. With few exceptions, therapeutically used drugs and their metabolites have much smaller molecular weights and can, therefore, undergo **glomerular filtration**, i.e., pass from blood into primary urine. Separating the capillary **endothelium** from the tubular **epithelium**, the **basal membrane** consists of charged glycoproteins and acts as a filtration barrier for high-molecular-weight substances. The relative density of this barrier depends on the electrical charge of molecules that attempt to permeate it.

Apart from **glomerular filtration** (**B**), drugs present in blood may pass into urine by **active secretion**. Certain cations and anions are secreted by the epithelium of the proximal tubules into the tubular fluid via special, energy-consuming transport systems. These transport systems have a limited capacity. When several substrates are present simultaneously, competition for the carrier may occur (see p. 268).

During passage down the renal tubule, urinary volume shrinks more than 100-fold; accordingly, there is a corresponding concentration of filtered drug or drug metabolites (**A**). The resulting concentration gradient between urine and interstitial fluid is preserved in the case of drugs incapable of permeating the tubular epithelium. However, with lipophilic drugs the concentration gradient will favor **reabsorption** of the filtered molecules. In this case, reabsorption is not based on an active process but results instead from passive diffusion. Accordingly, for protonated substances, the extent of reabsorption is dependent upon urinary pH or the degree of dissociation. The degree of dissociation varies as a function of the urinary pH and the pK_a, which represents the pH value at which half of the substance exists in protonated (or unprotonated) form. This relationship is graphically illustrated (**D**) with the example of a protonated amine having a pK_a of 7.0. In this case, at urinary pH 7.0, 50 % of the amine will be present in the protonated, hydrophilic, membrane-impermeant form (blue dots), whereas the other half, representing the uncharged amine (orange dots), can leave the tubular lumen in accordance with the resulting concentration gradient. If the pK_a of an amine is higher (pK_a = 7.5) or lower (pK_a = 6.5), a correspondingly smaller or larger proportion of the amine will be present in the uncharged, reabsorbable form. Lowering or raising urinary pH by half a pH unit would result in analogous changes for an amine having a pK_a of 7.0.

The same considerations hold for acidic molecules, with the important difference that alkalinization of the urine (increased pH) will promote the deprotonization of -COOH groups and thus impede reabsorption. Intentional alteration in urinary pH can be used in intoxications with proton-acceptor substances in order to hasten elimination of the toxin (alkalinization $\rightarrow$ phenobarbital; acidification $\rightarrow$ amphetamine).

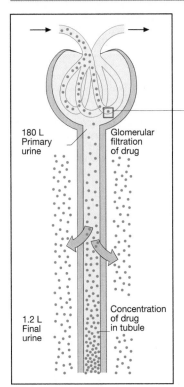

A. Filtration and concentration

180 L
Primary
urine

Glomerular
filtration
of drug

1.2 L
Final
urine

Concentration
of drug
in tubule

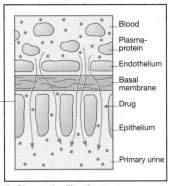

B. Glomerular filtration

Blood

Plasma-
protein

Endothelium

Basal
membrane

Drug

Epithelium

Primary urine

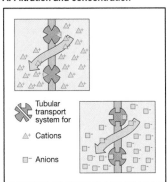

C. Active secretion

Tubular
transport
system for

△⁺ Cations

□⁻ Anions

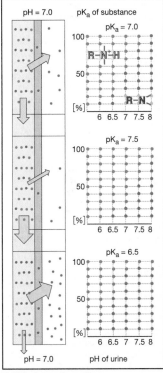

D. Tubular reabsorption

pH = 7.0

pK$_a$ of substance

pK$_a$ = 7.0

R–N⁺–H

R–N

[%]

6 6.5 7 7.5 8

pK$_a$ = 7.5

[%]

6 6.5 7 7.5 8

pK$_a$ = 6.5

[%]

6 6.5 7 7.5 8

pH = 7.0

pH of urine

Elimination of Lipophilic and Hydrophilic Substances

The terms **lipophilic** and **hydrophilic** (or hydro- and lipophobic) refer to the solubility of substances in media of low and high polarity, respectively. Blood plasma, interstitial fluid, and cytosol are highly polar aqueous media, whereas lipids — at least in the interior of the lipid bilayer membrane — and fat constitute apolar media. Most polar substances are readily dissolved in aqueous media (i.e., are hydrophilic) and lipophilic ones in apolar media. A **hydrophilic drug**, on reaching the bloodstream, probably after a partial, slow absorption (not illustrated), passes through the liver unchanged, because it either cannot, or will only slowly, permeate the lipid barrier of the hepatocyte membrane and thus will fail to gain access to hepatic biotransforming enzymes. The unchanged drug reaches the arterial blood and the kidneys, where it is filtered. With hydrophilic drugs, there is little binding to plasma proteins (protein binding increases as a function of lipophilicity), hence the entire amount present in plasma is available for glomerular filtration. A hydrophilic drug is not subject to tubular reabsorption and appears in the urine. Hydrophilic drugs undergo **rapid elimination**.

If a **lipophilic drug**, because of its chemical nature, cannot be converted into a polar product, despite having access to all cells, including metabolically active liver cells, it is likely to be retained in the organism. The portion filtered during glomerular passage will be reabsorbed from the tubules. Reabsorption will be nearly complete, because the free concentration of a lipophilic drug in plasma is low (lipophilic substances are usually largely protein-bound). The situation portrayed for a lipophilic non-metabolizable drug would seem undesirable because pharmacotherapeutic measures once initiated would be virtually irreversible (poor control over blood concentration).

Lipophilic drugs that are converted in the liver to **hydrophilic metabolites** permit better control, because the lipophilic agent can be eliminated in this manner. The speed of formation of hydrophilic metabolite determines the drug's length of stay in the body.

If hepatic conversion to a polar metabolite is rapid, only a portion of the absorbed drug enters the systemic circulation in unchanged form, the remainder having undergone **presystemic** (first-pass) **elimination**. When biotransformation is rapid, oral administration of the drug is impossible (e.g., glyceryl trinitate, p. 120). Parenteral or, alternatively, sublingual, intranasal, or transdermal administration is then required in order to bypass the liver. Irrespective of the route of administration, a portion of administered drug may be taken up into and transiently stored in lung tissue before entering the general circulation. This also constitutes presystemic elimination.

Presystemic elimination refers to the fraction of drug absorbed that is excluded from the general circulation by biotransformation or by first-pass binding.

Presystemic elimination diminishes the *bioavailability* of a drug after its oral administration. **Absolute bioavailability** = systemically available amount/dose administered; **relative bioavailability** = availability of a drug contained in a test preparation with reference to a standard preparation.

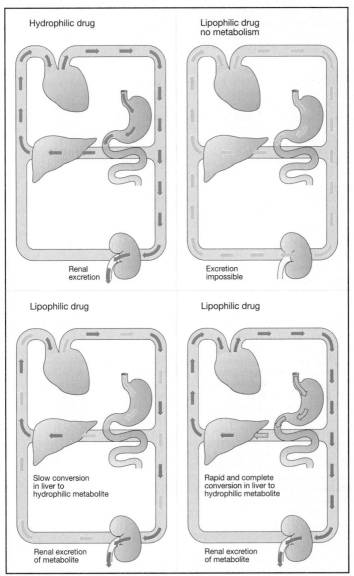

A. Elimination of hydrophilic and hydrophobic drugs

Drug Concentration in the Body as a Function of Time. First-Order (Exponential) Rate Processes

Processes such as drug absorption and elimination display exponential characteristics. As regards the former, this follows from the simple fact that the amount of drug being moved per unit of time depends on the concentration difference (gradient) between two body compartments (Fick's Law). In drug absorption from the alimentary tract, the intestinal contents and blood would represent the compartments containing an initially high and low concentration, respectively. In drug elimination via the kidney, excretion often depends on glomerular filtration, i.e., the filtered amount of drug present in primary urine. As the blood concentration falls, the amount of drug filtered per unit of time diminishes. The resulting exponential decline is illustrated in (**A**). The exponential time course implies constancy of the interval during which the concentration decreases by one-half. This interval represents the half-life ($t_{1/2}$) and is related to the elimination rate constant k by the equation $t_{1/2} = \ln 2/k$. The two parameters, together with the initial concentration c_0, describe a first-order (exponential) rate process.

The constancy of the process permits calculation of the plasma volume that would be cleared of drug, if the remaining drug were not to assume a homogeneous distribution in the total volume (a condition not met in reality). This **notional plasma volume freed of drug per unit of time** is termed the **clearance**. Depending on whether plasma concentration falls as a result of urinary excretion or metabolic alteration, clearance is considered to be renal or hepatic. Renal and hepatic clearances add up to total clearance (Cl_{tot}) in the case of drugs that are eliminated unchanged via the kidney and biotransformed in the liver. Cl_{tot} represents the sum of all processes contributing to elimination; it is related to the half-life

($t_{1/2}$) and the apparent volume of distribution V_{app} (p. 28) by the equation:

$$t_{1/2} = \ln 2 \times \frac{V_{app}}{Cl_{tot}}$$

The smaller the volume of distribution or the larger the total clearance, the shorter is the half-life.

In the case of drugs renally eliminated in unchanged form, the half-life of elimination can be calculated from the cumulative excretion in urine; the final total amount eliminated corresponds to the amount absorbed.

Hepatic elimination obeys exponential kinetics because metabolizing enzymes operate in the quasilinear region of their concentration-activity curve; hence the amount of drug metabolized per unit of time diminishes with decreasing blood concentration.

The best-known exception to exponential kinetics is the elimination of alcohol (ethanol), which obeys a *linear* time course (zero-order kinetics), at least at blood concentrations > 0.02 %. It does so because the rate-limiting enzyme, alcohol dehydrogenase, achieves half-saturation at very low substrate concentrations, i.e., at about 80 mg/L (0.008 %). Thus, reaction velocity reaches a plateau at blood ethanol concentrations of about 0.02 %, and the amount of drug eliminated per unit of time remains constant at concentrations above this level.

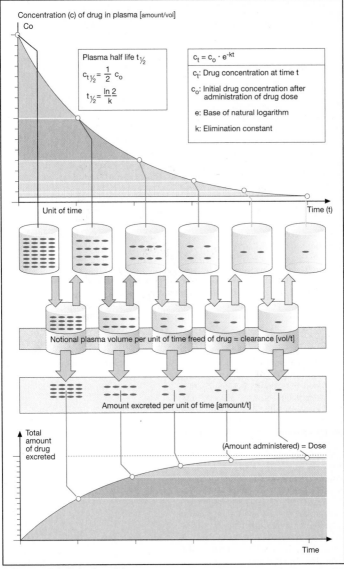

Concentration (c) of drug in plasma [amount/vol]

C_0

Plasma half life $t_{1/2}$

$c_{t_{1/2}} = \frac{1}{2} c_0$

$t_{1/2} = \frac{\ln 2}{k}$

$c_t = c_0 \cdot e^{-kt}$

c_t: Drug concentration at time t

c_0: Initial drug concentration after administration of drug dose

e: Base of natural logarithm

k: Elimination constant

Unit of time

Time (t)

Notional plasma volume per unit of time freed of drug = clearance [vol/t]

Amount excreted per unit of time [amount/t]

Total amount of drug excreted

(Amount administered) = Dose

Time

A. Exponential elimination of drug

Time Course of Drug Concentration in Plasma

A. Drugs are taken up into and eliminated from the body by various routes. The body thus represents an open system wherein the actual drug concentration reflects the interplay of intake (ingestion) and egress (elimination). When an orally administered drug is absorbed from the stomach and intestine, speed of uptake depends on many factors, including the speed of drug dissolution (in the case of solid dosage forms) and of gastrointestinal transit; the membrane penetrability of the drug; its concentration gradient across the mucosa-blood barrier; and mucosal blood flow. **Absorption** from the intestine causes the drug concentration in blood to increase. Transport in blood conveys the drug to different organs (**distribution**), into which it is taken up to a degree compatible with its chemical properties and rate of blood flow through the organ. For instance, well-perfused organs such as the brain receive a greater proportion than do less well-perfused ones. Uptake into tissue causes the blood concentration to fall. Absorption from the gut diminishes as the mucosa-blood gradient decreases. Plasma concentration reaches a peak when the drug amount leaving the blood per unit of time equals that being absorbed.

Drug entry into hepatic and renal tissue constitutes movement into the **organs of elimination**. The characteristic phasic time course of drug concentration in plasma represents the sum of the constituent processes of **absorption, distribution,** and **elimination**, which overlap in time. When distribution takes place significantly faster than elimination, there is an initial rapid and then a greatly retarded fall in the plasma level, the former being designated the α-phase (distribution phase), the latter the β-phase (elimination phase). When the drug is distributed faster than it is absorbed, the time course of the plasma level can be described in mathematically simplified form by the Bate-man function (k_1 and k_2 represent the rate constants for absorption and elimination, respectively).

B. The velocity of absorption depends on the route of administration. The more rapid the administration, the shorter will be the time (t_{max}) required to reach the peak plasma level (c_{max}), the higher will be the c_{max}, and the earlier the plasma level will begin to fall again.

The *area under the plasma level time curve* (AUC) is independent of the route of administration, provided the doses and bioavailability are the same (Dost's law of corresponding areas). The AUC can thus be used to determine the **bioavailability F** of a drug. The ratio of AUC values determined after oral or intravenous administration of a given dose of a particular drug corresponds to the proportion of drug entering the systemic circulation after oral administration. The determination of plasma levels affords a comparison of different proprietary preparations containing the same drug in the same dosage. Identical plasma level time-curves of different manufacturers' products with reference to a standard preparation indicate **bioequivalence** of the preparation under investigation with the standard.

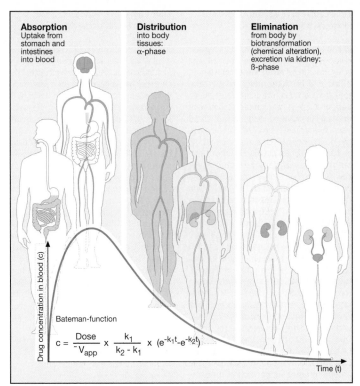

Absorption
Uptake from stomach and intestines into blood

Distribution
into body tissues: α-phase

Elimination
from body by biotransformation (chemical alteration), excretion via kidney: ß-phase

Drug concentration in blood (c)

Bateman-function

$$c = \frac{Dose}{\tilde{V}_{app}} \times \frac{k_1}{k_2 - k_1} \times (e^{-k_1 t} - e^{-k_2 t})$$

Time (t)

A. Time course of drug concentration

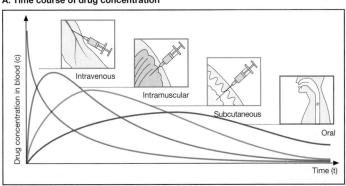

Drug concentration in blood (c)

Intravenous

Intramuscular

Subcutaneous

Oral

Time (t)

B. Mode of application and time course of drug concentration

Time Course of Drug Plasma Levels During Repeated Dosing (A)

When a drug is administered at regular intervals over a prolonged period, the rise and fall of drug concentration in blood will be determined by the relationship between the half-life of elimination and the time interval between doses. If the drug amount administered in each dose has been eliminated before the next dose is applied, repeated intake at constant intervals will result in similar plasma levels. If intake occurs before the preceding dose has been eliminated completely, the next dose will add on to the residual amount still present in the body, i.e., the drug **accumulates**. The shorter the dosing interval relative to the elimination half-life, the larger will be the residual amount of drug to which the next dose is added and the more extensively will the drug accumulate in the body. However, at a given dosing frequency, the drug does not accumulate infinitely and a **steady state** (C_{ss}) or **accumulation equilibrium** is eventually reached. This is so because the activity of elimination processes is concentration-dependent. The higher the drug concentration rises, the greater is the amount eliminated per unit of time. After several doses, the concentration will have climbed to a level at which the amounts eliminated and taken in per unit of time become equal, i.e., a steady state is reached. Within this concentration range, the plasma level will continue to rise (peak) and fall (trough) as dosing is continued at a regular interval. The height of the steady state (C_{ss}) depends upon the amount (D) administered per dosing interval (τ) and the clearance (Cl_{tot}):

$$C_{ss} = \frac{D}{(\tau \cdot Cl_{tot})}$$

The speed at which the steady state is reached corresponds to the speed of elimination of the drug. The time needed to reach 90 % of the concentration plateau is about 3 times the $t_{1/2}$ of elimination.

Time Course of Drug Plasma Levels During Irregular Intake (B)

In practice, it proves difficult to achieve a plasma level that undulates evenly around the desired effective concentration. For instance, if two successive doses are omitted, the plasma level will drop below the therapeutic range and a longer period will be required to regain the desired plasma level. In everyday life, patients will be apt to neglect drug intake at the scheduled time. **Patient compliance** means strict adherence to the prescribed regimen. Apart from poor compliance, the same problem may occur when the total daily dose is divided into three individual doses (tid) and the first dose is taken at breakfast, the second at lunch, and the third at supper. Under this condition, the nocturnal dosing interval will be twice the diurnal one. Consequently, plasma levels during the early morning hours may have fallen far below the desired or, possibly, urgently needed range.

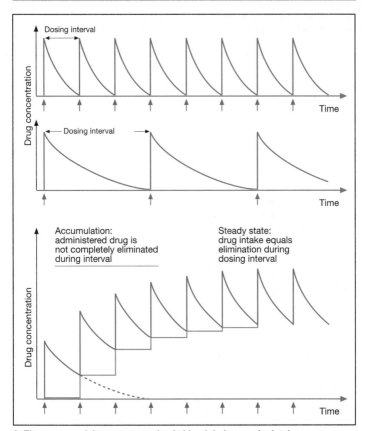

A. Time course of drug concentration in blood during regular intake

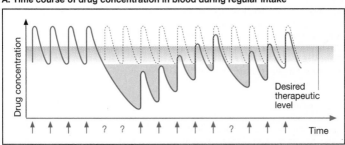

B. Time course of drug concentration with irregular intake

Accumulation: Dose, Dose Interval, and Plasma Level Fluctuation

Successful drug therapy in many illnesses is accomplished only if drug concentration is maintained at a steady high level. This requirement necessitates regular drug intake and a dosage schedule that ensures that the plasma concentration neither falls below the therapeutically effective range nor exceeds the minimal toxic concentration. A constant plasma level would, however, be undesirable if it accelerated a loss of effectiveness (development of tolerance), or if the drug were required to be present at specified times only.

A steady plasma level can be achieved by giving the drug in a constant intravenous infusion, the steady-state plasma level being determined by the infusion rate, dose D per unit of time τ, and the clearance, according to the equation:

$$C_{ss} = \frac{D}{(\tau \cdot Cl_{tot})}$$

This procedure is routinely used in intensive care hospital settings, but is otherwise impracticable. With oral administration, dividing the total daily dose into several individual ones, e.g., four, three, or two, offers a practical compromise.

When the daily dose is given in several divided doses, the mean plasma level shows little fluctuation. In practice, it is found that a regimen of frequent regular drug ingestion is not well adhered to by patients. The degree of fluctuation in plasma level over a given dosing interval can be reduced by use of a dosage form permitting slow (sustained) release (p. 10).

The time required to reach steady-state accumulation during multiple constant dosing depends on the rate of elimination. As a rule of thumb, a plateau is reached after approximately three elimination half-lives ($t_{1/2}$).

For slowly eliminated drugs, which tend to accumulate extensively (phenprocoumon, digitoxin, methadone), the optimal plasma level is attained only after a long period. Here, increasing the initial doses (loading dose) will speed up the attainment of equilibrium, which is subsequently maintained with a lower dose (maintenance dose).

Change in Elimination Characteristics During Drug Therapy (B)

With any drug taken regularly and accumulating to the desired plasma level, it is important to consider that conditions for biotransformation and excretion do not necessarily remain constant. Elimination may be hastened due to enzyme induction (p. 32) or to a change in urinary pH (p. 40). Consequently, the steady-state plasma level declines to a new value corresponding to the new rate of elimination. The drug effect may diminish or disappear. Conversely, when elimination is impaired (e.g., in progressive renal insufficiency), the mean plasma level of renally eliminated drugs rises and may enter a toxic concentration range.

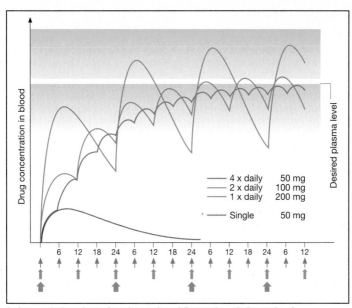

A. Accumulation: dose, dose interval, and fluctuation of plasma level

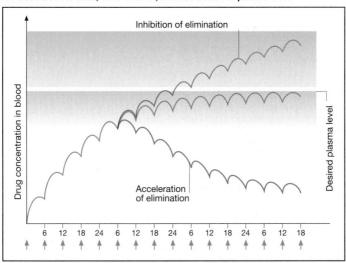

B. Changes in elimination kinetics in the course of drug therapy

Dose–Response Relationship

The effect of a substance depends on the amount administered, i.e., the dose. If the dose chosen is below the critical threshold (subliminal dosing), an effect will be absent. Depending on the nature of the effect to be measured, ascending doses may cause the effect to increase in intensity. Thus, the effect of an antipyretic or hypotensive drug can be quantified in a graded fashion, in that the extent of fall in body temperature or blood pressure is being measured. A dose-effect relationship is then encountered, as discussed on p. 54.

The dose-effect relationship may vary depending on the sensitivity of the individual person receiving the drug, i.e., for the same effect, different doses may be required in different individuals. Interindividual variation in sensitivity is especially obvious with effects of the "all-or-none" kind.

To illustrate this point, we consider an experiment in which the subjects individually respond in all-or-none fashion, as in the Straub tail phenomenon (**A**). Mice react to morphine with excitation, evident in the form of an abnormal posture of the tail and limbs. The dose dependence of this phenomenon is observed in groups of animals (e.g., 10 mice per group) injected with increasing doses of morphine. At the low dose, only the most sensitive, at increasing doses a growing proportion, at the highest dose all of the animals are affected (**B**). There is a relationship between the frequency of responding animals and the dose given. At 2 mg/kg, one out of 10 animals reacts; at 10 mg/kg, 5 out of 10 respond. The **dose-frequency relationship** results from the different sensitivity of individuals, which as a rule exhibits a log-normal distribution (**C**, graph at right, linear scale). If the cumulative frequency (total number of animals responding at a given dose) is plotted against the logarithm of the dose (abscissa), a sigmoidal curve results (**C**, graph at left, semilogarithmic scale). The inflection point of the curve lies at the dose at which one-half of the group has responded. The dose range encompassing the dose-frequency relationship reflects the variation in individual sensitivity to the drug. Although similar in shape, a dose-frequency relationship has, thus, a different meaning than does a dose-effect relationship. The latter can be evaluated in one individual and results from an intraindividual dependency of the effect on drug concentration.

The evaluation of a dose-effect relationship within a group of human subjects is compounded by interindividual differences in sensitivity. To account for the biological variation, measurements have to be carried out on a representative sample and the results averaged. Thus, recommended therapeutic doses will be appropriate for the majority of patients, but not necessarily for *each* individual.

The variation in sensitivity may be based on pharmacokinetic differences (same dose → different plasma levels) or on differences in target organ sensitivity (same plasma level → different effects).

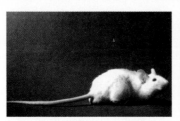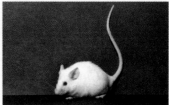

A. Abnormal posture in mouse given morphine

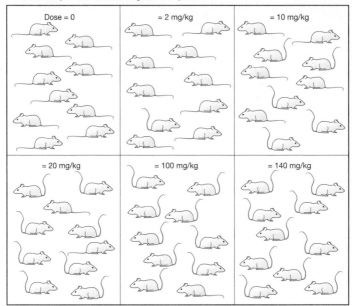

B. Incidence of effect as a function of dose

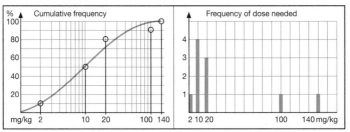

C. Dose-frequency relationship

Concentration-Effect Relationship (A)

The relationship between the concentration of a drug and its effect is determined in order to define the range of active drug concentrations (potency) and the maximum possible effect (efficacy). On the basis of these parameters, differences between drugs can be quantified. As a rule, the therapeutic effect or toxic action depends critically on the response of a single organ or a limited number of organs, e.g., blood flow is affected by a change in vascular luminal width. By isolating critical organs or tissues from a larger functional system, these actions can be studied with more accuracy; for instance, vasoconstrictor agents can be examined in isolated preparations from different regions of the vascular tree, e.g., the portal or saphenous vein, or the mesenteric, coronary, or basilar artery. In many cases, isolated organs or organ parts can be kept viable for hours in an appropriate nutrient medium sufficiently supplied with oxygen and held at a suitable temperature.

Responses of the preparation to a physiological or pharmacological stimulus can be determined by a suitable recording apparatus. Thus, narrowing of a blood vessel is recorded with the help of two clamps by which the vessel is suspended under tension.

Experimentation on isolated organs offers several *advantages:*
1. The drug concentration in the tissue is usually known.
2. Reduced complexity and ease of relating stimulus and effect.
3. It is possible to circumvent compensatory responses that may partially cancel the primary effect in the intact organism — e.g., the heart rate increasing action of norepinephrine cannot be demonstrated in the intact organism, because a simultaneous rise in blood pressure elicits a counter-regulatory reflex that slows cardiac rate.
4. The ability to examine a drug effect over its full rage of intensities — e.g.,

it would be impossible in the intact organism to follow negative chronotropic effects to the point of cardiac arrest.

Disadvantages are:
1. Unavoidable tissue injury during dissection.
2. Loss of physiological regulation of function in the isolated tissue.
3. The artificial milieu imposed on the tissue.

Concentration-Effect Curves (B)

As the concentration is raised by a constant factor, the *increment in effect* diminishes steadily and tends asymptotically towards zero the closer one comes to the maximally effective concentration. The concentration at which a maximal effect occurs cannot be measured accurately; however, that eliciting a half-maximal effect (EC_{50}) is readily determined. It typically corresponds to the inflection point of the concentration–response curve in a semilogarithmic plot (log concentration on abscissa). Full characterization of a concentration–effect relationship requires determination of the EC_{50}, the maximally possible effect (E_{max}), and the slope at the point of inflection.

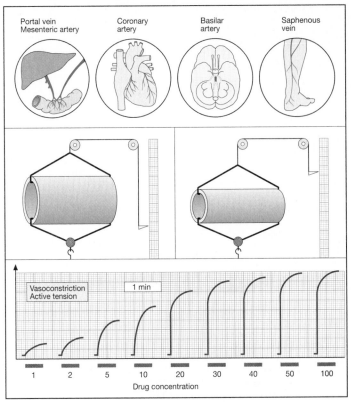

A. Measurement of effect as a function of concentration

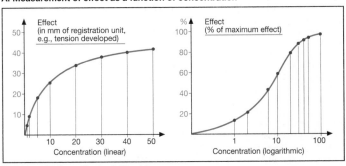

B. Concentration-effect relationship

Concentration-Binding Curves

In order to elicit their effect, drug molecules must be bound to the cells of the effector organ. Binding commonly occurs at specific cell structures, namely, the receptors. The analysis of drug binding to receptors aims to determine the affinity of ligands, the kinetics of interaction, and the characteristics of the binding site itself.

In studying the affinity and number of such binding sites, use is made of membrane suspensions of different tissues. This approach is based on the expectation that binding sites will retain their characteristic properties during cell homogenization. Provided that binding sites are freely accessible in the medium in which membrane fragments are suspended, drug concentration at the "site of action" would equal that in the medium. The drug under study is radiolabeled (enabling low concentrations to be measured quantitatively), added to the membrane suspension, and allowed to bind to receptors. Membrane fragments and medium are then separated, e.g., by filtration, and the amount of bound drug is measured. Binding increases in proportion to concentration as long as there is a negligible reduction in the number of *free* binding sites (c = 1 and B ≈ 10% of maximum binding; c = 2 and B ≈ 20%). As binding approaches saturation, the number of free sites decreases and the increment in binding is no longer proportional to the increase in concentration (in the example illustrated, an increase in concentration by 1 is needed to increase binding from 10 to 20%; however, an increase by 20 is needed to raise it from 70 to 80%).

The **law of mass action** describes the hyperbolic relationship between binding (B) and ligand concentration (c). This relationship is characterized by the drug's affinity ($1/K_D$) and the maximum binding (B_{max}), i.e., the total number of binding sites per unit of weight of membrane homogenate.

$$B = B_{max} \cdot \frac{c}{c + K_D}$$

K_D is the equilibrium dissociation constant and corresponds to that ligand concentration at which 50% of binding sites are occupied. The values given in (**A**) and used for plotting the concentration-binding graph (**B**) result when $K_D = 10$.

The differing affinity of different ligands for a binding site can be demonstrated elegantly by binding assays. Although simple to perform, these binding assays pose the difficulty of correlating unequivocally the binding sites concerned with the pharmacological effect; this is particularly difficult when more than one population of binding sites is present. Therefore, receptor binding must not be implied until it can be shown that

- binding is saturable (*saturability*);
- the only substances bound are those possessing the same pharmacological mechanism of action (*specificity*);
- binding *affinity* of different substances is *correlated* with their pharmacological *potency*.

Binding assays provide information about the affinity of ligands, but they do not give any clue as to whether a ligand is an agonist or antagonist (p. 60). Use of radiolabeled drugs bound to their receptors may be of help in purifying and analyzing further the receptor protein.

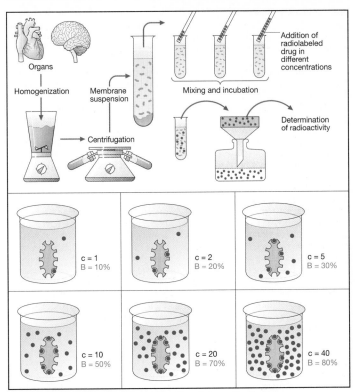

A. Measurement of binding (B) as a function of concentration (c)

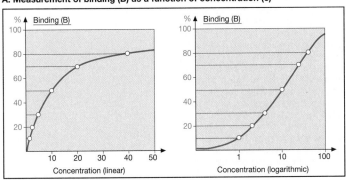

B. Concentration-binding relationship

Types of Binding Forces

Unless a drug comes into contact with intrinsic structures of the body, it cannot affect body function.

Covalent bond. Two atoms enter a covalent bond if each donates an electron to a shared electron pair (cloud). This state is depicted in structural formulas by a dash. The covalent bond is "firm", that is, not reversible or only poorly so. Few drugs are covalently bound to biological structures. The bond, and possibly the effect, persist for a long time after intake of a drug has been discontinued, making therapy difficult to control. Examples include alkylating cytostatics (p. 298) or organophosphates (p. 102). Conjugation reactions occurring in biotransformation also represent a covalent linkage (e.g., to glucuronic acid, p. 38).

Noncovalent bond. There is no formation of a shared electron pair. The bond is reversible and typical of most drug-receptor interactions. Since a drug usually attaches to its site of action by multiple contacts, several of the types of bonds described below may participate.

Electrostatic attraction (A). A positive and negative charge attract each other.

Ionic interaction: An ion is a particle charged either positively (cation) or negatively (anion), i.e., the atom lacks or has surplus electrons, respectively. Attraction between ions of opposite charge is inversely proportional to the square of the distance between them; it is the initial force drawing a charged drug to its binding site. Ionic bonds have a relatively high stability.

Dipole-ion interaction: When bond electrons are asymmetrically distributed over both atomic nuclei, one atom will bear a negative (δ^-), and its partner a positive (δ^+) partial charge. The molecule thus presents a positive and a negative pole, i.e., has *polarity* or a *dipole.* A partial charge can interact electrostatically with an ion of opposite charge.

Dipole-dipole interaction is the electrostatic attraction between opposite partial charges. When a hydrogen atom bearing a partial positive charge bridges two atoms bearing a partial negative charge, a hydrogen bond is created.

A **van der Waals' bond (B)** is formed between apolar molecular groups that have come into close proximity. Spontaneous transient distortion of electron clouds (momentary faint dipole, $\delta\delta$) may induce an opposite dipole in the neighboring molecule. The van der Waals' bond, therefore, is a form of electrostatic attraction, albeit of very low strength (inversely proportional to the seventh power of the distance).

Hydrophobic interaction (C). The attraction between the dipoles of water is strong enough to hinder intercalation of any apolar (uncharged) molecules. By tending towards each other, H_2O molecules squeeze apolar particles from their midst. Accordingly, in the organism, apolar particles have an increased probability of staying in nonaqueous, apolar surroundings, such as fatty acid chains of cell membranes or apolar regions of a receptor.

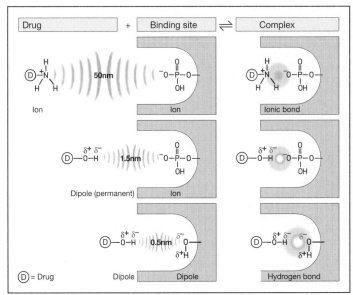

A. Electrostatic attraction

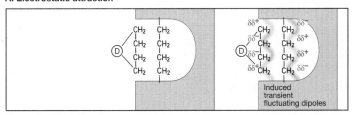

B. van der Waals' bond

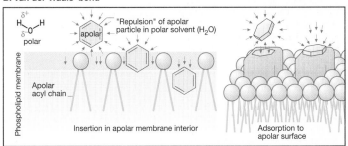

C. Hydrophobic interaction

Agonists – Antagonists

An **agonist** has affinity (binding avidity) for its receptor and alters the receptor protein in such a manner as to generate a stimulus that elicits a change in cell function: **"intrinsic activity"**. The biological effect of the agonist, i.e., the change in cell function, depends on the efficiency of signal transduction steps (p. 64, 66) initiated by the activated receptor. Some agonists attain a maximal effect even when they occupy only a small fraction of receptors (**B**, agonist A). Other ligands (agonist B), possessing equal affinity for the receptor but lower activating capacity (lower intrinsic activity), are unable to produce a full maximal response even when all receptors are occupied: lower **efficacy**. Ligand B is a *partial agonist*. The **potency** of an agonist can be expressed in terms of the concentration (EC_{50}) at which the effect reaches one-half of its respective maximum.

Antagonists (A) attenuate the effect of agonists, that is, their action is "anti-agonistic".

Competitive antagonists possess affinity for receptors, but binding to the receptor does not lead to a change in cell function (*zero* intrinsic activity).

When an agonist and a competitive antagonist are present simultaneously, affinity and concentration of the two rivals will determine the relative amount of each that is bound. Thus, although the antagonist is present, increasing the concentration of the agonist can restore the full effect (**C**). However, in the presence of the antagonist, the concentration-response curve of the agonist is shifted to higher concentrations ("rightward shift").

Molecular Models of Agonist/Antagonist Action (A)

Agonist induces active conformation. The *agonist* binds to the inactive receptor and thereby causes a change from the resting conformation to the active state. The *antagonist* binds to the inactive receptor without causing a conformational change.

Agonist stabilizes spontaneously occurring active conformation. The receptor can spontaneously "flip" into the active conformation. However, the statistical probability of this event is usually so small that the cells do not reveal signs of spontaneous receptor activation. Selective binding of the *agonist* requires the receptor to be in the active conformation, thus promoting its existence. The *"antagonist"* displays affinity only for the inactive state and stabilizes the latter. When the system shows minimal spontaneous activity, application of an antagonist will not produce a measurable effect. When the system has high spontaneous activity, the antagonist may cause an effect that is the opposite of that of the agonist: *inverse* agonist.

A "true" antagonist lacking intrinsic activity ("neutral antagonist") displays equal affinity for both the active and inactive states of the receptor and does not alter basal activity of the cell.
According to this model, a *partial* agonist shows lower selectivity for the active state and, to some extent, also binds to the receptor in its inactive state.

Other Forms of Antagonism

Allosteric antagonism. The antagonist is bound outside the receptor agonist binding site proper and induces a *decrease* in affinity of the agonist. It is also possible that the allosteric deformation of the receptor *increases* affinity for an agonist, resulting in an **allosteric synergism**.

Functional antagonism. Two agonists affect the same parameter (e.g., bronchial diameter) via different receptors in the opposite direction (epinephrine → dilation; histamine → constriction).

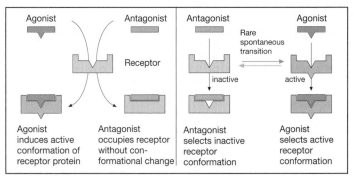

A. Molecular mechanisms of drug-receptor interaction

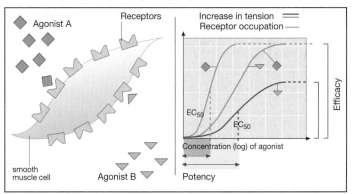

B. Potency and Efficacy of agonists

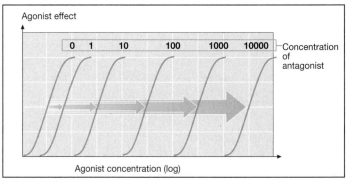

C. Competitive antagonism

Enantioselectivity of Drug Action

Many drugs are racemates, including β-blockers, nonsteroidal anti-inflammatory agents, and anticholinergics (e.g., benzetimide **A**). A **racemate** consists of a molecule and its corresponding mirror image which, like the left and right hand, cannot be superimposed. Such **chiral** ("handed") pairs of molecules are referred to as **enantiomers**. Usually, chirality is due to a carbon atom (C) linked to four different substituents (*"asymmetric center"*). Enantiomerism is a special case of stereoisomerism. Nonchiral stereoisomers are called **diastereomers** (e.g., quinidine/quinine).

Bond lengths in enantiomers, but not in diastereomers, are the same. Therefore, enantiomers possess **similar physicochemical properties** (e.g., solubility, melting point) and both forms are usually obtained in equal amounts by chemical synthesis. As a result of enzymatic activity, however, only one of the enantiomers is usually found in nature.

In solution, enantiomers **rotate the wave plane of linearly polarized light in opposite directions**; hence they are refered to as *"dextro"- or "levo-rotatory"*, designated by the prefixes *d* or (+) and *l* or (-), respectively. The direction of rotation gives no clue concerning the spatial structure of enantiomers. The absolute configuration, as determined by certain rules, is described by the prefixes S and R. In some compounds, designation as the D- and L-form is possible by reference to the structure of D- and L-glyceraldehyde.

For drugs to exert biological actions, contact with reaction partners in the body is required. When the reaction favors one of the enantiomers, enantioselectivity is observed.

Enantioselectivity of affinity. If a receptor has sites for three of the substituents (symbolized in **B** by a cone, a sphere, and a cube) on the asymmetric carbon to attach to, only one of the enantiomers will have optimal fit. Its affinity will then be higher. Thus, *dexetimide* displays an affinity at the musca-

rinic ACh receptors almost 10000 times (p. 98) that of *levetimide*; and at β-adrenoceptors, S(-)-propranolol has an affinity 100 times that of the R(+)-form.

Enantioselectivity of intrinsic activity. The mode of attachment at the receptor also determines whether an effect is elicited and whether or not a substance has intrinsic activity, i.e., acts as an agonist or antagonist. For instance, (-) *dobutamine* is an agonist at α-adrenoceptors whereas the (+)-enantiomer is an antagonist.

Inverse enantioselectivity at another receptor. An enantiomer may possess an unfavorable configuration at one receptor that may, however, be optimal for interaction with another receptor. In the case of *dobutamine*, the (+)-enantiomer has affinity at β-adrenoceptors 10 times higher than that of the (-)-enantiomer, both having agonist activity. However, the α-adrenoceptor stimulant action is due to the (-)-form (see above).

As described for receptor interactions, enantioselectivity may also be manifested in drug interactions with **enzymes** and **transport proteins**. Enantiomers may display different affinities and reaction velocities.

Conclusion: The enantiomers of a racemate can differ sufficiently in their pharmacodynamic and pharmacokinetic properties to constitute two distinct drugs.

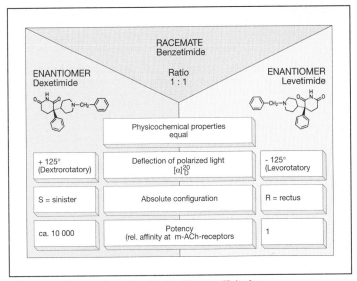

ENANTIOMER Dexetimide		ENANTIOMER Levetimide
RACEMATE Benzetimide	Ratio 1 : 1	
	Physicochemical properties equal	
+ 125° (Dextrorotatory)	Deflection of polarized light $[\alpha]_D^{20}$	- 125° (Levorotatory
S = sinister	Absolute configuration	R = rectus
ca. 10 000	Potency (rel. affinity at m-ACh-receptors	1

A. Example of an enantiomeric pair with different affinity for a stereoselective receptor

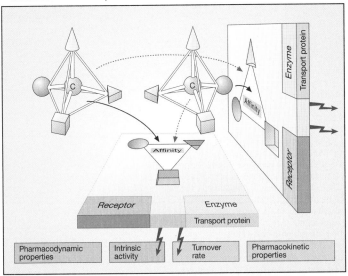

Pharmacodynamic properties	Intrinsic activity	Turnover rate	Pharmacokinetic properties

B. Reasons for different pharmacological properties of enantiomers

Receptor Types

Receptors are macromolecules that bind mediator substances and transduce this binding into an effect, i.e., a change in cell function. Receptors differ in terms of their structure and the manner in which they translate occupancy by a ligand into a cellular response (**signal transduction**).

G-protein-coupled receptors (A) consist of an amino acid chain that weaves in and out of the membrane in serpentine fashion. The extramembranal loop regions of the molecule may possess sugar residues at different N-glycosylation sites. The seven α-helical membrane-spanning domains probably form a circle around a central pocket that carries the attachment sites for the mediator substance. Binding of the mediator molecule or of a structurally related agonist molecule induces a change in the conformation of the receptor protein, enabling the latter to interact with a G-protein (= guanyl nucleotide-binding protein). G-proteins lie at the inner leaf of the plasmalemma and consist of three subunits designated α, β, and γ. There are various G-proteins that differ mainly with regard to their α-unit. Association with the receptor activates the G-protein, leading in turn to activation of another protein (enzyme, ion channel). A large number of mediator substances act via G-protein-coupled receptors (see p. 66 for more details).

An example of a **ligand-gated ion channel (B)** is the nicotinic cholinoceptor of the motor endplate. The receptor complex consists of five subunits, each of which contains four transmembrane domains. Simultaneous binding of two acetylcholine (ACh) molecules to the two α-subunits results in opening of the ion channel, with entry of Na^+ (and exit of some K^+), membrane depolarization, and triggering of an action potential (p. 82). The ganglionic N-cholinoceptors apparently consist only of α and β subunits ($α_2β_2$). Some of the receptors for the transmitter γ-aminobutyric acid (GABA) belong to this receptor family:

the $GABA_A$ subtype is linked to a chloride channel (and also to a benzodiazepine-binding site, see p. 227). Glutamate and glycine both act via ligand-gated ion channels.

The insulin receptor protein represents a **ligand-operated enzyme (C)**, a catalytic receptor. When insulin binds to the extracellular attachment site, a tyrosine kinase activity is "switched on" at the intracellular portion. Protein phosphorylation leads to altered cell function via the assembly of other signal proteins. Receptors for growth hormones also belong to the catalytic receptor class.

Protein synthesis-regulating receptors (D) for steroids, thyroid hormone, and retinoic acid are found in the cytosol and in the cell nucleus, respectively.

Binding of hormone exposes a normally hidden domain of the receptor protein, thereby permitting the latter to bind to a particular nucleotide sequence on a gene and to regulate its transcription. Transcription is usually initiated or enhanced, rarely blocked.

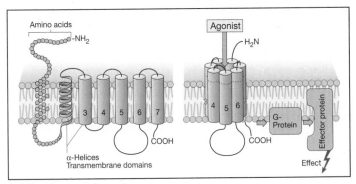

A. G-Protein-coupled receptor

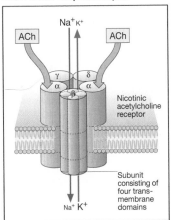

B. Ligand-gated ion channel

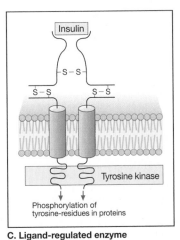

C. Ligand-regulated enzyme

D. Protein synthesis-regulating receptor

Mode of Operation of G-Protein-Coupled Receptors

Signal transduction at G-protein-coupled receptors uses essentially the same basic mechanisms (**A**). Agonist binding to the receptor leads to a change in receptor protein conformation. This change propagates to the G-protein: the α-subunit exchanges GDP for GTP, then dissociates from the two other subunits, associates with an effector protein, and alters its functional state. The α-subunit slowly hydrolyzes bound GTP to GDP. G_α-GDP has no affinity for the effector protein and reassociates with the β and γ subunits (**A**). G-proteins can undergo lateral diffusion in the membrane; they are not assigned to individual receptor proteins. However, a relation exists between receptor types and G-protein types (**B**). Furthermore, the α-subunits of individual G-proteins are distinct in terms of their affinity for different effector proteins, as well as the kind of influence exerted on the effector protein. G_α-GTP of the G_S-protein stimulates adenylate cyclase, whereas G_α-GTP of the G_i-protein is inhibitory. The G-protein-coupled receptor family includes muscarinic cholinoceptors, adrenoceptors for norepinephrine and epinephrine, receptors for dopamine, histamine, serotonin, glutamate, GABA, morphine, prostaglandins, leukotrienes, and many other mediators and hormones.

Major effector proteins for G-protein-coupled receptors include **adenylate cyclase** (ATP $\rightarrow$ intracellular messenger **cAMP**), **phospholipase C** (phosphatidylinositol $\rightarrow$ intracellular messengers **inositol trisphosphate** and **diacylglycerol**), as well as ion channel proteins. Numerous cell functions are regulated by cellular cAMP concentration, because cAMP enhances activity of protein kinase A, which catalyzes the transfer of phosphate groups onto functional proteins. Elevation of cAMP levels *inter alia* leads to relaxation of smooth muscle tonus and enhanced contractility of cardiac muscle, as well as increased glycogenolysis and lipolysis (p.

84). Phosphorylation of cardiac calcium-channel proteins increases the probability of channel opening during membrane depolarization. It should be noted that cAMP is inactivated by phosphodiesterase. Inhibitors of this enzyme elevate intracellular cAMP concentration and elicit effects resembling those of epinephrine.

The receptor protein itself may undergo phosphorylation, with a resultant loss of its ability to activate the associated G-protein. This is one of the mechanisms that contributes to a decrease in sensitivity of a cell during prolonged receptor stimulation by an agonist (*desensitization*).

Activation of phospholipase C leads to cleavage of the membrane phospholipid phosphatidylinositol-4,5 bisphosphate into **inositol trisphosphate** (IP_3) and **diacylglycerol** (DAG). IP_3 promotes release of Ca^{2+} from storage organelles, whereby contraction of smooth muscle cells, breakdown of glycogen, or exocytosis may be initiated. Diacylglycerol stimulates protein kinase C, which phosphorylates certain serine- or threonine-containing enzymes.

The α-subunit of some G-proteins may induce opening of a **channel protein**. In this manner, K^+ channels can be activated (e.g., ACh effect on sinus node, p. 100; opioid action on neural impulse transmission, p. 210).

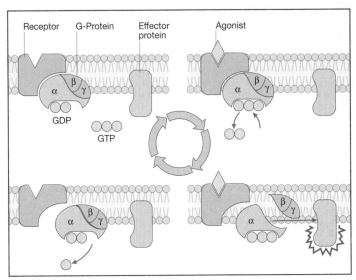

A. G-Protein-mediated effect of an agonist

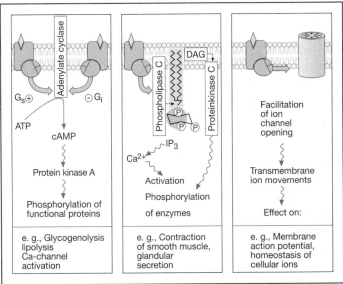

B. G-Proteins, cellular messenger substances, and effects

Time Course of Plasma Concentration and Effect

After the administration of a drug, its concentration in plasma rises, reaches a peak, and then declines gradually to the starting level, due to the processes of distribution and elimination (p. 46). Plasma concentration at a given point in time depends on the dose administered. Many drugs exhibit a linear relationship between plasma concentration and dose within the therapeutic range (**dose-linear kinetics**; (**A**); note different scales on ordinate). However, the same does not apply to drugs whose elimination processes are already sufficiently activated at therapeutic plasma levels so as to preclude further proportional increases in the rate of elimination when the concentration is increased further. Under these conditions, a smaller proportion of the dose administered is eliminated per unit of time.

The time course of the *effect* and of the *concentration* in plasma are not identical, because the **concentration-effect relationships** obeys a hyperbolic function (**B**; cf. also p. 54). This means that the time course of the effect exhibits dose dependence also in the presence of dose-linear kinetics (**C**).

In the lower dose range (example 1), the plasma level passes through a concentration range ($0 \rightarrow 0.9$) in which the concentration effect relationship is quasi-linear. The respective time courses of plasma concentration and effect (A and C, left graphs) are very similar. However, if a high dose (100) is applied, there is an extended period of time during which the plasma level will remain in a concentration range (between 90 and 20) in which a change in concentration does not cause a change in the size of the effect. Thus, at high doses (100), the time-effect curve exhibits a kind of plateau. The effect declines only when the plasma level has returned (below 20) into the range where a change in plasma level causes a change in the intensity of the effect.

The dose dependence of the time course of the drug effect is exploited when the duration of the effect is to be prolonged by administration of a dose in excess of that required for the effect. This is done in the case of penicillin G (p. 268), when a dosing interval of 8 h is being recommended, although the drug is eliminated with a half-life of 30 min. This procedure is, of course, feasible only if supramaximal dosing is not associated with toxic effects.

Futhermore it follows that a nearly constant effect can be achieved, although the plasma level may fluctuate greatly during the interval between doses.

The hyperbolic relationship between plasma concentration and effect explains why the time course of the effect, unlike that of the plasma concentration, cannot be described in terms of a simple exponential function. A half-life can be given for the processes of drug absorption and elimination, hence for the change in plasma levels, but generally not for the onset or decline of the effect.

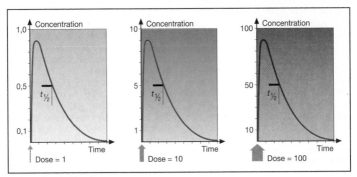

A. Dose-linear kinetics

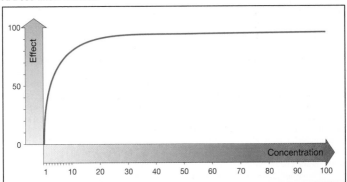

B. Concentration-effect relationship

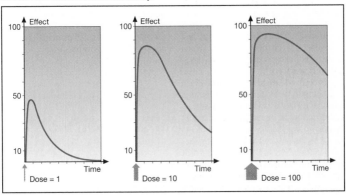

C. Dose dependence of the time course of effect

Adverse Drug Effects

The desired (or intended) principal effect of any drug is to modify body function in such a manner as to alleviate symptoms caused by the patient's illness. In addition, a drug may also cause unwanted effects that can be grouped into minor or "side" effects and major or adverse effects. These, in turn, may give rise to complaints or illness, or may even cause death.

Causes of adverse effects: overdosage (A). The drug is administered in a higher dose than is required for the principal effect; this directly or indirectly affects other body functions. For instances, morphine (p. 210), given in the appropriate dose, affords excellent pain relief by influencing nociceptive pathways in the CNS. In excessive doses, it inhibits the respiratory center and makes apnea imminent. The dose dependence of both effects can be graphed in the form of dose-response curves (DRC). The distance between both DRCs indicates the difference between the therapeutic and toxic doses. This *margin of safety* indicates the risk of toxicity when standard doses are exceeded.

"The dose alone makes the poison" (Paracelsus). This holds true for both medicines and environmental poisons. *No substance as such is toxic!* In order to assess the risk of toxicity, knowledge is required of: 1) the effective dose during exposure; 2) the dose level at which damage is likely to occur; 3) the duration of exposure.

Increased Sensitivity (B). If certain body functions develop hyperreactivity, unwanted effects can occur even at normal dose levels. Increased sensitivity of the respiratory center to morphine is found in patients with chronic lung disease, in neonates, or during concurrent exposure to other respiratory depressant agents. The DRC is shifted to the left and a smaller dose of morphine is sufficient to paralyze respiration. Genetic anomalies of metabolism may also lead to hypersensitivity. Thus, several drugs (aspirin, antimalarials, etc.) can provoke premature breakdown of red blood cells (hemolysis) in subjects with a glucose-6-phosphate dehydrogenase deficiency. The discipline of *pharmacogenetics* deals with the importance of the genotype for reactions to drugs.

The above forms of hypersensitivity must be distinguished from allergies involving the immune system (p. 72).

Lack of selectivity (C). Despite appropriate dosing and normal sensitivity, undesired effects can occur because the drug does not specifically act on the targeted (diseased) tissue or organ. For instance, the anticholinergic, atropine, is bound only to acetylcholine receptors of the muscarinic type; however, these are present in many different organs.

Moreover, the neuroleptic, chlorpromazine, formerly used as a neuroleptic, is able to interact with several different receptor types. Thus, its action is neither organ-specific nor receptor-specific.

The consequences of lack of selectivity can often be avoided if the drug does not require the blood route to reach the target organ, but is, instead, applied locally, as in the administration of parasympatholytics in the form of eye drops or in an aerosol for inhalation.

With every drug use, unwanted effects must be taken into account. Before prescribing a drug, the physician should therefore assess the **risk: benefit ratio**. In this, knowledge of principal and adverse effects is a prerequisite.

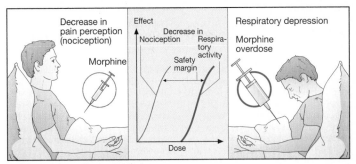

A. Adverse drug effect: overdosing

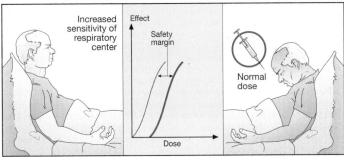

B. Adverse drug effect: increased sensitivity

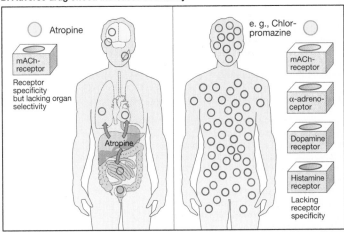

C. Adverse drug effect: lacking selectivity

Drug Allergy

The immune system normally functions to rid the organism of invading foreign particles, such as bacteria. Immune responses can occur without appropriate cause or with exaggerated intensity and may harm the organism, for instance, when allergic reactions are caused by drugs (active ingredient or pharmaceutical excipients). Only a few drugs, e.g. (heterologous) proteins, have a molecular mass (>10,000) large enough to act as effective **antigens** or **immunogens,** capable by themselves of initiating an immune response. Most drugs or their metabolites (so-called **haptens**) must first be converted to an antigen by linkage to a body protein. In the case of penicillin G, a cleavage product (penicilloyl residue) probably undergoes covalent binding to protein. During **initial contact** with the drug, the immune system is sensitized: antigen-specific lymphocytes of the T-type and B-type (antibody formation) proliferate in lymphatic tissue and some of them remain as so-called memory cells. Usually, these processes remain clinically silent. During the **second contact**, antibodies are already present and memory cells proliferate rapidly. A detectable immune response, the allergic reaction, occurs. This can be of severe intensity, even at a low dose of the antigen. Four types of reactions can be distinguished:

Type 1, anaphylactic reaction. Drug-specific antibodies of the *IgE type* combine via their F_c moiety with receptors on the surface of *mast cells.* Binding of the drug provides the stimulus for the release of histamine and other mediators. In the most severe form, a life-threatening anaphylactic shock develops, accompanied by hypotension, bronchospasm (asthma attack), laryngeal edema, urticaria, stimulation of gut musculature, and spontaneous bowel movements (p. 326).

Type 2, cytotoxic reaction. *Drug-antibody (IgG) complexes* adhere to the *surface of blood cells,* where either circulating drug molecules or complexes already formed in blood accumulate. These complexes mediate the *activation of complement,* a family of proteins that circulate in the blood in an inactive form, but can be activated in a cascade-like succession by an appropriate stimulus. "Activated complement" normally directed against microorganisms, can *destroy the cell membranes* and thereby cause cell death; it also promotes phagocytosis, attracts neutrophil granulocytes (chemotaxis), and stimulates other inflammatory responses. Activation of complement on blood cells results in their destruction, evidenced by hemolytic anemia, agranulocytosis, and thrombocytopenia.

Type 3, immune complex vasculitis (serum sickness, Arthus reaction). *Drug-antibody complexes* precipitate on *vascular walls, complement* is activated, and an *inflammatory reaction* is triggered. Attracted *neutrophils,* in a futile attempt to phagocytose the complexes, liberate lysosomal enzymes that damage the vascular walls (inflammation, vasculitis). Symptoms may include fever, exanthema, swelling of lymph nodes, arthritis, nephritis, and neuropathy.

Type 4, contact dermatitis. A cutaneously applied drug is bound to the surface of *T-lymphocytes* directed specifically against it. The lymphocytes release signal molecules (*lymphokines*) into their vicinity that activate macrophages and provoke an inflammatory reaction.

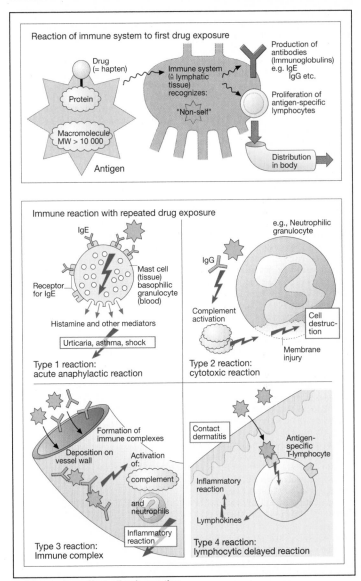

A. Adverse drug effect: allergic reaction

Drug Toxicity in Pregnancy and Lactation

Drugs taken by the mother can be passed on transplacentally or via breast milk and adversely affect the unborn or the neonate.

Pregnancy (A)

Limb malformations induced by the hypnotic, thalidomide, first focused attention on the potential of drugs to cause malformations (*teratogenicity*). Drug effects on the unborn fall into two basic categories:

1. Predictable effects that derive from the known pharmacological drug properties. Examples are: masculinization of the female fetus by androgenic hormones; brain hemorrhage due to oral anticoagulants; bradycardia due to β-blockers.

2. Effects that specifically affect the developing organism and that cannot be predicted on the basis of the known pharmacological activity profile.

In assessing the risks attending drug use during pregnancy, the following points have to be considered:

a) *Time of drug use.* The possible sequelae of exposure to a drug depend on the stage of fetal development, as shown in A. Thus, the hazard posed by a drug with a specific action is limited in time, as illustrated by the tetracyclines, which produce effects on teeth and bones only after the third month of gestation, when mineralization begins.

b) *Transplacental passage.* Most drugs can pass in the placenta from the maternal into the fetal circulation. The fused cells of the syncytiotrophoblast form the major diffusion barrier. They possess a higher permeability to drugs than is suggested by the term "placental barrier".

c) *Teratogenicity.* Statistical risk estimates are available for familiar, frequently used drugs. For many drugs, teratogenic potency cannot be demonstrated; however, in the case of novel drugs it is usually not yet possible to define their teratogenic hazard.

Drugs with established human teratogenicity include derivatives of vitamin A (etretinate, isotretinoin [used internally in skin diseases]), and oral anticoagulants. A peculiar type of damage results from the synthetic estrogenic agent, diethylstilbestrol, following its use during pregnancy; daughters of treated mothers have an increased incidence of cervical and vaginal carcinoma at the age of approx. 20.

In assessing the risk: benefit ratio, it is also necessary to consider the benefit for the child resulting from adequate therapeutic treatment of its mother. For instance, therapy with antiepileptic drugs is indispensable, because untreated epilepsy endangers the infant at least as much as does administration of anticonvulsants.

Lactation (B)

Drugs present in the maternal organism can be secreted in breast milk and thus be ingested by the infant. Evaluation of risk should be based on factors listed in **B**. In case of doubt, potential danger to the infant can be averted only by weaning.

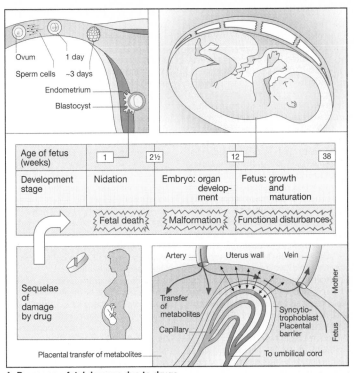

A. Pregnancy: fetal damage due to drugs

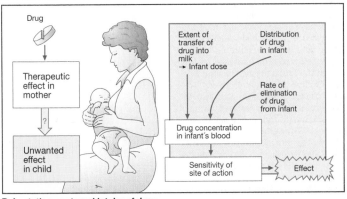

B. Lactation: maternal intake of drug

Placebo (A)

A placebo is a dosage form devoid of an active ingredient, a dummy medication. Administration of a placebo may elicit the desired effect (relief of symptoms) or undesired effects that reflect a change in the patient's psychological situation brought about by the therapeutic setting.

Physicians may consciously or unconsciously communicate to the patient whether or not they are concerned about the patient's problem, or certain about the diagnosis and about the value of prescribed therapeutic measures. In the care of a physician who projects personal warmth, competence, and confidence, the patient in turn feels comfortable and less anxious and optimistically anticipates recovery.

The physical condition determines the psychic disposition and vice versa. Consider gravely wounded combatants in war, oblivious to their injuries while fighting to survive, only to experience severe pain in the safety of the field hospital, or the patient with a peptic ulcer caused by emotional stress.

Clinical trials. In the individual case, it may be impossible to decide whether therapeutic success is attributable to the drug or to the therapeutic situation. What is therefore required is a comparison of the effects of a drug and of a placebo in matched groups of patients by means of statistical procedures, i.e., a *placebo-controlled trial.* A *prospective trial* is planned in advance, a *retrospective (case-control)* study follows patients backwards in time. Patients are *randomly allotted* to two groups, namely, the *placebo* and the *active* or test drug group. In a *double-blind* trial, neither the patients nor the treating physicians know which patient is given drug and which placebo. Finally, a switch from drug to placebo and vice versa can be made in a successive phase of treatment, the *cross-over trial.* In this fashion, drug vs. placebo comparisons can be made not only between two patient groups, but also within either group itself.

Homeopathy (B) is an alternative method of therapy, developed in the 1800s by Samuel Hahnemann. His idea was this: when given in normal (allopathic) dosage, a drug (in the sense of medicament) will produce a constellation of symptoms; however, in a patient whose disease symptoms resemble just this mosaic of symptoms, the same drug *(simile principle)* would effect a cure when given in a very low dosage *("potentiation").* The body's self-healing powers were to be properly activated only by minimal doses of the medicinal substance.

The homeopath's task is not to diagnose the causes of morbidity, but to find the drug with a "symptom profile" most closely resembling that of the patient's illness. This drug is then applied in very high dilution.

A direct action or effect on body functions cannot be demonstrated for homeopathic medicines. Therapeutic success is due to the suggestive powers of the homeopath and the expectancy of the patient. When an illness is strongly influenced by emotional (psychic) factors and cannot be treated well by allopathic means, a case can be made in favor of exploiting suggestion as a therapeutic tool. Homeopathy is one of several possible methods of doing so.

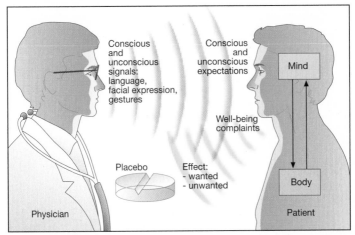

A. Therapeutic effects resulting from physician's power of suggestion

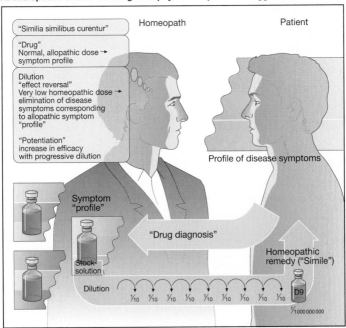

B. Homeopathy: concepts and procedure

Systems Pharmacology

Sympathetic Nervous System

In the course of phylogeny an efficient control system evolved that enabled the functions of individual organs to be orchestrated in increasingly complex life forms and permitted rapid adaptation to changing environmental conditions. This regulatory system consists of the CNS (brain plus spinal cord) and two separate pathways for two-way communication with peripheral organs, viz., the somatic and the autonomic nervous systems. The **somatic nervous system** comprising extero- and interoceptive afferents, special sense organs, and motor efferents, serves to perceive *external* states and to target appropriate body movement (sensory perception: threat → response: flight or attack). The **autonomic (vegetative) nervous system** (ANS), together with the endocrine system, controls the *milieu interieur.* It adjusts internal organ functions to the changing needs of the organism. Neural control permits very quick adaptation, whereas the endocrine system provides for a long-term regulation of functional states. The ANS operates largely beyond voluntary control; it functions autonomously. Its central components reside in the hypothalamus, brain stem, and spinal cord. The ANS also participates in the regulation of endocrine functions.

The ANS has **sympathetic** and **parasympathetic** branches. Both are made up of centrifugal (efferent) and centripetal (afferent) nerves. In many organs innervated by both branches, respective activation of the sympathetic and parasympathetic input evokes opposing responses.

In various disease states (organ malfunctions), drugs are employed with the intention of normalizing susceptible organ functions. To understand the biological effects of substances capable of inhibiting or exciting sympathetic or parasympathetic nerves, one must first envisage the functions subserved by the sympathetic and parasympathetic divisions (**A, Responses to sympathetic activation**). In simplistic terms, activation of the sympathetic division can be considered a means by which the body achieves a state of maximal work capacity as required in fight or flight situations.

In both cases, there is a need for vigorous activity of skeletal musculature. To ensure adequate supply of oxygen and nutrients, blood flow in skeletal muscle is increased; cardiac rate and contractility are enhanced, resulting in a larger blood volume being pumped into the circulation. Narrowing of splanchnic blood vessels diverts blood into vascular beds in muscle.

Because digestion of food in the intestinal tract is dispensable and only counterproductive, the propulsion of intestinal contents is slowed to the extent that peristalsis diminishes and sphincteric tonus increases. However, in order to increase nutrient supply to heart and musculature, glucose from the liver and free fatty acid from adipose tissue must be released into the blood. The bronchi are dilated, enabling tidal volume and alveolar oxygen uptake to be increased.

Sweat glands are also innervated by sympathetic fibers (wet palms due to excitement); however, these are exceptional as regards their neurotransmitter (ACh, p. 106).

Although the life styles of modern humans are different from those of hominid ancestors, biological functions have remained the same.

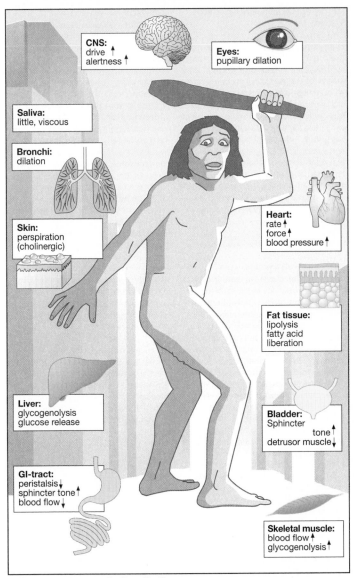

CNS:
drive ↑
alertness ↑

Eyes:
pupillary dilation

Saliva:
little, viscous

Bronchi:
dilation

Skin:
perspiration
(cholinergic)

Heart:
rate ↑
force ↑
blood pressure ↑

Fat tissue:
lipolysis
fatty acid
liberation

Liver:
glycogenolysis
glucose release

Bladder:
Sphincter
          tone ↑
detrusor muscle ↓

GI-tract:
peristalsis ↓
sphincter tone ↑
blood flow ↓

Skeletal muscle:
blood flow ↑
glycogenolysis ↑

A. Responses to sympathetic activation

Structure of the Sympathetic Nervous System

The sympathetic preganglionic neurons (first neurons) project from the intermediolateral column of the spinal gray matter to the *paired paravertebral ganglionic chain* lying alongside the vertebral column and to *unpaired prevertebral ganglia*. These **ganglia** represent sites of synaptic contact between **preganglionic axons** (1st neurons) and nerve cells (2nd neurons or sympathocytes) that emit **postganglionic axons** terminating on cells in various end organs. In addition, there are preganglionic neurons that project either to peripheral ganglia in end organs or to the adrenal medulla.

Sympathetic Transmitter Substances

Whereas **acetylcholine** (see p. 98) serves as the chemical transmitter at ganglionic synapses between **first and second neurons, norepinephrine (= noradrenaline)** is the mediator at synapses of the second neuron (**B**). This second neuron does not synapse with only a single cell in the effector organ; rather, it branches out, each branch making *en passant* contacts with several cells. At these junctions the nerve axons form enlargements (**varicosities**) resembling beads on a string. Thus, excitation of the neuron leads to activation of a larger aggregate of effector cells, although the action of released norepinephrine may be confined to the region of each junction. Excitation of preganglionic neurons innervating the adrenal medulla causes a liberation of acetylcholine. This, in turn, elicits a secretion of **epinephrine** (= adrenaline) into the blood, by which it is distributed to body tissues as a hormone (**A**).

Adrenergic Synapse

Within the varicosities, norepinephrine is stored in small membrane-enclosed vesicles (granules, 0.05 to 0.2 μm in diameter). In the axoplasm, L-tyrosine is converted via two intermediate steps to dopamine, which is taken up into the vesicles and there converted to norepinephrine by dopamine-β-hydroxylase. When stimulated electrically, the sympathetic nerve discharges the contents of part of its vesicles, including norepinephrine, into the extracellular space. Liberated **norepinephrine** reacts with **adrenoceptors** located postjunctionally on the membrane of effector cells or prejunctionally on the membrane of varicosities. Activation of presynaptic α_2-receptors inhibits norepinephrine release. By this negative feedback, release can be regulated.

The effect of released norepinephrine wanes quickly, because approx. 90% is actively transported back into the axoplasm, then into storage vesicles (**neuronal re-uptake**). Small portions of norepinephrine are inactivated by the enzyme **c**atechol-**O**-**m**ethyl**t**ransferase (COMT, present in the cytoplasm of postjunctional cells, to yield normetanephrine), and **m**ono**a**mine **o**xidase (MAO, present in mitochondria of nerve cells and postjunctional cells, to yield 3,4-dihydroxymandelic acid).

The liver is richly endowed with COMT and MAO; it therefore contributes significantly to the degradation of circulating norepinephrine and epinephrine. The end product of the combined actions of MAO and COMT is vanillylmandelic acid.

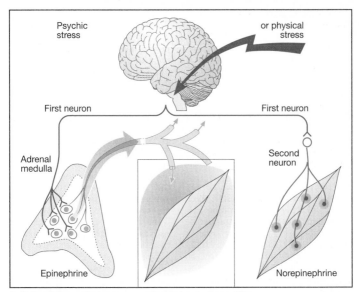

A. Epinephrine as hormone, norepinephrine as transmitter

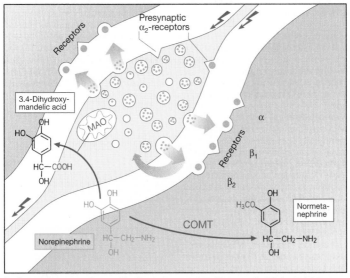

B. Second neuron of sympathetic system, varicosity, norepinephrine release

Adrenoceptor Subtypes and Catecholamine Actions

Adrenoceptors fall into three major groups, designated α_1, α_2, and β, within each of which further subtypes can be distinguished pharmacologically. The different adrenoceptors are differentially distributed according to region and tissue. Agonists at adrenoceptors (**direct sympathomimetics**) mimic the actions of the naturally occurring *catecholamines*, norepinephrine and epinephrine, and are used for various therapeutic effects.

Smooth muscle effects. The opposing effects on smooth muscle (**A**) of α-and β-adrenoceptor activation are due to differences in signal transduction (p. 66). This is exemplified by vascular smooth muscle (**A**). α_1-Receptor stimulation leads to intracellular release of Ca^{2+} via activation of the inositol trisphosphate (IP_3) pathway. In concert with the protein calmodulin, Ca^{2+} can activate myosin kinase, leading to a rise in tonus via phosphorylation of the contractile protein myosin. cAMP inhibits activation of myosin kinase. Via the former effector pathway, stimulation of α-receptors results in vasoconstriction; via the latter, β_2-receptors mediate vasodilation, particularly in skeletal muscle — an effect that has little therapeutic use.

Vasoconstriction. Local application of α-sympathomimetics can be employed in infiltration anesthesia (p. 204) or for nasal decongestion (naphazoline, tetrahydrozoline, xylometazoline; pp. 90, 324). Systemically administered epinephrine is important in the treatment of anaphylactic shock for combating hypotension.

Bronchodilation. β_2-Adrenoceptor-mediated *bronchodilation* (e.g., with terbutaline, fenoterol, or salbutamol) plays an essential part in the treatment of bronchial asthma (p. 328).

Tocolysis. The uterine relaxant effect of β_2-adrenoceptor agonists, such as terbutaline or fenoterol, can be used to prevent *premature labor*. Vasodilation with a resultant drop in systemic blood pressure results in reflex tachycardia, which is also due in part to the β_1-stimulant action of these drugs.

Cardiostimulation. By stimulating β_1-receptors, hence activation of adenylatcyclase (Ad-cyclase) and cAMP production, catecholamines augment all heart functions, including *systolic force* (positive inotropism), *velocity of shortening* (p. clinotropism), *sinoatrial rate* (p. chronotropism), *conduction velocity* (p. dromotropism), and *excitability* (p. bathmotropism). In pacemaker fibers, *diastolic depolarization* is hastened, so that the firing threshold for the action potential is reached sooner (positive chronotropic effect, **B**). The cardiostimulant effect of β-sympathomimetics such as epinephrine is exploited in the treatment of cardiac arrest. Use of β-sympathomimetics in heart failure carries the risk of cardiac arrhythmias.

Metabolic effects. β-Receptors mediate increased *conversion of glycogen* to glucose *(glycogenolysis)* in both liver and skeletal muscle. From the liver, glucose is released into the blood, In adipose tissue, triglycerides are hydrolyzed to fatty acids (*lipolysis,* mediated *by* β_3-receptors), which then enter the blood (**C**). The metabolic effects of catecholamines are not amenable to therapeutic use.

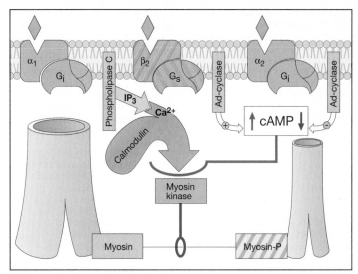

A. Vasomotor effects of catecholamines

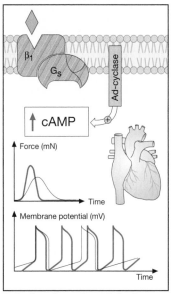

B. Cardiac effects of catecholamines

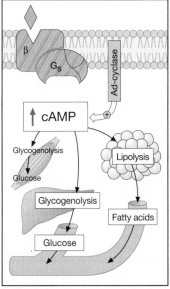

C. Metabolic effects of catecholamines

Structure – Activity Relationships of Sympathomimetics

Due to its equally high affinity for all α- and β-receptors, epinephrine does not permit selective activation of a particular receptor subtype. Like most catecholamines, it is also unsuitable for oral administration (catechol is a trivial name for o-hydroxyphenol). Norepinephrine differs from epinephrine by its high affinity for α-receptors and low affinity for β_2-receptors. In contrast, isoproterenol has high affinity for β-receptors, but virtually none for α-receptors (**A**).

norepinephrine $\rightarrow$ α, β_1
epinephrine $\rightarrow$ α, β_1, β_2
isoproterenol $\rightarrow$ β_1, β_2

Knowledge of **structure–activity relationships** has permitted the synthesis of sympathomimetics that display a high degree of selectivity at adrenoceptor subtypes.

Direct-acting sympathomimetics (i.e., adrenoceptor agonists) typically share a *phenylethylamine* structure. The *side chain β-hydroxyl group* confers affinity for α- and β-receptors. *Substitution on the amino group* reduces affinity for α-receptors, but increases it for β-receptors (exception: α-agonist phenylephrine), with optimal affinity being seen after the introduction of only one isopropyl group. Increasing the bulk of the amino substituent favors affinity for β_2-receptors (e.g., fenoterol, salbutamol). Both *hydroxyl groups* on the aromatic nucleus contribute to affinity; high activity at α-receptors is associated with hydroxyl groups at the 3 and 4 positions. Affinity for β-receptors is preserved in congeners bearing hydroxyl groups at positions 3 and 5 (orciprenaline, terbutaline, fenoterol).

The hydroxyl groups of catecholamines are responsible for the very low lipophilicity of these substances. Polarity is increased at physiological pH due to protonation of the amino group. Deletion of one or all hydroxyl groups improves membrane penetrability at the intestinal mucosa-blood and the blood-brain barriers. Accordingly, these non-catecholamine congeners can be given orally and can exert CNS actions; however, this structural change entails a loss in affinity.

Absence of one or both aromatic hydroxyl groups is associated with an increase in **indirect sympathomimetic activity**, denoting the ability of a substance to release norepinephrine from its neuronal stores without exerting an agonist action at the adrenoceptor (p. 88).

An altered position of aromatic hydroxyl groups (e.g., in orciprenaline, fenoterol, or terbutaline) or their substitution (e.g., salbutamol) protects against *inactivation* by COMT (p. 82). Indroduction of a small alkyl residue at the carbon atom adjacent to the amino group (ephedrine, methamphetamine) confers resistance to *degradation by MAO* (p. 80), as does replacement on the amino groups of the methyl residue with larger substituents (e.g., ethyl in etilefrine). Accordingly, the congeners are less subject to presystemic inactivation.

Since structural requirements for high affinity, on the one hand, and oral applicability, on the other, do not match, choosing a sympathomimetic is a matter of compromise. If the high affinity of epinephrine is to be exploited, absorbability from the intestine must be foregone (epinephrine, isoprenaline). If good bioavailability with oral administration is desired, losses in receptor affinity must be accepted (etilefrine).

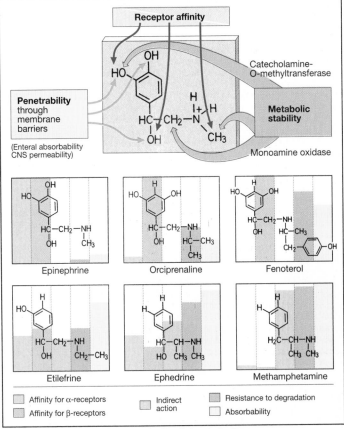

A. Chemical structure of catecholamines and affinity for α- and β-receptors

B. Structure-activity relationship of epinephrine derivatives

Indirect Sympathomimetics

Apart from **receptors**, adrenergic neurotransmission involves mechanisms for the **active re-uptake** and **re-storage** of released amine, as well as enzymatic breakdown by **monoamine oxidase** (**MAO**). Norepinephrine (NE) displays affinity for receptors, transport systems, and degradative enzymes. Chemical alterations of the catecholamine differentially affect these properties and result in substances with selective actions.

Inhibitors of MAO (A). The enzyme is located predominantly on mitochondria, and serves to scavenge axoplasmic free NE. Inhibition of the enzyme causes free NE concentrations to rise. Likewise, dopamine catabolism is impaired, making more of it available for NE synthesis. Consequently, the amount of NE stored in granular vesicles will increase, and with it the amount of amine released per nerve impulse.

In the CNS, inhibition of MAO affects neuronal storage not only of NE but also of dopamine and serotonin. These mediators probably play significant roles in CNS functions consistent with the stimulant effects of MAO inhibitors on mood and psychomotor drive and their use as antidepressants in the treatment of depression (**A**). *Tranylcypromine* is used to treat particular forms of depressive illness; as a covalently bound suicide substrate, it causes long-lasting inhibition of both MAO isozymes, (MAO_A, MAO_B). *Moclobemide* reversibly inhibits MAO_A and is also used as an antidepressant. The MAO_B inhibitor *selegiline* (deprenyl) retards the catobolism of dopamine, an effect used in the treatment of parkinsonism (p. 188).

Indirect sympathomimetics (**B**) are agents that elevate the concentration of NE at neuroeffector junctions, because they either inhibit re-uptake *(cocaine)*, facilitate release, or slow breakdown by MAO, or exert all three of these effects *(amphetamine, methamphetamine)*. The effectiveness of such indirect sympathomimetics diminishes or disappears (**tachyphylaxis**) when ve-sicular stores of NE close to the axolemma are depleted.

Indirect sympathomimetics can penetrate the blood-brain barrier and evoke such CNS effects as a feeling of well-being, enhanced physical activity and mood (**euphoria**), and decreased sense of hunger or fatigue. Subsequently, the user may feel tired and depressed. These after effects are partly responsible for the urge to re-administer the drug (high abuse potential). To prevent their misuse, these substances are subject to governmental regulations (e.g., Food and Drugs Act: Canada; Controlled Drugs Act: USA) restricting their prescription and distribution.

When amphetamine-like substances are misused to enhance athletic performance (*doping*), there is a risk of dangerous physical overexertion. Because of the absence of a sense of fatigue, a drugged athlete may be able to mobilize ultimate energy reserves. In extreme situations, cardiovascular failure may result (**B**).

Closely related chemically to amphetamine are the so-called appetite suppressants or anorexiants, such as fenfluramine, mazindole, and sibutramine. These may also cause dependence and their therapeutic value and safety are questionable.

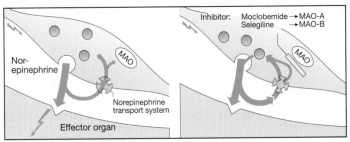

A. Monoamine oxidase inhibitor

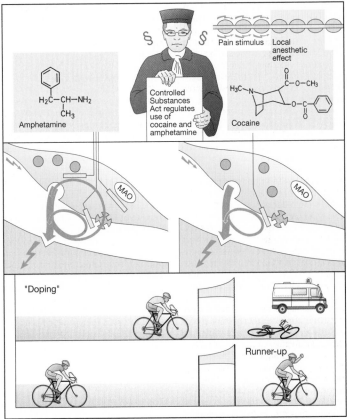

B. Indirect sympathomimetics with central stimulant activity and abuse potential

α-Sympathomimetics, α-Sympatholytics

α-Sympathomimetics can be used *systemically* in certain types of hypotension (p. 314) and *locally* for nasal or conjunctival decongestion (pp. 324, 326) or as adjuncts in infiltration anesthesia (p. 206) for the purpose of delaying the removal of local anesthetic. With local use, underperfusion of the vasoconstricted area results in a lack of oxygen (**A**). In the extreme case, local hypoxia can lead to tissue necrosis. The appendages (e.g., digits, toes, ears) are particularly vulnerable in this regard, thus precluding vasoconstrictor adjuncts in infiltration anesthesia at these sites.

Vasoconstriction induced by an α-sympathomimetic is followed by a phase of enhanced blood flow (**reactive hyperemia, A**). This reaction can be observed after the application of α-sympathomimetics (naphazoline, tetrahydrozoline, xylometazoline) to the nasal mucosa. Initially, vasoconstriction reduces mucosal blood flow and, hence, capillary pressure. Fluid exuded into the interstitial space is drained through the veins, thus shrinking the nasal mucosa. Due to the reduced supply of fluid, secretion of nasal mucus decreases. In coryza, nasal patency is restored. However, after vasoconstriction subsides, reactive hyperemia causes renewed exudation of plasma fluid into the interstitial space, the nose is "stuffy" again, and the patient feels a need to reapply decongestant. In this way, a vicious cycle threatens. Besides rebound congestion, persistent use of a decongestant entails the risk of atrophic damage caused by prolonged hypoxia of the nasal mucosa.

α-Sympatholytics (B). The interaction of norepinephrine with α-adrenoceptors can be inhibited by α-sympatholytics (α-adrenoceptor antagonists, α-blockers). This inhibition can be put to therapeutic use in antihypertensive treatment (vasodilation → peripheral resistance ↓, blood pressure ↓, p. 118). The first α-sympatholytics blocked the action of norepinephrine at both *post-* and *prejunctional* α-adrenoceptors (**non-selective α-blockers**, e.g., phenoxybenzamine, phentolamine).

Presynaptic α_2-adrenoceptors function like sensors that enable norepinephrine concentration outside the axolemma to be monitored, thus regulating its release via a local feedback mechanism. When presynaptic α_2-receptors are stimulated, further release of norepinephrine is inhibited. Conversely, their blockade leads to uncontrolled release of norepinephrine with an overt enhancement of sympathetic effects at β_1-adrenoceptor-mediated myocardial neuroeffector junctions, resulting in tachycardia and tachyarrhythmia.

Selective α-Sympatholytics

α-Blockers, such as prazosin, or the longer-acting terazosin and doxazosin, lack affinity for prejunctional α_2-adrenoceptors. They suppress activation of α_1-receptors without a concomitant enhancement of norepinephrine release.

α_1-Blockers may be used in hypertension (p. 312). Because they prevent reflex vasoconstriction, they are likely to cause postural hypotension with pooling of blood in lower limb capacitance veins during change from the supine to the erect position (orthostatic collapse: ↓ venous return, ↓ cardiac output, fall in systemic pressure, ↓ blood supply to CNS, syncope, p. 314).

In benign hyperplasia of the prostate, α-blockers (terazosin, alfuzosin) may serve to lower tonus of smooth musculature in the prostatic region and thereby facilitate micturition (p. 252).

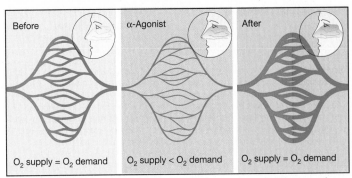

A. Reactive hyperemia due to α-sympathomimetics, e.g., following decongestion of nasal mucosa

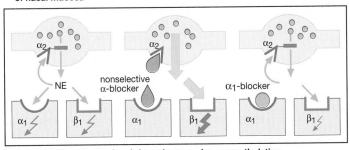

B. Autoinhibition of norepinephrine release and α-sympatholytics

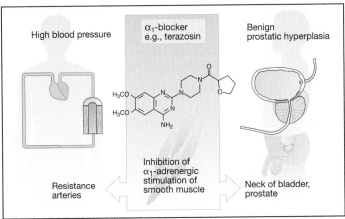

C. Indications for α₁-sympatholytics

β-Sympatholytics (β-Blockers)

β-Sympatholytics are antagonists of norepiphephrine and epinephrine at β-adrenoceptors; they lack affinity for α-receptors.

Therapeutic effects. β-Blockers protect the heart from the oxygen-wasting effect of sympathetic inotropism (p. 306) by blocking cardiac β-receptors; thus, cardiac work can no longer be augmented above basal levels (the heart is "coasting"). This effect is utilized prophylactically in angina pectoris to prevent myocardial stress that could trigger an ischemic attack (p. 308, 310). β-Blockers also serve to *lower cardiac rate* (sinus tachycardia, p. 134) and *elevated blood pressure* due to high cardiac output (p. 312). The mechanism underlying their *antihypertensive action* via reduction of peripheral resistance is unclear.

Applied topically to the eye, β-blockers are used in the management of *glaucoma;* they lower production of aqueous humor without affecting its drainage.

Undesired effects. The hazards of treatment with β-blockers become apparent particularly when continuous activation of β-receptors is needed in order to maintain the function of an organ.

Congestive heart failure: In myocardial insufficiency, the heart depends on a tonic sympathetic drive to maintain adequate cardiac output. Sympathetic activation gives rise to an increase in heart rate and systolic muscle tension, enabling cardiac output to be restored to a level comparable to that in a healthy subject. When sympathetic drive is eliminated during β-receptor blockade, stroke volume and cardiac rate decline, a latent myocardial insufficiency is unmasked, and overt insufficiency is exacerbated (**A**).

On the other hand, clinical evidence suggests that β-blockers produce favorable effects in certain forms of congestive heart failure (idiopathic dilated cardiomyopathy).

Bradycardia, A-V block: Elimination of sympathetic drive can lead to a marked fall in cardiac rate as well as to disorders of impulse conduction from the atria to the ventricles.

Bronchial asthma: Increased sympathetic activity prevents bronchospasm in patients disposed to paroxysmal constriction of the bronchial tree (bronchial asthma, bronchitis in smokers). In this condition, β_2-receptor blockade will precipitate acute respiratory distress (**B**).

Hypoglycemia in diabetes mellitus: When treatment with insulin or oral hypoglycemics in the diabetic patient lowers blood glucose below a critical level, epinephrine is released, which then stimulates hepatic glucose release via activation of β_2-receptors. β-Blockers suppress this counter-regulation; in addition, they mask other epinephrine-mediated warning signs of imminent hypoglycemia, such as tachycardia and anxiety, thereby enhancing the risk of hypoglycemic shock.

Altered vascular responses: When β_2-receptors are blocked, the vasodilating effect of epinephrine is abolished, leaving the α-receptor-mediated vasoconstriction unaffected: peripheral blood flow $\downarrow$ – "cold hands and feet".

β-Blockers exert an **"anxiolytic"** action that may be due to the suppression of somatic responses (palpitations, trembling) to epinephrine release that is induced by emotional stress; in turn, these would exacerbate "anxiety" or "stage fright". Because alertness is not impaired by β-blockers, these agents are occasionally taken by orators and musicians before a major performance (**C**). Stage fright, however, is not a disease requiring drug therapy.

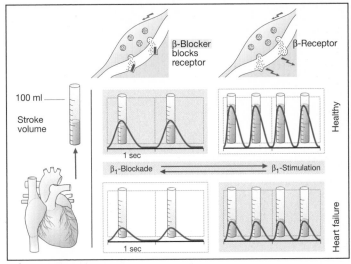

A. β-Sympatholytics: effect on cardiac function

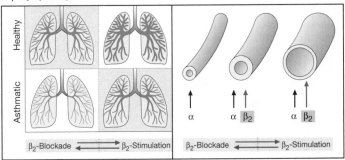

B. β-Sympatholytics: effect on bronchial and vascular tone

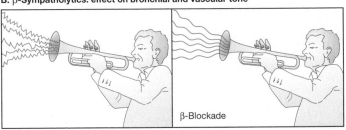

C. "Anxiolytic" effect of β-sympatholytics

Types of β-Blockers

The **basic structure** shared by most β-sympatholytics is the side chain of β-sympathomimetics (cf. isoproterenol with the β-blockers propranolol, pindolol, atenolol). As a rule, this basic structure is linked to an aromatic nucleus by a methylene and oxygen bridge. The side chain C-atom bearing the hydroxyl group forms the chiral center. With some exceptions (e.g., timolol, penbutolol), all β-sympatholytics are brought as racemates into the market (p. 62).

Compared with the dextrorotatory form, the levorotatory enantiomer possesses a greater than 100-fold higher affinity for the β-receptor and is, therefore, practically alone in contributing to the β-blocking effect of the racemate. The side chain and substituents on the amino group critically affect affinity for β-receptors, whereas the aromatic nucleus determines whether the compound possess **intrinsic sympathomimetic activity (ISA)**, that is, acts as a *partial* agonist (p. 60) or partial antagonist. In the presence of a partial agonist (e.g., pindolol), the ability of a full agonist (e.g., isoprenaline) to elicit a maximal effect would be attenuated, because binding of the full agonist is impeded. However, the β-receptor at which such partial agonism can be shown appears to be atypical (β_3 or β_4 subtype). Whether ISA confers a therapeutic advantage on a β-blocker remains an open question.

As cationic amphiphilic drugs, β-blockers can exert a **membrane-stabilizing effect**, as evidenced by the ability of the more lipophilic congeners to inhibit Na^+-channel function and impulse conduction in cardiac tissues. At the usual therapeutic dosage, the high concentration required for these effects will not be reached.

Some β-sympatholytics possess higher affinity for cardiac β_1-receptors than for β_2-receptors and thus display **cardioselectivity** (e.g., metoprolol, acebutolol, bisoprolol). None of these blockers is sufficiently selective to permit its use in patients with bronchial asthma or diabetes mellitus (p. 92).

The chemical structure of β-blockers also determines their **pharmacokinetic properties.** Except for hydrophilic representatives (atenolol), β-sympatholytics are completely absorbed from the intestines and subsequently undergo **presystemic elimination** to a major extent (**A**).

All the above differences are of little clinical importance. The abundance of commercially available congeners would thus appear all the more curious (**B**). Propranolol was the first β-blocker to be introduced into therapy in 1965. Thirty-five years later, about 20 different congeners are being marketed in different countries. This questionable development unfortunately is typical of any drug group that has major therapeutic relevance, in addition to a relatively fixed active structure. Variation of the molecule will create a new *patentable* chemical, not necessarily a drug with a novel action. Moreover, a drug no longer protected by patent is offered as a *generic* by different manufacturers under dozens of different proprietary names. Propranolol alone has been marketed by 13 manufacturers under 11 different names.

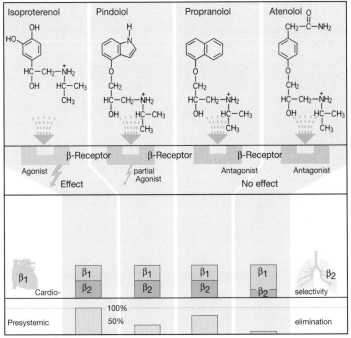

A. Types of β-sympatholytics

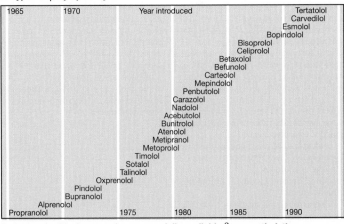

B. Avalanche-like increase in commercially available β-sympatholytics

Antiadrenergics

Antiadrenergics are drugs capable of lowering transmitter output from sympathetic neurons, i.e., "sympathetic tone". Their action is hypotensive (indication: hypertension, p. 312); however, being poorly tolerated, they enjoy only limited therapeutic use.

Clonidine is an α_2-agonist whose high lipophilicity (dichlorophenyl ring) permits rapid penetration through the blood-brain barrier. The activation of *postsynaptic* α_2-receptors dampens the activity of vasomotor neurons in the medulla oblongata, resulting in a resetting of systemic arterial pressure at a lower level. In addition, activation of presynaptic α_2-receptors in the periphery (pp. 82, 90) leads to a decreased release of both norepinephrine (NE) and acetylcholine.

Side effects. Lassitude, dry mouth; rebound hypertension after abrupt cessation of clonidine therapy.

Methyldopa (dopa = **d**ihydr**o**xy-**p**hen**y**l**a**lanine), as an amino acid, is transported across the blood-brain barrier, decarboxylated in the brain to α-methyldopamine, and then hydroxylated to α-methyl-NE. The decarboxylation of methyldopa competes for a portion of the available enzymatic activity, so that the rate of conversion of L-dopa to NE (via dopamine) is decreased. The *false transmitter* α-methyl-NE can be stored; however, unlike the endogenous mediator, it has a higher affinity for α_2- than for α_1-receptors and therefore produces effects similar to those of clonidine. The same events take place in peripheral adrenergic neurons.

Adverse effects. Fatigue, orthostatic hypotension, extrapyramidal Parkinson-like symptoms (p. 88), cutaneous reactions, hepatic damage, immune-hemolytic anemia.

Reserpine, an alkaloid from the *Rauwolfia* plant, abolishes the vesicular storage of biogenic amines (NE, dopamine = DA, serotonin = 5-HT) by inhibiting an ATPase required for the vesicular amine pump. The amount of NE re-

leased per nerve impulse is decreased. To a lesser degree, release of epinephrine from the adrenal medulla is also impaired. At higher doses, there is irreversible damage to storage vesicles ("pharmacological sympathectomy"), days to weeks being required for their resynthesis. Reserpine readily enters the brain, where it also impairs vesicular storage of biogenic amines.

Adverse effects. Disorders of extrapyramidal motor function with development of pseudo-Parkinsonism (p. 88), sedation, depression, stuffy nose, impaired libido, and impotence; increased appetite. These adverse effects have rendered the drug practically obsolete.

Guanethidine possesses high affinity for the axolemmal and vesicular amine transporters. It is stored instead of NE, but is unable to mimic the functions of the latter. In addition, it stabilizes the axonal membrane, thereby impeding the propagation of impulses into the sympathetic nerve terminals. Storage and release of epinephrine from the adrenal medulla are not affected, owing to the absence of a re-uptake process. The drug does not cross the blood-brain barrier.

Adverse effects. Cardiovascular crises are a possible risk: emotional stress of the patient may cause sympathoadrenal activation with epinephrine release. The resulting rise in blood pressure can be all the more marked because persistent depression of sympathetic nerve activity induces supersensitivity of effector organs to circulating catecholamines.

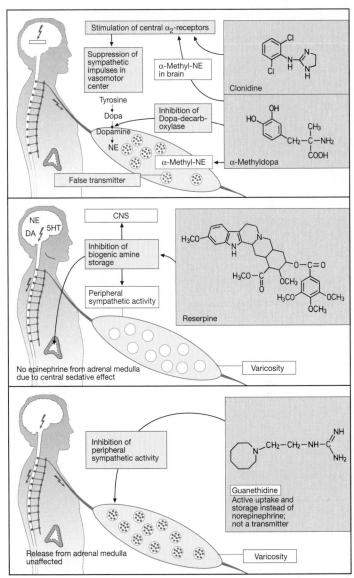

A. Inhibitors of sympathetic tone

Parasympathetic Nervous System

Responses to activation of the parasympathetic system. Parasympathetic nerves regulate processes connected with energy assimilation (food intake, digestion, absorption) and storage. These processes operate when the body is at rest, allowing a decreased tidal volume (increased bronchomotor tone) and decreased cardiac activity. Secretion of saliva and intestinal fluids promotes the digestion of foodstuffs; transport of intestinal contents is speeded up because of enhanced peristaltic activity and lowered tone of sphincteric muscles. To empty the urinary bladder (micturition), wall tension is increased by detrusor activation with a concurrent relaxation of sphincter tonus.

Activation of ocular parasympathetic fibers (see below) results in narrowing of the pupil and increased curvature of the lens, enabling near objects to be brought into focus (accommodation).

Anatomy of the parasympathetic system. The cell bodies of parasympathetic preganglionic neurons are located in the brainstem and the sacral spinal cord. Parasympathetic outflow is channelled from the brainstem (1) through the third cranial nerve (oculomotor n.) via the ciliary ganglion to the eye; (2) through the seventh cranial nerve (facial n.) via the pterygopalatine and submaxillary ganglia to lacrimal glands and salivary glands (sublingual, submandibular), respectively; (3) through the ninth cranial nerve (glossopharyngeal n.) via the otic ganglion to the parotid gland; and (4) via the tenth cranial nerve (vagus n.) to thoracic and abdominal viscera. Approximately 75 % of all parasympathetic fibers are contained within the vagus nerve. The neurons of the sacral division innervate the distal colon, rectum, bladder, the distal ureters, and the external genitalia.

Acetylcholine (ACh) as a transmitter. ACh serves as mediator at terminals of all postganglionic parasympathetic fibers, in addition to fulfilling its transmitter role at ganglionic synapses within both the sympathetic and parasympathetic divisions and the motor endplates on striated muscle. However, different types of receptors are present at these synaptic junctions:

Localization	Agonist	Antagonist	Receptor Type
Target tissues of 2nd parasympathetic neurons	ACh Muscarine	Atropine	Muscarinic (M) cholinoceptor; G-protein-coupled-receptor protein with 7 transmembrane domains
Sympathetic & parasympathetic ganglia	ACh Nicotine	Trimethaphan	Ganglionic type ($\alpha3\ \beta4$) Nicotinic (N) cholinoceptor ligand-gated cation channel formed by five transmembrane subunits
Motor endplate	ACh Nicotine	d-Tubocurarine	muscular type ($\alpha1_2\beta1\gamma\delta$)

The existence of distinct cholinoceptors at different cholinergic synapses allows selective pharmacological interventions.

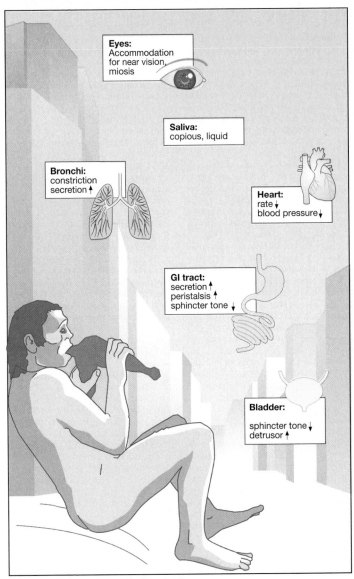

Eyes:
Accommodation for near vision, miosis

Saliva:
copious, liquid

Bronchi:
constriction
secretion ↑

Heart:
rate ↓
blood pressure ↓

GI tract:
secretion ↑
peristalsis ↑
sphincter tone ↓

Bladder:
sphincter tone ↓
detrusor ↑

A. Responses to parasympathetic activation

Cholinergic Synapse

Acetylcholine (ACh) is the transmitter at postganglionic synapses of parasympathetic nerve endings. It is highly concentrated in synaptic storage vesicles densely present in the axoplasm of the terminal. ACh is formed from **choline** and activated acetate (**acetylcoenzyme A**), a reaction catalyzed by the enzyme **choline acetyltransferase**. The highly polar choline is actively transported into the axoplasm. The specific choline transporter is localized exclusively to membranes of cholinergic axons and terminals. The mechanism of transmitter release is not known in full detail. The vesicles are anchored via the protein synapsin to the cytoskeletal network. This arrangement permits clustering of vesicles near the presynaptic membrane, while preventing fusion with it. During activation of the nerve membrane, Ca^{2+} is thought to enter the axoplasm through voltage-gated channels and to activate protein kinases that phosphorylate synapsin. As a result, vesicles close to the membrane are detached from their anchoring and allowed to fuse with the presynaptic membrane. During fusion, vesicles discharge their contents into the synaptic gap. ACh quickly diffuses through the synaptic gap (the acetylcholine molecule is a little longer than 0.5 nm; the synaptic gap is as narrow as 30–40 nm). At the postsynaptic effector cell membrane, ACh reacts with its **receptors.** Because these receptors can also be activated by the alkaloid muscarine, they are referred to as **muscarinic (M-)cholinoceptors.** In contrast, at ganglionic (p. 108) and motor endplate (p. 184) cholinoceptors, the action of ACh is mimicked by nicotine and they are, therefore, said to be **nicotinic cholinoceptors.**

Released ACh is rapidly hydrolyzed and inactivated by a specific **acetylcholinesterase,** present on pre- and postjunctional membranes, or by a less specific serum cholinesterase (butyryl cholinesterase), a soluble enzyme present in serum and interstitial fluid.

M-cholinoceptors can be classified into subtypes according to their molecular structure, signal transduction, and ligand affinity. Here, the M_1, M_2, and M_3 subtypes are considered. M_1 receptors are present on nerve cells, e.g., in ganglia, where they mediate a facilitation of impulse transmission from preganglionic axon terminals to ganglion cells. M_2 receptors mediate acetylcholine effects on the heart: opening of K^+ channels leads to slowing of diastolic depolarization in sinoatrial pacemaker cells and a decrease in heart rate. M_3 receptors play a role in the regulation of smooth muscle tone, e.g., in the gut and bronchi, where their activation causes stimulation of phospholipase C, membrane depolarization, and increase in muscle tone. M_3 receptors are also found in glandular epithelia, which similarly respond with activation of phospholipase C and increased secretory activity. In the CNS, where all subtypes are present, cholinoceptors serve diverse functions, including regulation of cortical excitability, memory, learning, pain processing, and brain stem motor control. The assignment of specific receptor subtypes to these functions has yet to be achieved.

In blood vessels, the relaxant action of ACh on muscle tone is indirect, because it involves stimulation of M_3-cholinoceptors on endothelial cells that respond by liberating NO (= endothelium-derived relaxing factor). The latter diffuses into the subjacent smooth musculature, where it causes a relaxation of active tonus (p. 121).

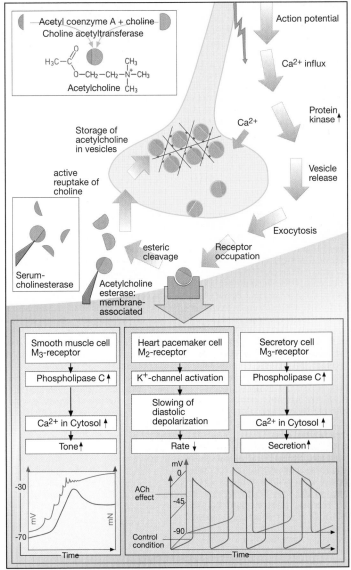

A. Acetylcholine: release, effects, and degradation

Parasympathomimetics

Acetylcholine (ACh) is too rapidly hydrolyzed and inactivated by acetylcholinesterase (AChE) to be of any therapeutic use; however, its action can be mimicked by other substances, namely direct or indirect parasympathomimetics.

Direct Parasympathomimetics. The choline ester, *carbachol,* activates M-cholinoceptors, but is not hydrolyzed by AChE. Carbachol can thus be effectively employed for local application to the eye (glaucoma) and systemic administration (bowel atonia, bladder atonia). The alkaloids, *pilocarpine* (from *Pilocarpus jaborandi*) and *arecoline* (from *Areca catechu;* betel nut) also act as direct parasympathomimetics. As tertiary amines, they moreover exert central effects. The central effect of muscarine-like substances consists of an enlivening, mild stimulation that is probably the effect desired in betel chewing, a widespread habit in South Asia. Of this group, only pilocarpine enjoys therapeutic use, which is limited to local application to the eye in glaucoma.

Indirect Parasympathomimetics. AChE can be inhibited selectively, with the result that ACh released by nerve impulses will accumulate at cholinergic synapses and cause prolonged stimulation of cholinoceptors. Inhibitors of AChE are, therefore, indirect parasympathomimetics. Their action is evident at all cholinergic synapses. Chemically, these agents include esters of carbamic acid (**carbamates** such as *physostigmine, neostigmine*) and of phosphoric acid (**organophosphates** such as para-oxon = E600 and *nitrostigmine* = parathion = E605, its prodrug).

Members of both groups react like ACh with AChE and can be considered false substrates. The esters are hydrolyzed upon formation of a complex with the enzyme. The rate-limiting step in ACh hydrolysis is deacetylation of the enzyme, which takes only milliseconds, thus permitting a high turnover rate and activity of AChE. **Decarbaminoylation** following hydrolysis of a carba-

mate takes hours to days, the enzyme remaining inhibited as long as it is carbaminoylated. Cleavage of the phosphate residue, i.e. **dephosphorylation,** is practically impossible; enzyme inhibition is irreversible.

Uses. The quaternary carbamate neostigmine is employed as an indirect parasympathomimetic in postoperative atonia of the bowel or bladder. Furthermore, it is needed to overcome the relative ACh-deficiency at the motor endplate in myasthenia gravis or to reverse the neuromuscular blockade (p. 184) caused by nondepolarizing muscle relaxants (decurarization before discontinuation of anesthesia). The tertiary carbamate physostigmine can be used as an antidote in poisoning with parasympatholytic drugs, because it has access to AChE in the brain. Carbamates (neostigmine, pyridostigmine, physostigmine) and organophosphates (paraoxon, ecothiopate) can also be applied locally to the eye in the treatment of glaucoma; however, their long-term use leads to cataract formation. Agents from both classes also serve as insecticides. Although they possess high acute toxicity in humans, they are more rapidly degraded than is DDT following their emission into the environment.

Tacrine is not an ester and interferes only with the choline-binding site of AChE. It is effective in alleviating symptoms of dementia in some subtypes of Alzheimer's disease.

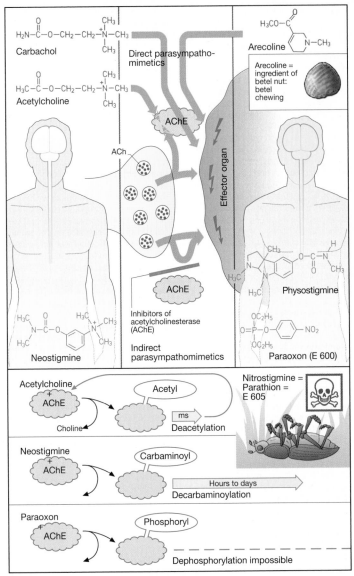

A. Direct and indirect parasympathomimetics

Parasympatholytics

Excitation of the parasympathetic division of the autonomic nervous system causes release of acetylcholine at neuroeffector junctions in different target organs. The major effects are summarized in **A** (blue arrows). Some of these effects have therapeutic applications, as indicated by the clinical uses of parasympathomimetics (p. 102).

Substances acting antagonistically at the M-cholinoceptor are designated **parasympatholytics** (prototype: the alkaloid **atropine**; actions shown in red in the panels). Therapeutic use of these agents is complicated by their low organ selectivity. Possibilities for a targeted action include:

- local application
- selection of drugs with either good or poor membrane penetrability as the situation demands
- administration of drugs possessing receptor subtype selectivity.

Parasympatholytics are employed for the following purposes:

1. Inhibition of exocrine glands
Bronchial secretion. **Premedication** with atropine before inhalation anesthesia prevents a possible hypersecretion of bronchial mucus, which cannot be expectorated by coughing during intubation (anesthesia).

Gastric secretion. Stimulation of gastric acid production by vagal impulses involves an M-cholinoceptor subtype (M_1-receptor), probably associated with enterochromaffin cells. *Pirenzepine* (p. 106) displays a preferential affinity for this receptor subtype. Remarkably, the HCl-secreting parietal cells possess only M_3-receptors. M_1-receptors have also been demonstrated in the brain; however, these cannot be reached by pirenzepine because its lipophilicity is too low to permit penetration of the blood-brain barrier. Pirenzepine was formerly used in the treatment of **gastric and duodenal ulcers** (p. 166).

2. Relaxation of smooth musculature
Bronchodilation can be achieved by the use of ipratropium in conditions of increased airway resistance (**chronic obstructive bronchitis,** bronchial asthma). When administered by inhalation, this quaternary compound has little effect on other organs because of its low rate of systemic absorption.

Spasmolysis by N-butylscopolamine in **biliary** or **renal colic** (p. 126). Because of its quaternary nitrogen, this drug does not enter the brain and requires parenteral administration. Its spasmolytic action is especially marked because of additional ganglionic blocking and direct muscle-relaxant actions.

Lowering of pupillary sphincter tonus and pupillary dilation by local administration of homatropine or tropicamide (**mydriatics**) allows observation of the ocular fundus. For diagnostic uses, only short-term pupillary dilation is needed. The effect of both agents subsides quickly in comparison with that of atropine (duration of several days).

3. Cardioacceleration
Ipratropium is used in bradycardia and AV-block, respectively, to raise **heart rate** and to facilitate cardiac *impulse conduction.* As a quaternary substance, it does not penetrate into the brain, which greatly reduces the risk of CNS disturbances (see below). Relatively high oral doses are required because of an inefficient intestinal absorption.

Atropine may be given to prevent **cardiac arrest** resulting from vagal reflex activation, incident to anesthetic induction, gastric lavage, or endoscopic procedures.

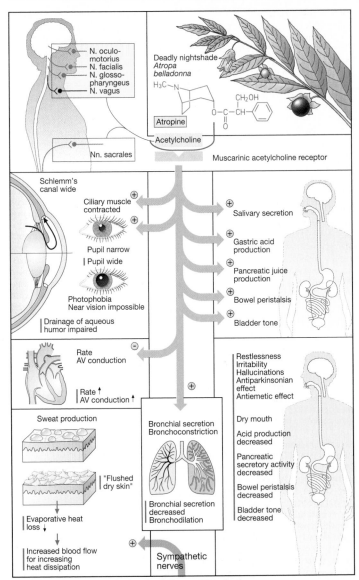

A. Effects of parasympathetic stimulation and blockade

4. CNS-dampening effects

Scopolamine is effective in the *prophylaxis of kinetosis* (motion sickness, **sea sickness**, see p. 330); it is well absorbed transcutaneously. Scopolamine (pK_a = 7.2) penetrates the blood-brain barrier faster than does atropine (pK_a = 9), because at physiologic pH a larger proportion is present in the neutral, membrane-permeant form.

In **psychotic excitement** (agitation), sedation can be achieved with scopolamine. Unlike atropine, scopolamine exerts a calming and amnesiogenic action that can be used to advantage in anesthetic premedication.

Symptomatic treatment in parkinsonism for the purpose of restoring a dopaminergic-cholinergic balance in the corpus striatum. Antiparkinsonian agents, such as benzatropine (p. 188), readily penetrate the blood-brain barrier. At centrally equi-effective dosage, their peripheral effects are less marked than are those of atropine.

Contraindications for parasympatholytics

Glaucoma: Since drainage of aqueous humor is impeded during relaxation of the pupillary sphincter, intraocular pressure rises.

Prostatic hypertrophy with impaired micturition: loss of parasympathetic control of the detrusor muscle exacerbates difficulties in voiding urine.

Atropine poisoning

Parasympatholytics have a wide therapeutic margin. Rarely life-threatening, poisoning with atropine is characterized by the following peripheral and central effects:

Peripheral: **tachycardia; dry mouth; hyperthermia** secondary to the inhibition of sweating. Although sweat glands are innervated by sympathetic fibers, these are cholinergic in nature. When sweat secretion is inhibited, the body loses the ability to dissipate metabolic heat by evaporation of sweat (p. 202). There is a compensatory vasodilation in the skin allowing increased heat exchange through increased cutaneous blood flow. Decreased peristaltic activity of the intestines leads to **constipation.**

Central: Motor restlessness, progressing to maniacal agitation, psychic disturbances, **disorientation**, and **hallucinations**. Elderly subjects are more sensitive to such central effects. In this context, the diversity of drugs producing atropine-like side effects should be borne in mind: e.g., tricyclic antidepressants, neuroleptics, antihistamines, antiarrhythmics, antiparkinsonian agents.

Apart from symptomatic, general measures (gastric lavage, cooling with ice water), therapy of severe **atropine intoxication** includes the administration of the indirect parasympathomimetic physostigmine (p. 102). The most common instances of "atropine" intoxication are observed after ingestion of the berry-like fruits of belladonna (children) or intentional overdosage with tricyclic antidepressants in attempted suicide.

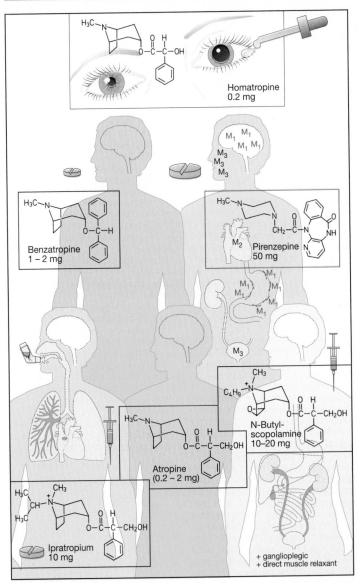

A. Parasympatholytics

Ganglionic Transmission

Whether sympathetic or parasympathetic, all efferent visceromotor nerves are made up of two serially connected neurons. The point of contact (synapse) between the first and second neurons occurs mainly in **ganglia**; therefore, the first neuron is referred to as *preganglionic* and efferents of the second as *postganglionic*.

Electrical excitation (action potential) of the first neuron causes the release of acetylcholine (ACh) within the ganglia. ACh stimulates receptors located on the subsynaptic membrane of the second neuron. Activation of these receptors causes the nonspecific cation channel to open. The resulting influx of Na^+ leads to a membrane depolarization. If a sufficient number of receptors is activated simultaneously, a threshold potential is reached at which the membrane undergoes rapid depolarization in the form of a propagated action potential. Normally, not all preganglionic impulses elicit a propagated response in the second neuron. The ganglionic synapse acts like a frequency filter (**A**). The effect of ACh elicited at receptors on the ganglionic neuronal membrane can be imitated by nicotine; i.e., it involves **nicotinic cholinoceptors.**

Ganglionic action of nicotine. If a small dose of nicotine is given, the ganglionic cholinoceptors are activated. The membrane depolarizes partially, but fails to reach the firing threshold. However, at this point an amount of released ACh smaller than that normally required will be sufficient to elicit a propagated action potential. *At a low concentration*, nicotine acts as a ganglionic stimulant; it alters the filter function of the ganglionic synapse, allowing action potential frequency in the second neuron to approach that of the first (**B**). *At higher concentrations*, nicotine acts to block ganglionic transmission. Simultaneous activation of many nicotinic cholinoceptors depolarizes the ganglionic cell membrane to such an extent that generation of action potentials is no longer possible, even in the face of an intensive and synchronized release of ACh (**C**).

Although nicotine mimics the action of ACh at the receptors, it cannot duplicate the time course of intrasynaptic agonist concentration required for appropriate high-frequency ganglionic activation. The concentration of nicotine in the synaptic cleft can neither build up as rapidly as that of ACh released from nerve terminals nor can nicotine be eliminated from the synaptic cleft as quickly as ACh.

The ganglionic effects of ACh can be blocked by tetraethylammonium, hexamethonium, and other substances (**ganglionic blockers**). None of these has intrinsic activity, that is, they fail to stimulate ganglia even at low concentration; some of them (e.g., hexamethonium) actually block the cholinoceptor-linked ion channel, but others (mecamylamine, trimethaphan) are typical receptor antagonists.

Certain sympathetic preganglionic neurons project without interruption to the chromaffin cells of the adrenal medulla. The latter are embryologic homologues of ganglionic sympathocytes. Excitation of preganglionic fibers leads to release of ACh in the adrenal medulla, whose chromaffin cells then respond with a release of epinephrine into the blood (**D**). Small doses of nicotine, by inducing a partial depolarization of adrenomedullary cells, are effective in liberating epinephrine (pp. 110, 112).

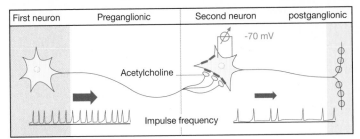

A. Ganglionic transmission: normal state

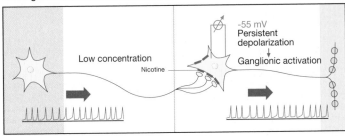

B. Ganglionic transmission: excitation by nicotine

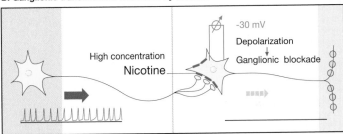

C. Ganglionic transmission: blockade by nicotine

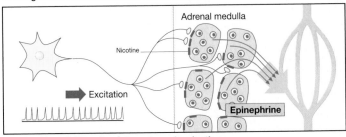

D. Adrenal medulla: epinephrine release by nicotine

Effects of Nicotine on Body Functions

At a low concentration, the tobacco alkaloid nicotine acts as a ganglionic stimulant by causing a partial depolarization via activation of ganglionic cholinoceptors (p. 108). A similar action is evident at diverse other neural sites, considered below in more detail.

Autonomic ganglia. Ganglionic stimulation occurs in both the sympathetic and parasympathetic divisions of the autonomic nervous system. Parasympathetic activation results in increased production of gastric juice (smoking ban in peptic ulcer) and enhanced bowel motility ("laxative" effect of the first morning cigarette: defecation; diarrhea in the novice).

Although stimulation of parasympathetic cardioinhibitory neurons would tend to lower *heart rate,* this response is overridden by the simultaneous stimulation of sympathetic cardioaccelerant neurons and the adrenal medulla. Stimulation of sympathetic nerves resulting in release of norepinephrine gives rise to *vasoconstriction*; peripheral resistance rises.

Adrenal medulla. On the one hand, release of epinephrine elicits cardiovascular effects, such as increases in *heart rate* und *peripheral vascular resistance.* On the other, it evokes metabolic responses, such as glycogenolysis and lipolysis, that generate energy-rich substrates. The sensation of hunger is suppressed. The metabolic state corresponds to that associated with physical exercise – "silent stress".

Baroreceptors. Partial depolarization of baroreceptors enables activation of the reflex to occur at a relatively smaller rise in blood pressure, leading to decreased sympathetic vasoconstrictor activity.

Neurohypophysis. Release of vasopressin (antidiuretic hormone) results in lowered urinary output (p. 164). Levels of vasopressin necessary for vasoconstriction will rarely be produced by nicotine.

Carotid body. Sensitivity to arterial pCO_2 increases; increased afferent input augments *respiratory rate and depth.*

Receptors for pressure, temperature, and pain. Sensitivity to the corresponding stimuli is enhanced.

Area postrema. Sensitization of chemoceptors leads to *excitation of the medullary emetic center.*

At low concentration, nicotine is also able to augment the excitability of the **motor endplate**. This effect can be manifested in heavy smokers in the form of muscle cramps (calf musculature) and soreness.

The central nervous actions of nicotine are thought to be mediated largely by presynaptic receptors that facilitate transmitter release from excitatory aminoacidergic (glutamatergic) nerve terminals in the cerebral cortex. Nicotine increases vigilance and the ability to concentrate. The effect reflects an enhanced readiness to perceive external stimuli (attentiveness) and to respond to them.

The multiplicity of its effects makes nicotine ill-suited for therapeutic use.

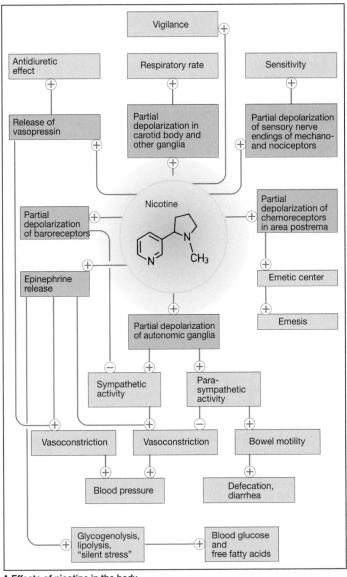

A. Effects of nicotine in the body

Consequences of Tobacco Smoking

The dried and cured leaves of the night-shade plant *Nicotiana tabacum* are known as tobacco. Tobacco is mostly smoked, less frequently chewed or taken as dry snuff. Combustion of tobacco generates approx. 4000 chemical compounds in detectable quantities. The xenobiotic burden on the smoker depends on a range of parameters, including tobacco quality, presence of a filter, rate and temperature of combustion, depth of inhalation, and duration of breath holding.

Tobacco contains 0.2–5 % nicotine. In tobacco smoke, nicotine is present as a constituent of small tar particles. It is rapidly absorbed through bronchi and lung alveoli, and is detectable in the brain only 8 s after the first inhalation. Smoking of a single cigarette yields peak plasma levels in the range of 25–50 ng/mL. The effects described on p. 110 become evident. When intake stops, nicotine concentration in plasma shows an initial rapid fall, reflecting distribution into tissues, and a terminal elimination phase with a half-life of 2 h. Nicotine is degraded by oxidation.

The enhanced **risk of vascular disease** (coronary stenosis, myocardial infarction, and central and peripheral ischemic disorders, such as stroke and intermittent claudication) is likely to be a consequence of chronic exposure to nicotine. Endothelial impairment and hence dysfunction has been proven to result from smoking, and nicotine is under discussion as a factor favoring the progression of arteriosclerosis. By releasing epinephrine, it elevates plasma levels of glucose and free fatty acids in the absence of an immediate physiological need for these energy-rich metabolites. Furthermore, it promotes platelet aggregability, lowers fibrinolytic activity of blood, and enhances coagulability.

The health risks of tobacco smoking are, however, attributable not only to nicotine, but also to various other ingredients of tobacco smoke, some of which possess demonstrable **carcinogenic** properties.

Dust particles inhaled in tobacco smoke, together with bronchial mucus, must be removed from the airways by the ciliated epithelium. Ciliary activity, however, is depressed by tobacco smoke; mucociliary transport is impaired. This depression favors bacterial infection and contributes to the chronic bronchitis associated with regular smoking. Chronic injury to the bronchial mucosa could be an important causative factor in increasing the risk in smokers of death from bronchial carcinoma.

Statistical surveys provide an impressive correlation between the number of cigarettes smoked a day and the risk of death from coronary disease or lung cancer. Statistics also show that, on cessation of smoking, the increased risk of death from coronary infarction or other cardiovascular disease declines over 5–10 years almost to the level of non-smokers. Similarly, the risk of developing bronchial carcinoma is reduced.

Abrupt cessation of regular smoking is not associated with severe physical withdrawal symptoms. In general, subjects complain of increased nervousness, lack of concentration, and weight gain.

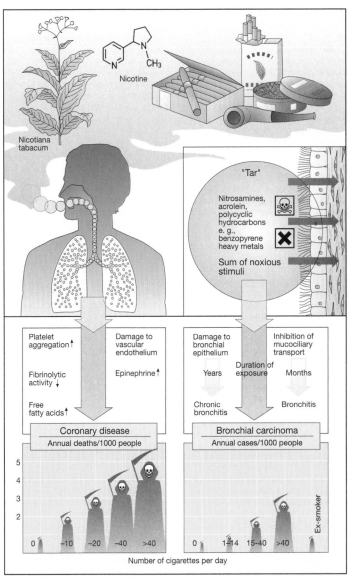

A. Sequelae of tobacco smoking

Biogenic Amines — Actions and Pharmacological Implications

Dopamine A. As the precursor of norepinephrine and epinephrine (p. 184), dopamine is found in sympathetic (adrenergic) neurons and adrenomedullary cells. In the CNS, dopamine itself serves as a neuromediator and is implicated in neostriatal motor programming (p. 188), the elicitation of emesis at the level of the area postrema (p. 330), and inhibition of prolactin release from the anterior pituitary (p. 242).

Dopamine receptors are coupled to G-proteins and exist as different subtypes. D_1-receptors (comprising subtypes D_1 and D_5) and D_2-receptors (comprising subtypes D_2, D_3, and D_4). The aforementioned actions are mediated mainly by D_2 receptors. When given by infusion, dopamine causes dilation of renal and splanchnic arteries. This effect is mediated by D_1 receptors and is utilized in the treatment of cardiovascular shock and hypertensive emergencies by infusion of dopamine and fenoldopam, respectively. At higher doses, β_1-adrenoceptors and, finally, α-receptors are activated, as evidenced by cardiac stimulation and vasoconstriction, respectively.

Dopamine is not to be confused with dobutamine which stimulates α- and β-adrenoceptors but not dopamine receptors (p. 62).

Dopamine-mimetics. Administration of the precursor L-dopa promotes endogenous synthesis of dopamine (indication: parkinsonian syndrome, p. 188). The ergolides, bromocriptine, pergolide, and lisuride, are ligands at D-receptors whose therapeutic effects are probably due to stimulation of D_2 receptors (indications: parkinsonism, suppression of lactation, infertility, acromegaly, p. 242). Typical adverse effects of these substances are nausea and vomiting. As indirect dopamine-mimetics, (+)-amphetamine and ritaline augment dopamine release.

Inhibition of the enzymes involved in dopamine degradation, catecholamine-oxygen-methyl-transferase (COMT) and monoamineoxidase (MAO), is another means to increase actual available dopamine concentration (COMT-inhibitors, p. 188), MAO_B-inhibitors, p. 88, 188).

Dopamine antagonist activity is the hallmark of classical neuroleptics. The antihypertensive agents, reserpine (obsolete) and α-methyldopa, deplete neuronal stores of the amine. A common adverse effect of dopamine antagonists or depletors is parkinsonism.

Histamine (B). Histamine is stored in basophils and tissue mast cells. It plays a role in inflammatory and allergic reactions (p. 72, 326) and produces bronchoconstriction, increased intestinal peristalsis, and dilation and increased permeability of small blood vessels. In the gastric mucosa, it is released from enterochromaffin-like cells and stimulates acid secretion by the parietal cells. In the CNS, it acts as a neuromodulator. Two receptor subtypes (G-protein-coupled), H_1 and H_2, are of therapeutic importance; both mediate vascular responses. Prejunctional H_3 receptors exist in brain and the periphery.

Antagonists. Most of the so-called *H_1-antihistamines* also block other receptors, including M-cholinoceptors and D-receptors. H_1-antihistamines are used for the symptomatic relief of allergies (e.g., bamipine, chlorpheniramine, clemastine, dimethindene, mebhydroline pheniramine); as antiemetics (meclizine, dimenhydrinate, p. 330), as over-the-counter hypnotics (e.g., diphenhydramine, p. 222). Promethazine represents the transition to the neuroleptic phenothiazines (p. 236). Unwanted effects of most H_1-antihistamines are lassitude (impaired driving skills) and atropine-like reactions (e.g., dry mouth, constipation). At the usual therapeutic doses, astemizole, cetrizine, fexofenadine, and loratidine are practically devoid of sedative and anticholinergic effects. H_2-antihistamines (cimetidine, ranitidine, famotidine, nizatidine) inhibit gastric acid secretion, and thus are useful in the treatment of peptic ulcers.

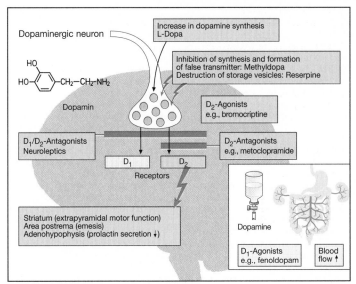

A. Dopamine actions as influenced by drugs

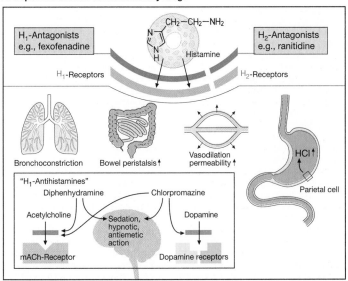

B. Histamine actions as influenced by drugs

Inhibitors of histamine release: One of the effects of the so-called mast cell stabilizers cromoglycate (cromolyn) and nedocromil is to decrease the release of histamine from mast cells (p. 72, 326). Both agents are applied topically. Release of mast cell mediators can also be inhibited by some H_1 antihistamines, e.g., oxatomide and ketotifen, which are used systemically.

Serotonin

Occurrence. Serotonin (5-hydroxytryptamine, 5-HT) is synthesized from L-tryptophan in enterochromaffin cells of the intestinal mucosa. 5-HT-synthesizing neurons occur in the enteric nerve plexus and the CNS, where the amine fulfills a neuromediator function. Blood platelets are unable to synthesize 5HT, but are capable of taking up, storing, and releasing it.

Serotonin receptors. Based on biochemical and pharmacological criteria, seven receptor classes can be distinguished. Of major pharmacotherapeutic importance are those designated 5-HT_1, 5-HT_2, 5-HT_4, and 5-HT_7, all of which are G-protein-coupled, whereas the 5-HT_3 subtype represents a ligand-gated nonselective cation channel.

Serotonin actions. The **cardiovascular** effects of 5-HT are complex, because multiple, in part opposing, effects are exerted via the different receptor subtypes. Thus, 5-HT_{2A} and 5-HT_7 receptors on vascular smooth muscle cells mediate direct vasoconstriction and vasodilation, respectively. Vasodilation and lowering of blood pressure can also occur by several indirect mechanisms: 5-HT_{1A} receptors mediate sympathoinhibition ($\rightarrow$ decrease in neurogenic vasoconstrictor tonus) both centrally and peripherally; 5-HT_{2B} receptors on vascular endothelium promote release of vasorelaxant mediators (NO, p. 120; prostacyclin, p. 196) 5-HT released from platelets plays a role in thrombogenesis, hemostasis, and the pathogenesis of preeclamptic hypertension.

Ketanserin is an antagonist at 5-HT_{2A} receptors and produces antihypertensive effects, as well as inhibition of thrombocyte aggregation. Whether 5-HT antagonism accounts for its antihypertensive effect remains questionable, because ketanserin also blocks α-adrenoceptors.

Sumatriptan and other triptans are antimigraine drugs that possess agonist activity at 5-HT_1 receptors of the B, D and F subtypes and may thereby alleviate this type of headache (p. 322).

Gastrointestinal tract. Serotonin released from myenteric neurons or enterochromaffin cells acts on 5-HT_3 and 5-HT_4 receptors to enhance bowel motility and enteral fluid secretion. *Cisapride* is a **prokinetic agent** that promotes propulsive motor activity in the stomach and in small and large intestines. It is used in motility disorders. Its mechanism of action is unclear, but stimulation of 5HT_4 receptors may be important.

Central Nervous System. Serotoninergic neurons play a part in various brain functions, as evidenced by the effects of drugs likely to interfere with serotonin. *Fluoxetine* is an antidepressant that, by blocking re-uptake, inhibits inactivation of released serotonin. Its activity spectrum includes significant psychomotor stimulation, depression of appetite, and anxiolysis. *Buspirone* also has anxiolytic properties thought to be mediated by central presynaptic 5-HT_{1A} receptors. *Ondansetron,* an antagonist at the 5-HT_3 receptor, possesses striking effectiveness against cytotoxic drug-induced emesis, evident both at the start of and during cytostatic therapy. *Tropisetron* and *granisetron* produce analogous effects.

Psychedelics *(LSD)* and other psychotomimetics such as *mescaline* and *psilocybin* can induce states of altered awareness, or induce hallucinations and anxiety, probably mediated by 5-HT_{2A} receptors. Overactivity of these receptors may also play a role in the genesis of negative symptoms in schizophrenia (p. 238) and sleep disturbances.

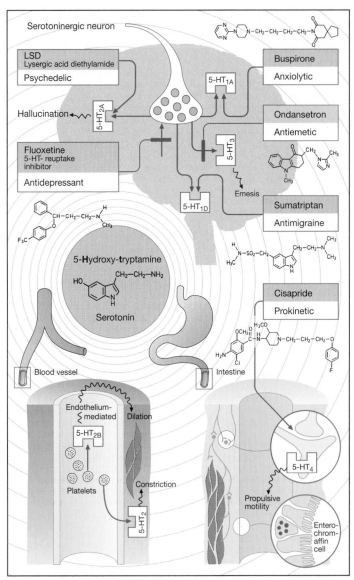

A. Serotonin receptors and actions

Vasodilators–Overview

The distribution of blood within the circulation is a function of vascular caliber. Venous tone regulates the volume of blood returned to the heart, hence, stroke volume and cardiac output. The luminal diameter of the arterial vasculature determines peripheral resistance. Cardiac output and peripheral resistance are prime determinants of arterial blood pressure (p. 314).

In **A,** the clinically most important vasodilators are presented in the order of approximate frequency of therapeutic use. Some of these agents possess different efficacy in affecting the venous and arterial limbs of the circulation (width of beam).

Possible uses. *Arteriolar vasodilators* are given to lower blood pressure in hypertension (p. 312), to reduce cardiac work in angina pectoris (p. 308), and to reduce ventricular afterload (pressure load) in cardiac failure (p. 132). *Venous vasodilators* are used to reduce venous filling pressure (preload) in angina pectoris (p. 308) or cardiac failure (p. 132). Practical uses are indicated for each drug group.

Counter-regulation in acute hypotension due to vasodilators (B). Increased *sympathetic* drive raises heart rate (reflex tachycardia) and cardiac output and thus helps to elevate blood pressure. Patients experience palpitations. Activation of the *renin-angiotensin-aldosterone (RAA) system* serves to increase blood volume, hence cardiac output. Fluid retention leads to an increase in body weight and, possibly, edemas. These counter-regulatory processes are susceptible to pharmacological inhibition (β-blockers, ACE inhibitors, AT1-antagonists, diuretics).

Mechanisms of action. The tonus of vascular smooth muscle can be decreased by various means. ACE inhibitors, antagonists at AT1-receptors and antagonists at α-adrenoceptors protect against the effects of excitatory mediators such as angiotensin II and norepinephrine, respectively. Prostacyclin an-

alogues such as iloprost, or prostaglandin E_1 analogues such as alprostanil, mimic the actions of relaxant mediators. Ca^{2+} antagonists reduce depolarizing inward Ca^{2+} currents, while K^+-channel activators promote outward (hyperpolarizing) K^+ currents. Organic nitrovasodilators give rise to NO, an endogenous activator of guanylate cyclase.

Individual vasodilators. Nitrates (p. 120) Ca^{2+}-antagonists (p. 122). α_1-antagonists (p. 90), ACE-inhibitors, AT1-antagonists (p. 124); and sodium nitroprusside (p. 120) are discussed elsewhere.

Dihydralazine and minoxidil (via its sulfate-conjugated metabolite) dilate arterioles and are used in antihypertensive therapy. They are, however, unsuitable for monotherapy because of compensatory circulatory reflexes. The mechanism of action of dihydralazine is unclear. Minoxidil probably activates K^+ channels, leading to hyperpolarization of smooth muscle cells. Particular adverse reactions are lupus erythematosus with dihydralazine and hirsutism with minoxidil—used topically for the treatment of baldness (alopecia androgenetica).

Diazoxide given i.v. causes prominent arteriolar dilation; it can be employed in hypertensive crises. After its oral administration, insulin secretion is inhibited. Accordingly, diazoxide can be used in the management of insulin-secreting pancreatic tumors. Both effects are probably due to opening of (ATP-gated) K^+ channels.

The methylxanthine theophylline (p. 326), the phosphodiesterase inhibitor amrinone (p. 132), prostacyclins (p. 197), and nicotinic acid derivatives (p. 156) also possess vasodilating activity.

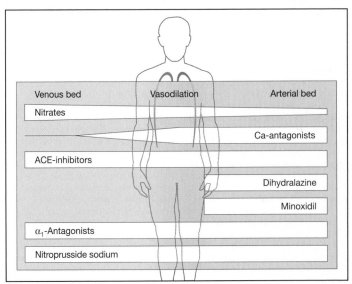

A. Vasodilators

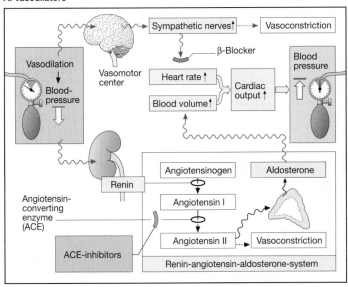

B. Counter-regulatory responses in hypotension due to vasodilators

Organic Nitrates

Various esters of nitric acid (HNO_3) and polyvalent alcohols relax vascular smooth muscle, e.g., nitroglycerin (glyceryltrinitrate) and isosorbide dinitrate. *The effect is more pronounced in venous than in arterial beds.*

These vasodilator effects produce hemodynamic consequences that can be put to therapeutic use. Due to a decrease in both venous return (preload) and arterial afterload, cardiac work is decreased (p. 308). As a result, the cardiac oxygen balance improves. Spasmodic constriction of larger coronary vessels (coronary spasm) is prevented.

Uses. Organic nitrates are used chiefly in *angina pectoris* (p. 308, 310), less frequently in severe forms of chronic and acute congestive heart failure. Continuous intake of higher doses with maintenance of steady plasma levels leads to loss of efficacy, inasmuch as the organism becomes refractory (tachyphylactic). This "nitrate tolerance" can be avoided if a daily "nitrate-free interval" is maintained, e.g., overnight.

At the start of therapy, **unwanted reactions** occur frequently in the form of a throbbing headache, probably caused by dilation of cephalic vessels. This effect also exhibits tolerance, even when daily "nitrate pauses" are kept. Excessive dosages give rise to hypotension, reflex tachycardia, and circulatory collapse.

Mechanism of action. The reduction in vascular smooth muscle tone is presumably due to activation of guanylate cyclase and elevation of cyclic GMP levels. The causative agent is most likely nitric oxide (NO) generated from the organic nitrate. NO is a physiological messenger molecule that endothelial cells release onto subjacent smooth muscle cells ("endothelium-derived relaxing factor," EDRF). Organic nitrates would thus utilize a pre-existing pathway, hence their high efficacy. The generation of NO within the smooth muscle cell depends on a supply of free sulfhydryl (-SH) groups; "nitrate-tolerance" has been attributed to a cellular exhaustion of SH-donors but this may be not the only reason.

Nitroglycerin (NTG) is distinguished by high membrane penetrability and very low stability. It is the drug of choice in the treatment of angina pectoris attacks. For this purpose, it is administered as a spray, or in sublingual or buccal tablets for transmucosal delivery. The onset of action is between 1 and 3 min. Due to a nearly complete presystemic elimination, it is poorly suited for oral administration. Transdermal delivery (nitroglycerin patch) also avoids presystemic elimination. **Isosorbide dinitrate (ISDN)** penetrates well through membranes, is more stable than NTG, and is partly degraded into the weaker, but much longer acting, 5-isosorbide mononitrate (ISMN). ISDN can also be applied sublingually; however, it is mainly administered orally in order to achieve a prolonged effect. **ISMN** is not suitable for sublingual use because of its higher polarity and slower rate of absorption. Taken orally, it is absorbed and is not subject to first-pass elimination.

Molsidomine itself is inactive. After oral intake, it is slowly converted into an active metabolite. Apparently, there is little likelihood of "nitrate tolerance".

Sodium nitroprusside contains a nitroso (-NO) group, but is not an ester. It dilates venous and arterial beds equally. It is administered by infusion to achieve controlled *hypotension* under continuous close monitoring. Cyanide ions liberated from nitroprusside can be inactivated with sodium thiosulfate ($Na_2S_2O_3$) (p. 304).

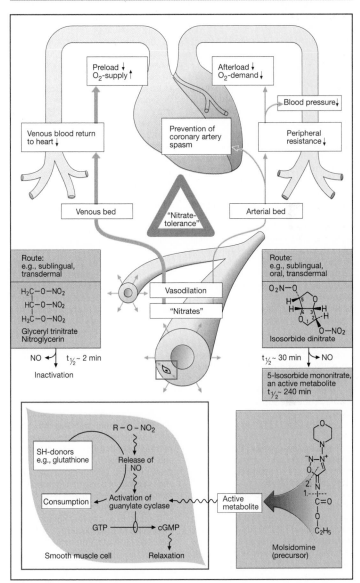

A. Vasodilators: Nitrates

Calcium Antagonists

During electrical excitation of the cell membrane of heart or smooth muscle, different ionic currents are activated, including an inward Ca^{2+} current. The term Ca^{2+} antagonist is applied to drugs that inhibit the influx of Ca^{2+} ions without affecting inward Na^+ or outward K^+ currents to a significant degree. Other labels are *Ca-entry blocker* or *Ca-channel blocker*. Therapeutically used Ca^{2+} antagonists can be divided into three groups according to their effects on heart and vasculature.

I. Dihydropyridine derivatives. The dihydropyridines, e.g., nifedipine, are uncharged hydrophobic substances. They induce a *relaxation* of vascular smooth muscle in *arterial beds*. An effect on cardiac function is practically absent at therapeutic dosage. (However, in pharmacological experiments on isolated cardiac muscle preparations a clear negative inotropic effect is demonstrable.) They are thus regarded as *vasoselective Ca^{2+} antagonists.* Because of the dilatation of resistance vessels, blood pressure falls. Cardiac afterload is diminished (p. 306) and, therefore, also oxygen demand. Spasms of coronary arteries are prevented.

Indications for nifedipine include *angina pectoris* (p. 308) and, − when applied as a sustained release preparation, − hypertension (p. 312). In angina pectoris, it is effective when given either prophylactically or during acute attacks. **Adverse effects** are palpitation (reflex tachycardia due to hypotension), headache, and pretibial edema.

Nitrendipine and *felodipine* are used in the treatment of hypertension. *Nimodipine* is given prophylactically after subarachnoidal hemorrhage to prevent vasospasms due to depolarization by excess K^+ liberated from disintegrating erythrocytes or blockade of NO by free hemoglobin.

II. Verapamil and other catamphilic Ca^{2+} antagonists. Verapamil contains a nitrogen atom bearing a positive charge at physiological pH and thus represents a *cationic amphiphilic molecule.* It exerts inhibitory effects not only on *arterial smooth muscle,* but also on *heart muscle.* In the heart, Ca^{2+} inward currents are important in generating depolarization of sinoatrial node cells (impulse generation), in impulse propagation through the AV- junction (atrioventricular conduction), and in electromechanical coupling in the ventricular cardiomyocytes. Verapamil thus produces negative chrono-, dromo-, and inotropic effects.

Indications. Verapamil is used as an antiarrhythmic drug in supraventricular tachyarrhythmias. In atrial flutter or fibrillation, it is effective in reducing ventricular rate by virtue of inhibiting AV-conduction. Verapamil is also employed in the prophylaxis of *angina pectoris attacks* (p. 308) and the treatment of hypertension (p. 312). **Adverse effects:** Because of verapamil's effects on the sinus node, a drop in blood pressure fails to evoke a reflex tachycardia. Heart rate hardly changes; bradycardia may even develop. AV-block and myocardial insufficiency can occur. Patients frequently complain of constipation.

Gallopamil (= methoxyverapamil) is closely related to verapamil in both structure and biological activity.

Diltiazem is a catamphiphilic benzothiazepine derivative with an activity profile resembling that of verapamil.

III. T-channel selective blockers. Ca^{2+}-channel blockers, such as verapamil and mibefradil, may block both L- and T-type Ca^{2+} channels. Mibefradil shows relative selectivity for the latter and is devoid of a negative inotropic effect; its therapeutic usefulness is compromised by numerous interactions with other drugs due to inhibition of cytochrome P_{450}-dependent enzymes (CYP 1A2, 2D6 and, especially, 3A4).

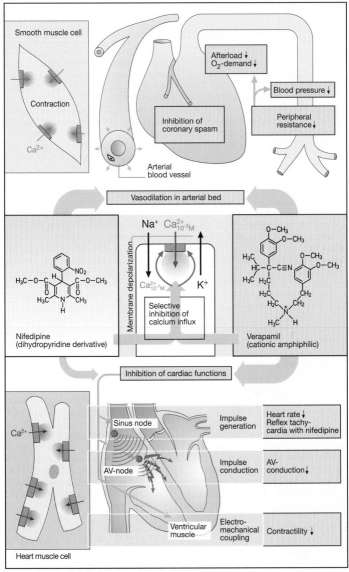

Smooth muscle cell

Contraction

Ca^{2+}

Afterload ↓
O_2-demand ↓

Inhibition of
coronary spasm

Arterial
blood vessel

Blood pressure ↓

Peripheral
resistance ↓

Vasodilation in arterial bed

Na^+ $Ca^{2+}_{10^{-3}M}$

Membrane depolarization

$Ca^{2+}_{10^{-7}M}$ K^+

Selective
inhibition of
calcium influx

Nifedipine
(dihydropyridine derivative)

Verapamil
(cationic amphiphilic)

Inhibition of cardiac functions

Ca^{2+}

Sinus node

AV-node

Ventricular
muscle

Impulse
generation

Impulse
conduction

Electro-
mechanical
coupling

Heart rate ↓
Reflex tachy-
cardia with nifedipine

AV-
conduction ↓

Contractility ↓

Heart muscle cell

A. Vasodilators: calcium antagonists

Inhibitors of the RAA System

Angiotensin-converting enzyme (ACE) is a component of the antihypotensive renin-angiotensin-aldosterone (RAA) system. Renin is produced by specialized cells in the wall of the afferent arteriole of the renal glomerulus. These cells belong to the juxtaglomerular apparatus of the nephron, the site of contact between afferent arteriole and distal tubule, and play an important part in controlling nephron function. Stimuli eliciting *release of renin* are: a drop in renal perfusion pressure, decreased rate of delivery of Na^+ or Cl^- to the distal tubules, as well as β-adrenoceptor-mediated sympathoactivation. The glycoprotein renin enzymatically cleaves the decapeptide angiotensin I from its circulating precursor substrate angiotensinogen. ACE, in turn, produces biologically active angiotensin II (ANG II) from angiotensin I (ANG I).

ACE is a rather nonspecific peptidase that can cleave C-terminal dipeptides from various peptides (dipeptidyl carboxypeptidase). As "kininase II," it contributes to the inactivation of kinins, such as bradykinin. ACE is also present in blood plasma; however, enzyme localized in the luminal side of vascular endothelium is primarily responsible for the formation of angiotensin II. The lung is rich in ACE, but kidneys, heart, and other organs also contain the enzyme.

Angiotensin II can raise blood pressure in different ways, including (1) vasoconstriction in both the arterial and venous limbs of the circulation; (2) stimulation of aldosterone secretion, leading to increased renal reabsorption of NaCl and water, hence an increased blood volume; (3) a central increase in sympathotonus and, peripherally, enhancement of the release and effects of norepinephrine.

ACE inhibitors, such as *captopril* and *enalaprilat,* the active metabolite of enalapril, occupy the enzyme as false substrates. Affinity significantly influences efficacy and rate of elimination. Enalaprilat has a stronger and longer-

lasting effect than does captopril. **Indications** are *hypertension* and *cardiac failure.*

Lowering of an elevated blood pressure is predominantly brought about by diminished production of angiotensin II. Impaired degradation of kinins that exert vasodilating actions may contribute to the effect.

In heart failure, cardiac output rises again because ventricular afterload diminishes due to a fall in peripheral resistance. Venous congestion abates as a result of (1) increased cardiac output and (2) reduction in venous return (decreased aldosterone secretion, decreased tonus of venous capacitance vessels).

Undesired effects. The magnitude of the antihypertensive effect of ACE inhibitors depends on the functional state of the RAA system. When the latter has been activated by loss of electrolytes and water (resulting from treatment with diuretic drugs), cardiac failure, or renal arterial stenosis, administration of ACE inhibitors may initially cause an excessive fall in blood pressure. In renal arterial stenosis, the RAA system may be needed for maintaining renal function and ACE inhibitors may precipitate renal failure. Dry cough is a fairly frequent side effect, possibly caused by reduced inactivation of kinins in the bronchial mucosa. Rarely, disturbances of taste sensation, exanthema, neutropenia, proteinuria, and angioneurotic edema may occur. In most cases, ACE inhibitors are well tolerated and effective. Newer analogues include lisinopril, perindopril, ramipril, quinapril, fosinopril, benazepril, cilazapril, and trandolapril.

Antagonists at angiotensin II receptors. Two receptor subtypes can be distinguished: AT1, which mediates the above actions of AT II; and AT2, whose physiological role is still unclear. The sartans (candesartan, eprosartan, irbesartan, losartan, and valsartan) are AT1 antagonists that reliably lower high blood pressure. They do not inhibit degradation of kinins and cough is not a frequent side-effect.

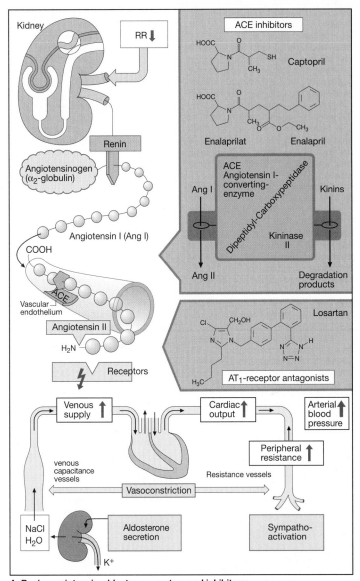

A. Renin-angiotensin-aldosterone system and inhibitors

Drugs Used to Influence Smooth Muscle Organs

Bronchodilators. Narrowing of bronchioles raises airway resistance, e.g., in bronchial or bronchitic asthma. Several substances that are employed as *bronchodilators* are described elsewhere in more detail: β_2-sympathomimetics (p. 84, given by pulmonary, parenteral, or oral route), the methylxanthine *theophylline* (p. 326, given parenterally or orally), as well as the parasympatholytic *ipratropium* (pp. 104, 107, given by inhalation).

Spasmolytics. N-Butylscopolamine (p. 104) is used for the relief of painful spasms of the biliary or ureteral ducts. Its poor absorption (N.B. quaternary N; absorption rate <10%) necessitates parenteral administration. Because the therapeutic effect is usually weak, a potent analgesic is given concurrently, e.g., the opioid meperidine. Note that some spasms of intestinal musculature can be effectively relieved by organic nitrates (in biliary colic) or by nifedipine (esophageal hypertension and achalasia).

Myometrial relaxants (Tocolytics). β_2-Sympathomimetics such as fenoterol or ritodrine, given orally or parenterally, can prevent premature labor or interrupt labor in progress when dangerous complications necessitate cesarean section. Tachycardia is a side effect produced reflexly because of β_2-mediated vasodilation or direct stimulation of cardiac β_1-receptors. Magnesium sulfate, given i.v., is a useful alternative when β-mimetics are contraindicated, but must be carefully titrated because its nonspecific calcium antagonism leads to blockade of cardiac impulse conduction and of neuromuscular transmission.

Myometrial stimulants. The neurohypophyseal hormone *oxytocin* (p. 242) is given parenterally (or by the nasal or buccal route) before, during, or after labor in order to prompt uterine contractions or to enhance them. Certain *prostaglandins* or analogues of them (p. 196; $F_{2\alpha}$: dinoprost; E_2: dinoprostone, misoprostol, sulprostone) are capable of inducing rhythmic uterine contractions and cervical relaxation at any time. They are mostly employed as abortifacients (oral or vaginal application of misoprostol in combination with mifepristone [p. 256]).

Ergot alkaloids are obtained from *Secale cornutum* (ergot), the sclerotium of a fungus *(Claviceps purpurea)* parasitizing rye. Consumption of flour from contaminated grain was once the cause of epidemic poisonings *(ergotism)* characterized by gangrene of the extremities (St. Anthony's fire) and CNS disturbances (hallucinations).

Ergot alkaloids contain lysergic acid (formula in **A** shows an amide). They act on uterine and vascular muscle. *Ergometrine* particularly stimulates the uterus. It readily induces a tonic contraction of the myometrium (tetanus uteri). This jeopardizes placental blood flow and fetal O_2 supply. The semisynthetic derivative methylergometrine is therefore used only *after* delivery for uterine contractions that are too weak.

Ergotamine, as well as the ergotoxine alkaloids (ergocristine, ergocryptine, ergocornine), have a predominantly vascular action. Depending on the initial caliber, constriction or dilation may be elicited. The mechanism of action is unclear; a mixed antagonism at α-adrenoceptors and agonism at 5-HT-receptors may be important. Ergotamine is used in the treatment of migraine (p. 322). Its congener, dihydroergotamine, is furthermore employed in orthostatic complaints (p. 314).

Other lysergic acid derivatives are the 5-HT antagonist methysergide, the dopamine agonists bromocriptine, pergolide, and cabergolide (pp. 114, 188), and the hallucinogen lysergic acid diethylamide (LSD, p. 240).

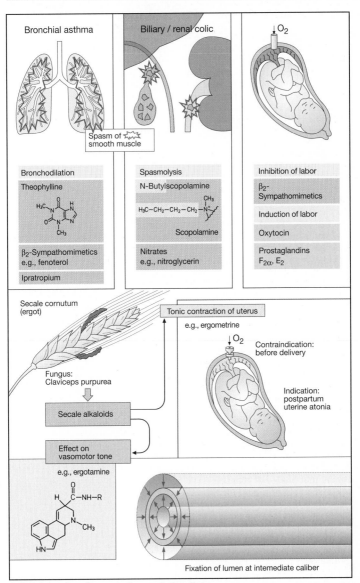

A. Drugs used to alter smooth muscle function

Overview of Modes of Action (A)

1. The pumping capacity of the heart is regulated by sympathetic and parasympathetic nerves (pp. 84, 105). Drugs capable of interfering with autonomic nervous function therefore provide a means of influencing cardiac performance. Thus, **anxiolytics** of the benzodiazepine type (p. 226), such as diazepam, can be employed in myocardial infarction to suppress sympathoactivation due to life-threatening distress. Under the influence of **antiadrenergic agents** (p. 96), used to lower an elevated blood pressure, cardiac work is decreased. **Ganglionic blockers** (p. 108) are used in managing hypertensive emergencies. Parasympatholytics (p. 104) and β-blockers (p. 92) prevent the transmission of autonomic nerve impulses to heart muscle cells by blocking the respective receptors.

2. An isolated mammalian heart whose extrinsic nervous connections have been severed will beat spontaneously for hours if it is supplied with a nutrient medium via the aortic trunk and coronary arteries (Langendorff preparation). In such a preparation, only those drugs that act directly on cardiomyocytes will alter contractile force and beating rate.

Parasympathomimetics and **sympathomimetics** act at membrane receptors for visceromotor neurotransmitters. The plasmalemma also harbors the sites of action of **cardiac glycosides** (the Na/K-ATPases, p. 130), of Ca^{2+} antagonists (Ca^{2+} channels, p. 122), and of **agents that block Na^+ channels** (local anesthetics; p. 134, p. 204). An intracellular site is the target for phosphodiesterase inhibitors (e.g., amrinone, p. 132).

3. Mention should also be made of the possibility of affecting cardiac function in angina pectoris (p. 306) or congestive heart failure (p. 132) by reducing venous return, peripheral resistance, or both, with the aid of vasodilators; and by reducing sympathetic drive applying β-blockers.

Events Underlying Contraction and Relaxation (B)

The signal triggering **contraction** is a propagated action potential (AP) generated in the sinoatrial node. Depolarization of the plasmalemma leads to a rapid *rise in cytosolic Ca^{2+} levels,* which causes the contractile filaments to shorten (**electromechanical coupling**). The level of Ca^{2+} concentration attained determines the degree of shortening, i.e., the force of contraction. Sources of Ca^{2+} are: a) extracellular Ca^{2+} entering the cell through voltage-gated *Ca^{2+} channels;* b) Ca^{2+} stored in membranous sacs of the *sarcoplasmic reticulum* (SR); c) Ca^{2+} bound to the inside of the plasmalemma. The plasmalemma of cardiomyocytes extends into the cell interior in the form of tubular invaginations (transverse tubuli).

The trigger signal for **relaxation** is the return of the membrane potential to its resting level. During repolarization, Ca^{2+} levels fall below the threshold for activation of the myofilaments (3×10^{-7} M), as the *plasmalemmal binding* sites regain their binding capacity; the SR pumps Ca^{2+} into its interior; and Ca^{2+} that entered the cytosol during systole is again extruded by plasmalemmal *Ca^{2+}-ATPases* with expenditure of energy. In addition, a carrier (antiporter), utilizing the transmembrane Na^+ gradient as energy source, transports Ca^{2+} out of the cell in exchange for Na^+ moving down its transmembrane gradient (*Na^+/Ca^{2+} exchange*).

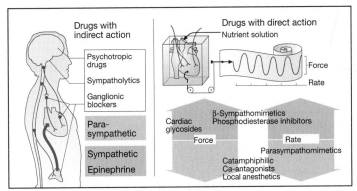

A. Possible mechanisms for influencing heart function

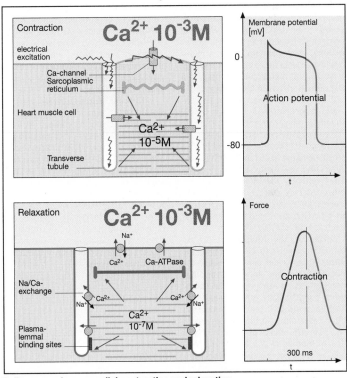

B. Processes in myocardial contraction and relaxation

Cardiac Glycosides

Diverse plants (**A**) are sources of sugar-containing compounds (glycosides) that also contain a steroid ring (structural formulas, p. 133) and augment the contractile force of heart muscle (**B**): *cardiotonic glycosides. cardiosteroids,* or *"digitalis."*

If the inotropic, "therapeutic" dose is exceeded by a small increment, signs of poisoning appear: arrhythmia and contracture (**B**). The *narrow therapeutic margin* can be explained by the **mechanism of action.**

Cardiac glycosides (CG) bind to the extracellular side of Na$^+$/K$^+$-ATPases of cardiomyocytes and inhibit enzyme activity. The Na$^+$/K$^+$-ATPases operate to pump out Na$^+$ leaked into the cell and to retrieve K$^+$ leaked from the cell. In this manner, they maintain the transmembrane gradients for K$^+$ and Na$^+$, the negative resting membrane potential, and the normal electrical excitability of the cell membrane. When part of the enzyme is occupied and inhibited by CG, the unoccupied remainder can increase its level of activity and maintain Na$^+$ and K$^+$ transport. The effective stimulus is a small elevation of intracellular Na$^+$ concentration (normally approx. 7 mM). Concomitantly, the amount of Ca^{2+} mobilized during systole and, thus, *contractile force,* increases. It is generally thought that the underlying cause is the decrease in the Na$^+$ transmembrane gradient, i.e., the driving force for the Na$^+$/Ca^{2+} exchange (p. 128), allowing the intracellular Ca^{2+} level to rise. When too many ATPases are blocked, K$^+$ and Na$^+$ homeostasis is deranged; the membrane potential falls, *arrhythmias* occur. Flooding with Ca^{2+} prevents relaxation during diastole, resulting in *contracture.*

The **CNS effects** of CG (**C**) are also due to binding to Na$^+$/K$^+$-ATPases. Enhanced vagal nerve activity causes a decrease in sinoatrial beating rate and velocity of atrioventricular conduction. In patients with heart failure, improved circulation also contributes to the reduction in heart rate. Stimulation of the area postrema leads to nausea and vomiting. Disturbances in color vision are evident.

Indications for CG are: (1) *chronic congestive heart failure;* and (2) *atrial fibrillation or flutter,* where inhibition of AV conduction protects the ventricles from excessive atrial impulse activity and thereby improves cardiac performance (**D**). Occasionally, sinus rhythm is restored.

Signs of intoxication are: (1) *cardiac arrhythmias,* which under certain circumstances are life-threatening, e.g., sinus bradycardia, AV-block, ventricular extrasystoles, ventricular fibrillation (ECG); (2) *CNS disturbances* — altered color vision (xanthopsia), agitation, confusion, nightmares, hallucinations; (3) *gastrointestinal* — anorexia, nausea, vomiting, diarrhea; (4) *renal* — loss of electrolytes and water, which must be differentiated from mobilization of accumulated edema fluid that occurs with therapeutic dosage.

Therapy of intoxication: administration of K$^+$, which *inter alia* reduces binding of CG, but may impair AV-conduction; administration of antiarrhythmics, such as *phenytoin or lidocaine* (p. 136); oral administration of *colestyramine* (p. 154, 156) for binding and preventing absorption of digitoxin present in the intestines (enterohepatic cycle); injection of *antibody (Fab) fragments* that bind and inactivate digitoxin and digoxin. Compared with full antibodies, fragments have superior tissue penetrability, more rapid renal elimination, and lower antigenicity.

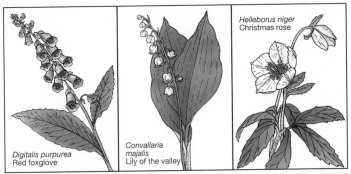

A. Plants containing cardiac glycosides

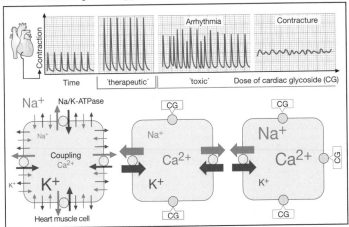

B. Therapeutic and toxic effects of cardiac glycosides (CG)

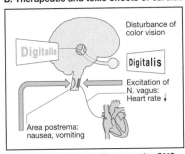

C. Cardiac glycoside effects on the CNS

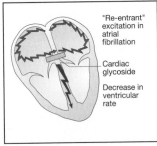

D. Cardiac glycoside effects in atrial fibrillation

Substance	Fraction absorbed %	Plasma concentr. (ng/mL) free	total	Digitalizing dose (mg)	Elimination %/d	Maintenance dose (mg)
Digitoxin	100	~1	~20	~1	10	~0.1
Digoxin	50–90	~1	~1.5	~1	30	~0.3
Ouabain	<1	~1	~1	0.5	no long-term use	

The **pharmacokinetics of cardiac glycosides (A)** are dictated by their polarity, i.e., the number of hydroxyl groups. Membrane penetrability is virtually nil in ouabain, high in digoxin, and very high in digitoxin. **Ouabain** (g-strophanthin) does not penetrate into cells, be they intestinal epithelium, renal tubular, or hepatic cells. At best, it is suitable for acute intravenous induction of glycoside therapy.

The absorption of **digoxin** depends on the kind of galenical preparation used and on absorptive conditions in the intestine. Preparations are now of such quality that the derivatives *methyldigoxin* and *acetyldigoxin* no longer offer any advantage. Renal reabsorption is incomplete; approx. 30% of the total amount present in the body (s.c. full "digitalizing" dose) is eliminated per day. When renal function is impaired, there is a risk of accumulation. **Digitoxin** undergoes virtually complete reabsorption in gut and kidneys. There is active hepatic biotransformation: cleavage of sugar moieties, hydroxylation at C12 (yielding digoxin), and conjugation to glucuronic acid. Conjugates secreted with bile are subject to enterohepatic cycling (p. 38); conjugates reaching the blood are renally eliminated. In renal insufficiency, there is no appreciable accumulation. When digitoxin is withdrawn following overdosage, its effect decays more slowly than does that of digoxin.

Other positive inotropic drugs. The **phosphodiesterase inhibitor amrinone** (cAMP elevation, p. 66) can be administered only parenterally for a maximum of 14 d because it is poorly tolerated. A closely related compound is *milrinone*. In terms of their positive inotropic effect, β-sympathomimetics, unlike dopamine (p. 114), are of little therapeutic use; they are also arrhythmogenic and the sensitivity of the β-receptor system declines during continuous stimulation.

Treatment Principles in Chronic Heart Failure

Myocardial insufficiency leads to a decrease in stroke volume and venous congestion with formation of edema. Administration of (thiazide) diuretics (p. 62) offers a therapeutic approach of proven efficacy that is brought about by a decrease in circulating blood volume (decreased venous return) and peripheral resistance, i.e., afterload. A similar approach is intended with ACE-inhibitors, which act by preventing the synthesis of angiotensin II (↓ vasoconstriction) and reducing the secretion of aldosterone (↓ fluid retention). In severe cases of myocardial insufficiency, cardiac glycosides may be added to augment cardiac force and to relieve the symptoms of insufficiency.

In more recent times β-blocker on a long term were found to improve cardiac performance — particularly in idiopathic dilating cardiomyopathy — probably by preventing sympathetic overdrive.

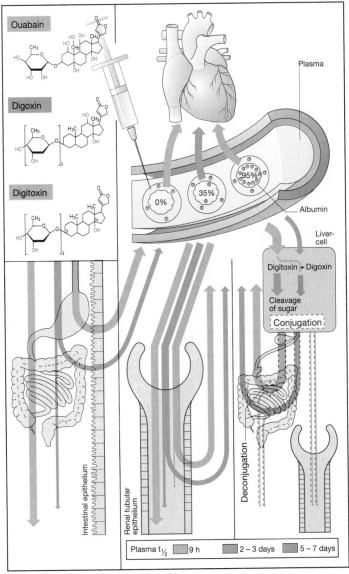

Ouabain

Digoxin

Digitoxin

Plasma

0%

35%

95%

Albumin

Liver-cell

Digitoxin → Digoxin

Cleavage of sugar

Conjugation

Intestinal epithelium

Renal tubular epithelium

Deconjugation

Plasma t$_{1/2}$ | 9 h | 2 – 3 days | 5 – 7 days

A. Pharmacokinetics of cardiac glycosides

Antiarrhythmic Drugs

The electrical impulse for contraction (propagated action potential; p. 136) originates in pacemaker cells of the sinoatrial node and spreads through the atria, atrioventricular (AV) node, and adjoining parts of the His-Purkinje fiber system to the ventricles (**A**). Irregularities of heart rhythm can interfere dangerously with cardiac pumping function.

I. Drugs for selective control of sinoatrial and AV nodes. In some forms of arrhythmia, certain drugs can be used that are capable of selectively facilitating and inhibiting (green and red arrows, respectively) the pacemaker function of sinoatrial or atrioventricular cells.

Sinus bradycardia. An abnormally low sinoatrial impulse rate (<60/min) can be raised by *parasympatholytics*. The quaternary *ipratropium* is preferable to atropine, because it lacks CNS penetrability (p. 107). Sympathomimetics also exert a positive chronotropic action; they have the disadvantage of increasing myocardial excitability (and automaticity) and, thus, promoting ectopic impulse generation (tendency to extrasystolic beats). In **cardiac arrest** *epinephrine* can be used to reinitiate heart beat.

Sinus tachycardia (resting rate >100 beats/min). β-Blockers eliminate sympathoexcitation and decrease cardiac rate.

Atrial flutter or fibrillation. An excessive ventricular rate can be decreased by *verapamil* (p. 122) or *cardiac glycosides* (p. 130). These drugs inhibit impulse propagation through the AV node, so that fewer impulses reach the ventricles.

II. Nonspecific drug actions on impulse generation and propagation. Impulses originating at loci outside the sinus node are seen in *supraventricular* or *ventricular extrasystoles, tachycardia, atrial* or *ventricular flutter,* and *fibrillation.* In these forms of rhythm disorders, **antiarrhythmics** of the **local anesthetic, Na⁺-channel blocking type (B)** are used for both prophylaxis and therapy. Local anesthetics inhibit electrical excitation of nociceptive nerve fibers (p. 204); concomitant cardiac inhibition *(cardiodepression)* is an unwanted effect. However, in certain types of arrhythmias (see above), this effect is useful. Local anesthetics are readily cleaved (arrows) and unsuitable for oral administration (procaine, lidocaine). Given judiciously, intravenous lidocaine is an effective antiarrhythmic. *Procainamide* and *mexiletine*, congeners endowed with greater metabolic stability, are examples of orally effective antiarrhythmics. The desired and undesired effects are inseparable. Thus, these antiarrhythmics not only depress electrical excitability of cardiomyocytes *(negative bathmotropism, membrane stabilization)*, but also lower sinoatrial rate *(neg. chronotropism)*, AV conduction *(neg. dromotropism)*, and force of contraction *(neg. inotropism)*. Interference with normal electrical activity can, not too paradoxically, also induce cardiac arrhythmias–*arrhythmogenic action.*

Inhibition of CNS neurons is the underlying cause of neurological effects such as vertigo, confusion, sensory disturbances, and motor disturbances (tremor, giddiness, ataxia, convulsions).

Na^+-channel blocking type (B) are

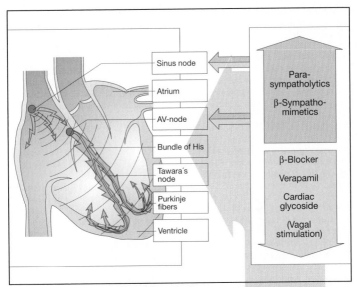

A. Cardiac impulse generation and conduction

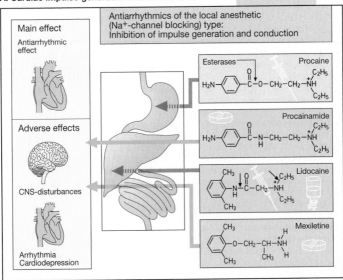

B. Antiarrhythmics of the Na⁺-channel blocking type

Electrophysiological Actions of Antiarrhythmics of the Na⁺-Channel Blocking Type

Action potential and ionic currents. The transmembrane electrical potential of cardiomyocytes can be recorded through an intracellular microelectrode. Upon electrical excitation, a characteristic change occurs in membrane potential—the action potential (AP). Its underlying cause is a sequence of transient ionic currents. During *rapid depolarization* (Phase 0), there is a short-lived *influx of Na⁺* through the membrane. A subsequent *transient influx of Ca²⁺* (as well as of Na⁺) maintains the depolarization (Phase 2, *plateau of AP*). A delayed *efflux of K⁺* returns the membrane potential (Phase 3, *repolarization*) to its resting value (Phase 4). The velocity of depolarization determines the speed at which the AP propagates through the myocardial syncytium.

Transmembrane ionic currents involve proteinaceous *membrane pores:* Na⁺, Ca²⁺, and K⁺ channels. In **A**, the phasic change in the functional state of Na⁺ channels during an action potential is illustrated.

Effects of antiarrhythmics. Antiarrhythmics of the Na⁺-channel blocking type *reduce the probability that Na⁺ channels* will open upon membrane depolarization **("membrane stabilization").** The potential consequences are (**A**, bottom): 1) a reduction in the velocity of depolarization and a decrease in the speed of impulse propagation; aberrant impulse propagation is impeded. 2) *Depolarization is entirely absent;* pathological impulse generation, e.g., in the marginal zone of an infarction, is suppressed. 3) The time required until a new depolarization can be elicited, i.e., *the refractory period, is increased;* prolongation of the AP (see below) contributes to the increase in refractory period. Consequently, premature excitation with risk of fibrillation is prevented.

Mechanism of action. Na⁺-channel blocking antiarrhythmics resemble most local anesthetics in being cationic amphiphilic molecules (p. 208, exception: phenytoin, p. 190). Possible molecular mechanisms of their inhibitory effects are outlined on p. 204 in more detail. Their low structural specificity is reflected by a low selectivity towards different cation channels. Besides the Na⁺ channel, *Ca²⁺ and K⁺ channels* are also likely to be *blocked.* Accordingly, cationic amphiphilic antiarrhythmics affect both the depolarization and repolarization phases. Depending on the substance, AP duration can be increased (Class IA), decreased (Class IB), or remain the same (Class IC).

Antiarrhythmics representative of these categories include: Class IA—quinidine, procainamide, ajmaline, disopyramide, propafenone; Class IB—lidocaine, mexiletine, tocainide, as well as phenytoin; Class IC—flecainide.

Note: With respect to classification, β-blockers have been assigned to Class II, and the Ca²⁺-channel blockers verapamil and diltiazem to Class IV.

Commonly listed under a separate rubric (Class III) are amiodarone and the β-blocking agent sotalol, which both inhibit K⁺-channels and which both cause marked prolongation of the AP with a lesser effect on Phase 0 rate of rise.

Therapeutic uses. Because of their *narrow therapeutic margin,* these antiarrhythmics are only employed when rhythm disturbances are of such severity as to impair the pumping action of the heart, or when there is a threat of other complications. The choice of drug is empirical. If the desired effect is not achieved, another drug is tried. Combinations of antiarrhythmics are not customary. Amiodarone is reserved for special cases.

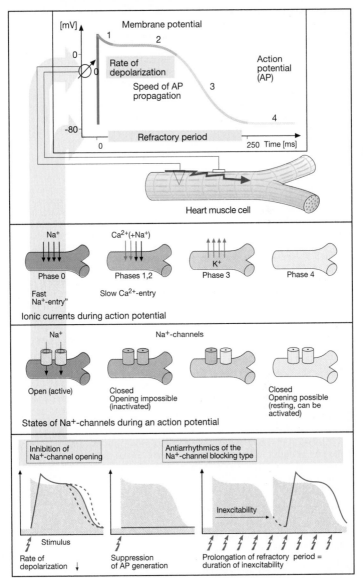

A. Effects of antiarrhythmics of the Na⁺-channel blocking type

Drugs for the Treatment of Anemias

Anemia denotes a reduction in red blood cell count, hemoglobin content, or both. Oxygen (O_2) transport capacity is decreased.

Erythropoiesis (A). Blood corpuscles develop from stem cells through several cell divisions. Hemoglobin is then synthesized and the cell nucleus is extruded. Erythropoiesis is stimulated by the hormone **erythropoietin** (a glycoprotein), which is released from the kidneys when renal O_2 tension declines.

Given an adequate production of erythropoietin, a **disturbance** of erythropoiesis is due to two principal causes: 1. **Cell multiplication is inhibited** because DNA synthesis is insufficient. This occurs in deficiencies of *vitamin B_{12}* or *folic acid* (macrocytic hyperchromic anemia). 2. **Hemoglobin synthesis is impaired.** This situation arises in **iron deficiency,** since Fe^{2+} is a constituent of hemoglobin (microcytic hypochromic anemia).

Vitamin B_{12} (B)

Vitamin B_{12} **(cyanocobalamin)** is produced by bacteria; B_{12} generated in the colon, however, is unavailable for absorption (see below). Liver, meat, fish, and milk products are rich sources of the vitamin. The **minimal requirement** is about 1 µg/d. Enteral absorption of vitamin B_{12} requires so-called **"intrinsic factor"** from parietal cells of the stomach. The complex formed with this glycoprotein undergoes endocytosis in the ileum. Bound to its transport protein, transcobalamin, vitamin B_{12} is destined for storage in the liver or uptake into tissues.

A frequent **cause of vitamin B_{12} deficiency** is atrophic gastritis leading to a *lack of intrinsic factor.* Besides megaloblastic anemia, damage to mucosal linings and degeneration of myelin sheaths with neurological sequelae will occur **(pernicious anemia).**

Optimal **therapy** consists in **parenteral administration** of **cyanocobalamin** or **hydroxycobalamin** (Vitamin B_{12a}; exchange of -CN for -OH group). Adverse effects, in the form of hypersensitivity reactions, are very rare.

Folic Acid (B). Leafy vegetables and liver are rich in folic acid (FA). The **minimal requirement** is approx. 50 µg/d. Polyglutamine-FA in food is hydrolyzed to monoglutamine-FA prior to being absorbed. FA is heat labile. **Causes of deficiency** include: insufficient intake, malabsorption in gastrointestinal diseases, increased requirements during pregnancy. Antiepileptic drugs (phenytoin, primidone, phenobarbital) may decrease FA absorption, presumably by inhibiting the formation of monoglutamine-FA. Inhibition of dihydro-FA reductase (e.g., by methotrexate, p. 298) depresses the formation of the active species, tetrahydro-FA. *Symptoms* of deficiency are megaloblastic anemia and mucosal damage. **Therapy** consists in **oral administration of FA** or in folinic acid (p. 298) when deficiency is caused by inhibitors of dihydro—FA—reductase.

Administration of FA can mask a vitamin B_{12} deficiency. Vitamin B_{12} is required for the conversion of methyltetrahydro-FA to tetrahydro-FA, which is important for DNA synthesis **(B).** Inhibition of this reaction due to B_{12} deficiency can be compensated by increased FA intake. The anemia is readily corrected; however, nerve degeneration progresses unchecked and its cause is made more difficult to diagnose by the absence of hematological changes. Indiscriminate use of FA-containing multivitamin preparations can, therefore, be harmful.

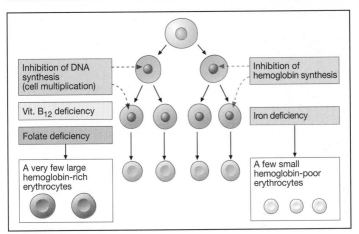

A. Erythropoiesis in bone marrow

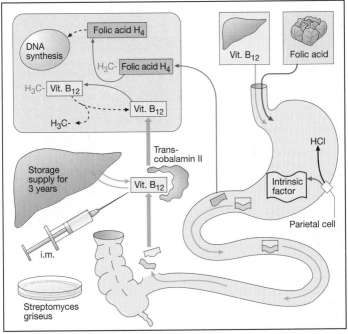

B. Vitamin B$_{12}$ and folate metabolism

Iron Compounds

Not all iron ingested in food is equally absorbable. Trivalent Fe^{3+} is virtually not taken up from the neutral milieu of the small bowel, where the divalent Fe^{2+} is markedly better absorbed. Uptake is particularly efficient in the form of heme (present in hemo- and myoglobin). Within the mucosal cells of the gut, iron is oxidized and either deposited as ferritin (see below) or passed on to the transport protein, transferrin, a β_1-glycoprotein. The amount absorbed does not exceed that needed to balance losses due to epithelial shedding from skin and mucosae or hemorrhage (so-called **"mucosal block"**). In men, this amount is approx. 1 mg/d; in women, it is approx. 2 mg/d (menstrual blood loss), corresponding to about 10% of the dietary intake. The transferrin-iron complex undergoes endocytotic uptake mainly into erythroblasts to be utilized for hemoglobin synthesis.

About 70% of the total body store of iron (~5 g) is contained within erythrocytes. When these are degraded by macrophages of the reticuloendothelial (mononuclear phagocyte) system, iron is liberated from hemoglobin. Fe^{3+} can be stored as ferritin (= protein apoferritin + Fe^{3+}) or returned to erythropoiesis sites via transferrin.

A frequent **cause of iron deficiency** is chronic blood loss due to gastric/intestinal ulcers or tumors. One liter of blood contains 500 mg of iron. Despite a significant increase in absorption rate (up to 50%), absorption is unable to keep up with losses and the body store of iron falls. Iron deficiency results in impaired synthesis of hemoglobin and **anemia** (p. 138).

The **treatment** of choice (after the cause of bleeding has been found and eliminated) consists of the **oral administration** of Fe^{2+} **compounds,** e.g., ferrous sulfate (daily dose 100 mg of iron equivalent to 300 mg of $FeSO_4$, divided into multiple doses). Replenishing of iron stores may take several months. Oral administration, however, is advantageous in that it is impossible to overload the body with iron through an intact mucosa because of its demand-regulated absorption (mucosal block).

Adverse effects. The frequent gastrointestinal complaints (epigastric pain, diarrhea, constipation) necessitate intake of iron preparations with or after meals, although absorption is higher from the empty stomach.

Interactions. Antacids inhibit iron absorption. Combination with ascorbic acid (Vitamin C), for protecting Fe^{2+} from oxidation to Fe^{3+}, is theoretically sound, but practically is not needed.

Parenteral administration of Fe^{3+} salts is indicated only when adequate oral replacement is not possible. There is a risk of overdosage with iron deposition in tissues **(hemosiderosis).** The binding capacity of transferrin is limited and free Fe^{3+} is toxic. Therefore, Fe^{3+} complexes are employed that can donate Fe^{3+} directly to transferrin or can be phagocytosed by macrophages, enabling iron to be incorporated into ferritin stores. Possible *adverse effects* are, with i.m. injection: persistent pain at the injection site and skin discoloration; with i.v. injection: flushing, hypotension, anaphylactic shock.

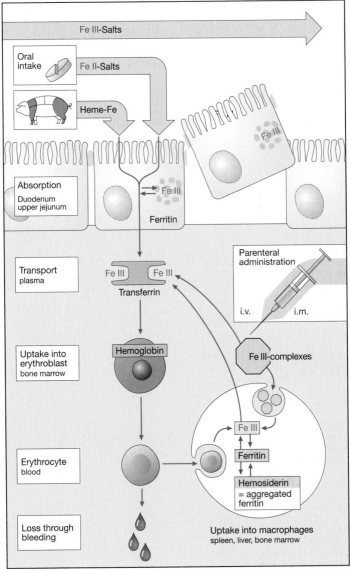

A. Iron: possible routes of administration and fate in the organism

Prophylaxis and Therapy of Thromboses

Upon vascular injury, the coagulation system is activated: thrombocytes and fibrin molecules coalesce into a "plug" (p. 148) that seals the defect and halts bleeding (**hemostasis**). Unnecessary formation of an intravascular clot – a **thrombosis** – can be life-threatening. If the clot forms on an atheromatous plaque in a coronary artery, myocardial infarction is imminent; a thrombus in a deep leg vein can be dislodged, carried into a lung artery, and cause complete or partial interruption of pulmonary blood flow (pulmonary embolism).

Drugs that *decrease the coagulability of blood,* such as **coumarins** and **heparin (A),** are employed for the **prophylaxis** of thromboses. In addition, attempts are directed at inhibiting the aggregation of blood platelets, which are prominently involved in intra-arterial thrombogenesis (p. 148). For the **therapy** of thrombosis, drugs are used that dissolve the fibrin meshwork→fibrinolytics (p. 146).

An overview of the **coagulation cascade** and sites of action for coumarins and heparin is shown in **A.** There are two ways to initiate the cascade (**B**): 1) conversion of factor XII into its active form (XII$_a$, intrinsic system) at intravascular sites denuded of endothelium; 2) conversion of factor VII into VII$_a$ (extrinsic system) under the influence of a tissue-derived lipoprotein (tissue thromboplastin). Both mechanisms converge via factor X into a common final pathway.

The **clotting factors** are protein molecules. "Activation" mostly means proteolysis (cleavage of protein fragments) and, with the exception of fibrin, conversion into protein-hydrolyzing enzymes *(proteases).* Some activated factors require the presence of phospholipids (PL) and Ca^{2+} for their proteolytic activity. Conceivably, Ca^{2+} ions cause the adhesion of factor to a phospholipid surface, as depicted in **C.** Phospholipids are contained in platelet factor 3 (PF3), which is released from ag-gregated platelets, and in tissue thromboplastin (**B**). The sequential activation of several enzymes allows the aforementioned reactions to "snowball", culminating in massive production of fibrin (p. 148).

Progression of the coagulation cascade can be inhibited as follows:

1) **coumarin derivatives** decrease the blood concentrations of inactive factors II, VII, IX, and X, by inhibiting their synthesis; 2) the complex consisting of **heparin** and antithrombin III neutralizes the protease activity of activated factors; 3) **Ca^{2+} chelators** prevent the enzymatic activity of Ca^{2+}-dependent factors; they contain COO-groups that bind Ca^{2+} ions (**C**): **citrate** and **EDTA** (ethylenediaminetetraacetic acid) form soluble complexes with Ca^{2+}; **oxalate** precipitates Ca^{2+} as insoluble calcium oxalate. Chelation of Ca^{2+} cannot be used for therapeutic purposes because Ca^{2+} concentrations would have to be lowered to a level incompatible with life (hypocalcemic tetany). These compounds (sodium salts) are, therefore, used only for rendering blood incoagulable outside the body.

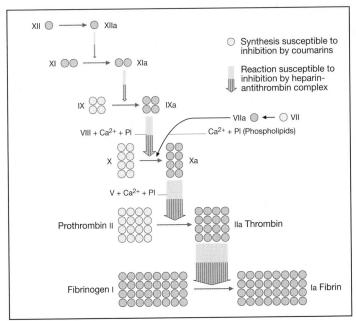

A. Inhibition of clotting cascade in vivo

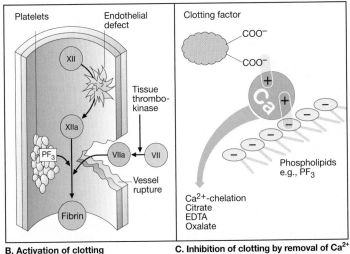

B. Activation of clotting

C. Inhibition of clotting by removal of Ca²⁺

Coumarin Derivatives (A)

Vitamin K promotes the hepatic γ-carboxylation of glutamate residues on the precursors of factors II, VII, IX, and X, as well as that of other proteins, e.g., protein C, protein S, or osteocalcin. Carboxyl groups are required for Ca^{2+}-mediated binding to phospholipid surfaces (p. 142). There are several vitamin K derivatives of different origins: K_1 (phytomenadione) from chlorophyllous plants; K_2 from gut bacteria; and K_3 (menadione) synthesized chemically. All are hydrophobic and require bile acids for absorption.

Oral anticoagulants. Structurally related to vitamin K, **4-hydroxycoumarins** act as "false" vitamin K and prevent regeneration of reduced (active) vitamin K from vitamin K epoxide, hence the synthesis of vitamin K-dependent clotting factors.

Coumarins are well absorbed after oral administration. Their duration of action varies considerably. Synthesis of clotting factors depends on the intrahepatocytic concentration ratio of coumarins to vitamin K. The dose required for an adequate anticoagulant effect must be determined individually for each patient *(one-stage prothrombin time)*. Subsequently, the patient must avoid changing dietary consumption of green vegetables (alteration in vitamin K levels), refrain from taking additional drugs likely to affect absorption or elimination of coumarins (alteration in coumarin levels), and not risk inhibiting platelet function by ingesting acetylsalicylic acid.

The **most important adverse effect is bleeding.** With coumarins, this can be counteracted by giving vitamin K_1. Coagulability of blood returns to normal only after hours or days, when the liver has resumed synthesis and restored sufficient blood levels of clotting factors. In urgent cases, deficient factors must be replenished directly (e.g., by transfusion of whole blood or of prothrombin concentrate).

Heparin (B)

A clotting factor is activated when the factor that precedes it in the clotting cascade splits off a protein fragment and thereby exposes an enzymatic center. The latter can again be inactivated physiologically by complexing with **antithrombin III (AT III)**, a circulating glycoprotein. Heparin acts to inhibit clotting by accelerating formation of this complex more than 1000-fold. Heparin is present (together with histamine) in the vesicles of mast cells; its physiological role is unclear. Therapeutically used heparin is obtained from porcine gut or bovine lung. Heparin molecules are chains of amino sugars bearing -COO$^-$ and -SO$_4$ groups; they contain approx. 10 to 20 of the units depicted in **(B)**; mean molecular weight, 20,000. Anticoagulant efficacy varies with chain length. The potency of a preparation is standardized in international units of activity (IU) by bioassay and comparison with a reference preparation.

The numerous negative charges are significant in several respects: (1) they contribute to the poor membrane penetrability—heparin is ineffective when applied by the oral route or topically onto the skin and must be injected; (2) attraction to positively charged lysine residues is involved in complex formation with ATIII; (3) they permit binding of heparin to its antidote, **protamine** (polycationic protein from salmon sperm).

If protamine is given in heparin-induced bleeding, the effect of heparin is immediately reversed.

For effective thromboprophylaxis, a low dose of 5000 IU is injected s.c. two to three times daily. With low dosage of heparin, the risk of bleeding is sufficiently small to allow the first injection to be given as early as 2 h prior to surgery. Higher daily i.v. doses are required to prevent growth of clots. Besides bleeding, other potential adverse effects are: allergic reactions (e.g., thrombocytopenia) and with chronic administration, reversible hair loss and osteoporosis.

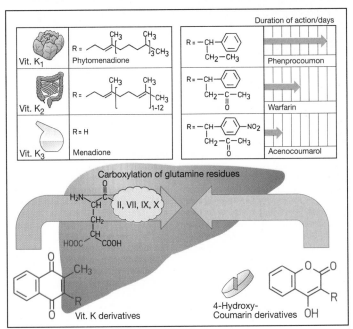

A. Vitamin K-antagonists of the coumarin type and vitamin K

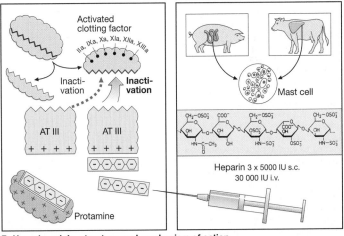

B. Heparin: origin, structure, and mechanism of action

Low-molecular-weight heparin (average MW ~5000) has a longer duration of action and needs to be given only once daily (e.g., *certoparin, dalteparin, enoxaparin, reviparin, tinzaparin*).

Frequent control of coagulability is not necessary with low molecular weight heparin and incidence of side effects (bleeding, heparin-induced thrombocytopenia) is less frequent than with unfractionated heparin.

Fibrinolytic Therapy (A)

Fibrin is formed from fibrinogen through thrombin (factor IIa)-catalyzed proteolytic removal of two oligopeptide fragments. Individual fibrin molecules polymerize into a fibrin mesh that can be split into fragments and dissolved by plasmin. Plasmin derives by proteolysis from an inactive precursor, plasminogen. Plasminogen activators can be infused for the purpose of dissolving clots (e.g., in myocardial infarction). Thrombolysis is not likely to be successful unless the activators can be given very soon after thrombus formation. Urokinase is an endogenous plasminogen activator obtained from cultured human kidney cells. Urokinase is better tolerated than is streptokinase. By itself, the latter is enzymatically inactive; only after binding to a plasminogen molecule does the complex become effective in converting plasminogen to plasmin. Streptokinase is produced by streptococcal bacteria, which probably accounts for the frequent adverse reactions. Streptokinase antibodies may be present as a result of prior streptococcal infections. Binding to such antibodies would neutralize streptokinase molecules.

With **alteplase**, another endogenous plasminogen activator (tissue plasminogen activator, tPA) is available. With physiological concentrations this activator preferentially acts on plasminogen bound to fibrin. In concentrations needed for therapeutic fibrinolysis this preference is lost and the risk of bleeding does not differ with alteplase and streptokinase. Alteplase is rather short-lived (inactivation by complexing with plasminogen activator inhibitor, PAI) and has to be applied by infusion. **Reteplase,** however, containing only the proteolytic active part of the alteplase molecule, allows more stable plasma levels and can be applied in form of two injections at an interval of 30 min.

Inactivation of the fibrinolytic system can be achieved by **"plasmin inhibitors,"** such as *ε-aminocaproic acid, p-aminomethylbenzoic acid (PAMBA), tranexamic acid,* and *aprotinin,* which also inhibits other proteases.

Lowering of blood fibrinogen concentration. Ancrod is a constituent of the venom from a Malaysian pit viper. It enzymatically cleaves a fragment from fibrinogen, resulting in the formation of a degradation product that cannot undergo polymerization. Reduction in blood fibrinogen level decreases the coagulability of the blood. Since fibrinogen (MW ~340 000) contributes to the viscosity of blood, an improved "fluidity" of the blood would be expected. Both effects are felt to be of benefit in the treatment of certain disorders of blood flow.

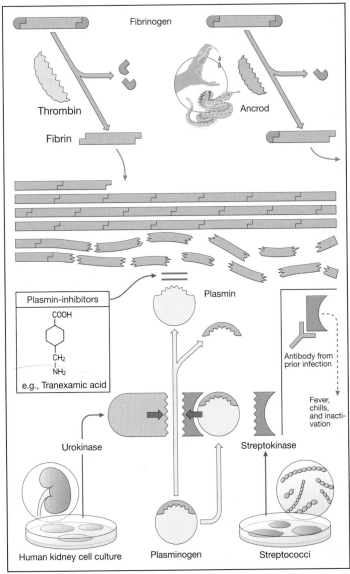

Fibrinogen

Thrombin

Ancrod

Fibrin

Plasmin-inhibitors

COOH

CH₂

NH₂

e.g., Tranexamic acid

Plasmin

Antibody from prior infection

Fever, chills, and inacti- vation

Urokinase

Streptokinase

Human kidney cell culture

Plasminogen

Streptococci

A. Activators and inhibitors of fibrinolysis; ancrod

Intra-arterial Thrombus Formation (A)

Activation of platelets, e.g., upon contact with collagen of the extracellular matrix after injury to the vascular wall, constitutes the immediate and decisive step in initiating the process of **primary hemostasis**, i.e., cessation of bleeding. However, in the absence of vascular injury, platelets can be activated as a result of damage to the endothelial cell lining of blood vessels. Among the multiple functions of the endothelium, the production of NO and prostacyclin plays an important role. Both substances inhibit the tendency of platelets to adhere to the endothelial surface (platelet adhesiveness). Impairment of endothelial function, e.g., due to chronic hypertension, cigarette smoking, chronic elevation of plasma LDL levels or of blood glucose, increases the probability of contact between platelets and endothelium. The adhesion process involves $GP_{IB/IX}$, a glycoprotein present in the platelet cell membrane and von Willebrandt's factor, an endothelial membrane protein. Upon endothelial contact, the platelet is activated with a resultant change in shape and affinity to fibrinogen. Platelets are linked to each other via fibrinogen bridges: they undergo **aggregation.**

Platelet aggregation increases like an avalanche because, once activated, platelets can activate other platelets. On the injured endothelial cell, a *platelet thrombus* is formed, which obstructs blood flow. Ultimately, the vascular lumen is occluded by the thrombus as the latter is solidified by a vasoconstriction produced by the release of serotonin and thromboxane A_2 from the aggregated platelets. When these events occur in a larger coronary artery, the consequence is a myocardial infarction; involvement of a cerebral artery leads to stroke.

The von Willebrandt's factor plays a key role in thrombogenesis. Lack of this factor causes *thrombasthenia*, a pathologically decreased platelet aggregation. Relative deficiency of the von Wille-brandt's factor can be temporarily overcome by the vasopressin anlogue desmopressin (p. 164), which increases the release of available factor from storage sites.

Formation, Activation, and Aggregation of Platelets (B)

Platelets originate by budding off from multinucleate precursor cells, the megakaryocytes. As the smallest formed element of blood (dia. 1–4 μm), they can be activated by various stimuli. Activation entails an alteration in shape and secretion of a series of highly active substances, including serotonin, platelet activating factor (PAF), ADP, and thromboxane A_2. In turn, all of these can activate other platelets, which explains the explosive nature of the process.

The primary consequence of activation is a conformational change of an integrin present in the platelet membrane, namely, GPIIB/IIIA. In its active conformation, GPIIB/IIIA shows high affinity for fibrinogen; each platelet contains up to 50,000 copies. The high plasma concentration of fibrinogen and the high density of integrins in the platelet membrane permit rapid cross-linking of platelets and formation of a platelet plug.

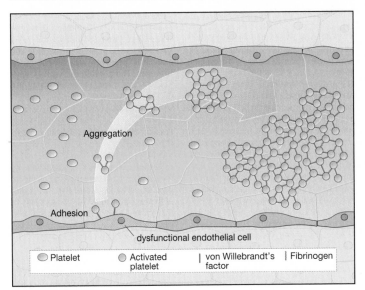

A. Thrombogenesis

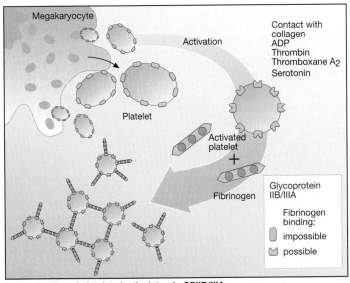

B. Aggregation of platelets by the integrin GPIIB/IIIA

Inhibitors of Platelet Aggregation (A)

Platelets can be activated by mechanical and diverse chemical stimuli, some of which, e.g., thromboxane A_2, thrombin, serotonin, and PAF, act via receptors on the platelet membrane. These receptors are coupled to G_q proteins that mediate activation of phospholipase C and hence a rise in cytosolic Ca^{2+} concentration. Among other responses, this rise in Ca^{2+} triggers a conformational change in GPIIB/IIIA, which is thereby converted to its fbrinogen-binding form. In contrast, ADP activates platelets by inhibiting adenylyl cyclase, thus causing internal cAMP levels to decrease. High cAMP levels would stabilize the platelet in its inactive state. Formally, the two messenger substances, Ca^{2+} and cAMP, can be considered functional antagonists.

Platelet aggregation can be inhibited by **acetylsalicylic acid** (ASA), which blocks thromboxane synthase, or by recombinant **hirudin** (originally harvested from leech salivary gland), which binds and inactivates thrombin. As yet, no drugs are available for blocking aggregation induced by serotonin or PAF. ADP-induced aggregation can be prevented by **ticlopidine** and **clopidogrel;** these agents are not classic receptor antagonists. ADP-induced aggregation is inhibited only *in vivo* but not *in vitro* in stored blood; moreover, once induced, inhibition is irreversible. A possible explanation is that both agents already interfere with elements of ADP receptor signal transduction at the megakaryocytic stage. The ensuing functional defect would then be transmitted to newly formed platelets, which would be incapable of reversing it.

The intra-platelet levels of cAMP can be stabilized by prostacyclin or its analogues (e.g., iloprost) or by **dipyridamole.** The former activates adenyl cyclase via a G-protein-coupled receptor; the latter inhibits a phosphodiesterase that breaks down cAMP.

The **integrin (GPIIB/IIIA)-antagonists** prevent cross-linking of platelets. Their action is independent of the aggregation-inducing stimulus. *Abciximab* is a chimeric human-murine monoclonal antibody directed against GPIIb/IIIa that blocks the fibrinogen-binding site and thus prevents attachment of fibrinogen. The peptide derivatives, *eptifibatide* and *tirofiban* block GPIIB/IIIA competitively, more selectively and have a shorter effect than does abciximab.

Presystemic Effect of Acetylsalicylic Acid (B)

Inhibition of platelet aggregation by ASA is due to a selective blockade of platelet cyclooxygenase (**B**). Selectivity of this action results from acetylation of this enzyme during the initial passage of the platelets through splanchnic blood vessels. Acetylation of the enzyme is irreversible. ASA present in the systemic circulation does not play a role in platelet inhibition. Since ASA undergoes extensive presystemic elimination, cyclooxygenases outside platelets, e.g., in endothelial cells, remain largely unaffected. With regular intake, selectivity is enhanced further because the anuclear platelets are unable to resynthesize new enzyme and the inhibitory effects of consecutive doses are added to each other. However, in the endothelial cells, de novo synthesis of the enzyme permits restoration of prostacyclin production.

Adverse Effects of Antiplatelet Drugs

All antiplatelet drugs increase the risk of bleeding. Even at the low ASA doses used to inhibit platelet function (100 mg/d), ulcerogenic and bronchoconstrictor (aspirin asthma) effects may occur. Ticlopidine frequently causes diarrhea and, more rarely, leukopenia, necessitating cessation of treatment. Clopidogrel reportedly does not cause hematological problems.

As peptides, hirudin and abciximab need to be injected; therefore their use is restricted to intensive-care settings.

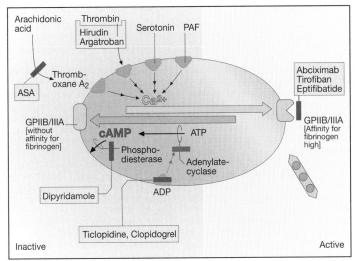

A. Inhibitors of platelet aggregation

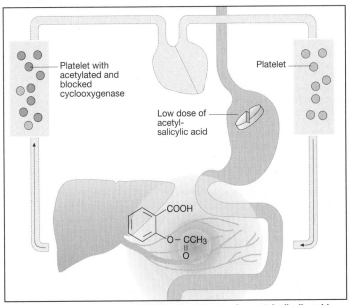

B. Presystemic inactivation of platelet cyclooxygenase by acetylsalicylic acid

Plasma Volume Expanders

Major blood loss entails the danger of life-threatening circulatory failure, i.e., hypovolemic shock. The immediate threat results not so much from the loss of erythrocytes, i.e., oxygen carriers, as from the reduction in volume of circulating blood.

To eliminate the threat of shock, replenishment of the circulation is essential. With moderate loss of blood, administration of a plasma volume expander may be sufficient. Blood plasma consists basically of water, electrolytes, and plasma proteins. However, a plasma substitute need not contain **plasma proteins.** These can be suitably **replaced** with **macromolecules** ("colloids") that, like plasma proteins, (1) *do not readily leave the circulation and are poorly filtrable in the renal glomerulus;* and (2) bind water along with its solutes due to their *colloid osmotic properties.* In this manner, they will maintain circulatory filling pressure for many hours. On the other hand, volume substitution is only transiently needed and therefore complete elimination of these colloids from the body is clearly desirable.

Compared with whole blood or plasma, plasma substitutes offer several *advantages:* they can be produced more easily and at lower cost, have a longer shelf life, and are free of pathogens such as hepatitis B or C or AIDS viruses.

Three colloids are currently employed as plasma volume expanders—the two polysaccharides, dextran and hydroxyethyl starch, as well as the polypeptide, gelatin.

Dextran is a glucose polymer formed by bacteria and linked by a $1{\to}6$ instead of the typical $1{\to}4$ bond. Commercial solutions contain dextran of a mean molecular weight of 70 kDa (**dextran 70**) or 40 kDa (**lower-molecular-weight dextran, dextran 40**). The chain length of single molecules, however, varies widely. Smaller dextran molecules can be filtered at the glomerulus and slowly excreted in urine; the larger ones are eventually taken up and degraded by cells of the reticuloendothelial system. Apart from restoring blood volume, dextran solutions are used for hemodilution in the management of blood flow disorders.

As for microcirculatory improvement, it is occasionally emphasized that low-molecular-weight dextran, unlike dextran 70, may directly reduce the aggregability of erythrocytes by altering their surface properties. With prolonged use, larger molecules will accumulate due to the more rapid renal excretion of the smaller ones. Consequently, the molecular weight of dextran circulating in blood will tend towards a higher mean molecular weight with the passage of time.

The most important adverse effect results from the antigenicity of dextrans, which may lead to an **anaphylactic reaction.**

Hydroxyethyl starch (hetastarch) is produced from starch. By virtue of its hydroxyethyl groups, it is metabolized more slowly and retained significantly longer in blood than would be the case with infused starch. Hydroxyethyl starch resembles dextrans in terms of its pharmacological properties and therapeutic applications.

Gelatin colloids consist of cross-linked peptide chains obtained from collagen. They are employed for blood replacement, but not for hemodilution, in circulatory disturbances.

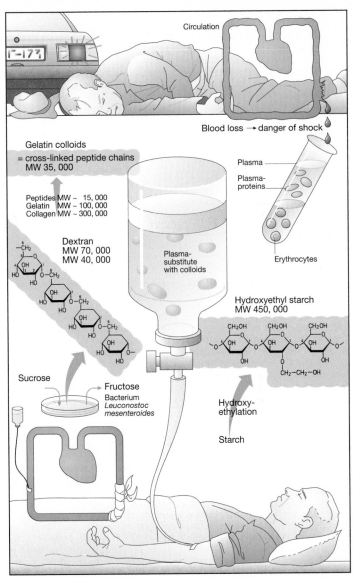

Circulation

Blood loss → danger of shock

Gelatin colloids
= cross-linked peptide chains
MW 35, 000

Plasma

Plasma-
proteins

Peptides MW ~ 15, 000
Gelatin   MW ~ 100, 000
Collagen MW ~ 300, 000

Dextran
MW 70, 000
MW 40, 000

Plasma-
substitute
with colloids

Erythrocytes

Hydroxyethyl starch
MW 450, 000

Sucrose

Fructose
Bacterium
*Leuconostoc
mesenteroides*

Hydroxy-
ethylation

Starch

A. Plasma substitutes

Lipid-Lowering Agents

Triglycerides and cholesterol are essential constituents of the organism. Among other things, triglycerides represent a form of energy store and cholesterol is a basic building block of biological membranes. Both lipids are water insoluble and require appropriate transport vehicles in the aqueous media of lymph and blood. To this end, small amounts of lipid are coated with a layer of phospholipids, embedded in which are additional proteins—the apolipoproteins (A). According to the amount and the composition of stored lipids, as well as the type of apolipoprotein, one distinguishes 4 transport forms:

	Origin	Density	Mean sojourn in blood plasma (h)	Diameter (nm)
Chylomicron	Gut epithelium	<1.006	0.2	500
VLDL particle	liver	0.95 –1.006	3	100–200
LDL particle	(blood)	1.006–1.063	50	25
HDL particle	liver	1.063–1.210	–	5–10

Lipoprotein metabolism. Enterocytes release absorbed lipids in the form of triglyceride-rich chylomicrons. Bypassing the liver, these enter the circulation mainly via the lymph and are hydrolyzed by extrahepatic endothelial lipoprotein lipases to liberate fatty acids. The remnant particles move on into liver cells and supply these with cholesterol of dietary origin.

The liver meets the larger part (60%) of its requirement for cholesterol by de novo synthesis from acetylcoenzyme-A. Synthesis rate is regulated at the step leading from hydroxymethylglutaryl CoA (HMG CoA) to mevalonic acid (p. 157A), with HMG CoA reductase as the rate-limiting enzyme.

The liver requires cholesterol for synthesizing VLDL particles and bile acids. Triglyceride-rich VLDL particles are released into the blood and, like the chylomicrons, supply other tissues with fatty acids. Left behind are LDL particles that either return into the liver or supply extrahepatic tissues with cholesterol.

LDL particles carry apolipoprotein B 100, by which they are bound to receptors that mediate uptake of LDL into the cells, including the hepatocytes (receptor-mediated endocytosis, p. 27).

HDL particles are able to transfer cholesterol from tissue cells to LDL particles. In this way, cholesterol is transported from tissues to the liver.

Hyperlipoproteinemias can be caused genetically (primary h.) or can occur in obesity and metabolic disorders (secondary h). Elevated LDL-cholesterol serum concentrations are associated with an increased risk of atherosclerosis, especially when there is a concomitant decline in HDL concentration (increase in LDL:HDL quotient).

Treatment. Various drugs are available that have different mechanisms of action and effects on LDL (cholesterol) and VLDL (triglycerides) (A). Their use is indicated in the therapy of primary hyperlipoproteinemias. In secondary hyperlipoproteinemias, the immediate goal should be to lower lipoprotein levels by dietary restriction, treatment of the primary disease, or both.

Drugs (B). Colestyramine and colestipol are nonabsorbable anion-exchange resins. By virtue of binding bile acids, they promote consumption of cholesterol for the synthesis of bile acids; the

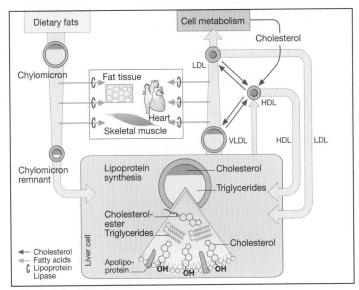

A. Lipoprotein metabolism

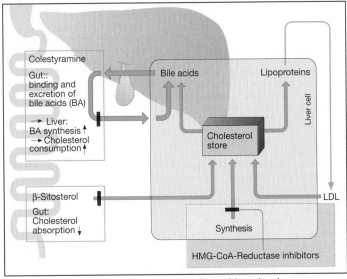

B. Cholesterol metabolism in liver cell and cholesterol-lowering drugs

liver meets its increased cholesterol demand by enhancing the expression of HMG CoA reductase and LDL receptors (negative feedback).

At the required dosage, the resins cause diverse gastrointestinal disturbances. In addition, they interfere with the absorption of fats and fat-soluble vitamins (A, D, E, K). They also adsorb and decrease the absorption of such drugs as digitoxin, vitamin K antagonists, and diuretics. Their gritty texture and bulk make ingestion an unpleasant experience.

The statins, *lovastatin* (L), *simvastatin* (S), *pravastatin* (P), *fluvastatin* (F), *cerivastatin,* and *atorvastatin,* inhibit HMG CoA reductase. The active group of L, S, P, and F (or their metabolites) resembles that of the physiological substrate of the enzyme **(A)**. L and S are lactones that are rapidly absorbed by the enteral route, subjected to extensive first-pass extraction in the liver, and there hydrolyzed into active metabolites. P and F represent the active form and, as acids, are actively transported by a specific anion carrier that moves bile acids from blood into liver and also mediates the selective hepatic uptake of the mycotoxin, amanitin **(A)**. *Atorvastatin* has the longest duration of action. Normally viewed as presystemic elimination, efficient hepatic extraction serves to confine the action of the statins to the liver. Despite the inhibition of HMG CoA reductase, hepatic cholesterol content does not fall, because hepatocytes compensate any drop in cholesterol levels by increasing the synthesis of LDL receptor protein (along with the reductase). Because the newly formed reductase is inhibited, too, the hepatocyte must meet its cholesterol demand by uptake of LDL from the blood **(B)**. Accordingly, the concentration of circulating LDL decreases, while its hepatic clearance from plasma increases. There is also a decreased likelihood of LDL being oxidized into its proatherosclerotic degradation product. The combination of a statin with an ion-exchange resin intensifies the decrease in LDL levels. A rare, but dangerous, side effect of the statins is damage to skeletal musculature. This risk is increased by combined use of fibric acid agents (see below).

Nicotinic acid and its derivatives *(pyridylcarbinol, xanthinol nicotinate, acipimox)* activate endothelial lipoprotein lipase and thereby lower triglyceride levels. At the start of therapy, a prostaglandin-mediated vasodilation occurs (flushing and hypotension) that can be prevented by low doses of acetylsalicylic acid.

Clofibrate and derivatives *(bezafibrate, etofibrate, gemfibrozil)* lower plasma lipids by an unknown mechanism. They may damage the liver and skeletal muscle (myalgia, myopathy, rhabdomyolysis).

Probucol lowers HDL more than LDL; nonetheless, it appears effective in reducing atherogenesis, possibly by reducing LDL oxidation.

ω_3-*Polyunsaturated fatty acids* (eicosapentaenoate, docosahexaenoate) are abundant in fish oils. Dietary supplementation results in lowered levels of triglycerides, decreased synthesis of VLDL and apolipoprotein B, and improved clearance of remnant particles, although total and LDL cholesterol are not decreased or are even increased. High dietary intake may correlate with a reduced incidence of coronary heart disease.

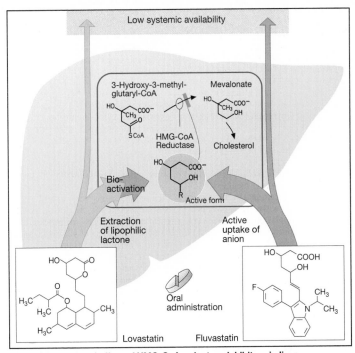

A. Accumulation and effect of HMG-CoA reductase inhibitors in liver

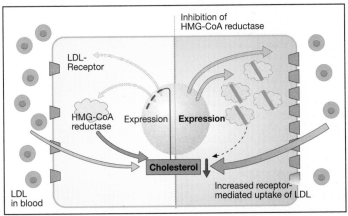

B. Regulation by cellular cholesterol concentration of HMG-CoA reductase and LDL-receptors

Diuretics – An Overview

Diuretics (saluretics) elicit increased production of urine (diuresis). In the strict sense, the term is applied to drugs with a direct renal action. The predominant action of such agents is to augment urine excretion by inhibiting the reabsorption of NaCl and water.

The most important **indications** for diuretics are:

Mobilization of edemas (A): In edema there is swelling of tissues due to accumulation of fluid, chiefly in the extracellular (interstitial) space. When a diuretic is given, increased renal excretion of Na^+ and H_2O causes a reduction in plasma volume with hemoconcentration. As a result, plasma protein concentration rises along with oncotic pressure. As the latter operates to attract water, fluid will shift from interstitium into the capillary bed. The fluid content of tissues thus falls and the edemas recede. The decrease in plasma volume and interstitial volume means a diminution of the extracellular fluid volume (EFV). Depending on the condition, use is made of: thiazides, loop diuretics, aldosterone antagonists, and osmotic diuretics.

Antihypertensive therapy. Diuretics have long been used as drugs of first choice for lowering elevated blood pressure (p. 312). Even at low dosage, they decrease peripheral resistance (without significantly reducing EFV) and thereby normalize blood pressure.

Therapy of congestive heart failure. By lowering peripheral resistance, diuretics aid the heart in ejecting blood (reduction in afterload, pp. 132, 306); cardiac output and exercise tolerance are increased. Due to the increased excretion of fluid, EFV and venous return decrease (reduction in preload, p. 306). Symptoms of venous congestion, such as ankle edema and hepatic enlargement, subside. The drugs principally used are thiazides (possibly combined with K^+-sparing diuretics) and loop diuretics.

Prophylaxis of renal failure. In circulatory failure (shock), e.g., secondary to massive hemorrhage, renal production of urine may cease (anuria). By means of diuretics an attempt is made to maintain urinary flow. Use of either osmotic or loop diuretics is indicated.

Massive use of diuretics entails a hazard of **adverse effects (A):** (1) the decrease in blood volume can lead to hypotension and *collapse;* (2) blood viscosity rises due to the increase in erythro- and thrombocyte concentration, bringing an increased risk of intravascular coagulation or *thrombosis.*

When depletion of NaCl and water (EFV reduction) occurs as a result of diuretic therapy, the body can initiate **counter-regulatory responses (B),** namely, activation of the renin-angiotensin-aldosterone system (p. 124). Because of the diminished blood volume, renal blood flow is jeopardized. This leads to release from the kidneys of the hormone, renin, which enzymatically catalyzes the formation of angiotensin I. Angiotensin I is converted to angiotensin II by the action of angiotensin-converting enzyme (ACE). Angiotensin II stimulates release of aldosterone. The mineralocorticoid promotes renal reabsorption of NaCl and water and thus counteracts the effect of diuretics. ACE inhibitors (p. 124) augment the effectiveness of diuretics by preventing this counter-regulatory response.

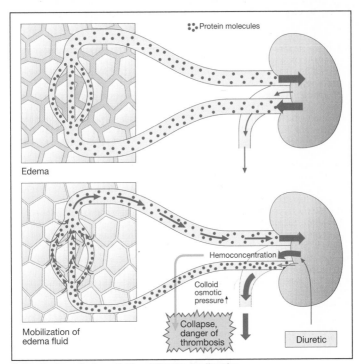

A. Mechanism of edema fluid mobilization by diuretics

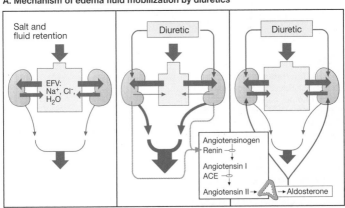

B. Possible counter-regulatory responses during long-term diuretic therapy

NaCl Reabsorption in the Kidney (A)

The smallest functional unit of the kidney is the **nephron.** In the glomerular capillary loops, ultrafiltration of plasma fluid into Bowman's capsule (BC) yields primary urine. In the proximal tubules (pT), approx. 70% of the ultrafiltrate is retrieved by isoosmotic reabsorption of NaCl and water. In the thick portion of the ascending limb of Henle's loop (HL), NaCl is absorbed unaccompanied by water. This is the prerequisite for the hairpin countercurrent mechanism that allows build-up of a very high NaCl concentration in the renal medulla. In the distal tubules (dT), NaCl and water are again jointly reabsorbed. At the end of the nephron, this process involves an aldosterone-controlled exchange of Na^+ against K^+ or H^+. In the collecting tubule (C), vasopressin (antidiuretic hormone, ADH) increases the epithelial permeability for water, which is drawn into the hyperosmolar milieu of the renal medulla and thus retained in the body. As a result, a concentrated urine enters the renal pelvis.

Na^+ transport through the tubular cells basically occurs in similar fashion in all segments of the nephron. The intracellular concentration of Na^+ is significantly below that in primary urine. This concentration gradient is the driving force for entry of Na^+ into the cytosol of tubular cells. A carrier mechanism moves Na^+ across the membrane. Energy liberated during this influx can be utilized for the coupled outward transport of another particle against a gradient. From the cell interior, Na^+ is moved with expenditure of energy (ATP hydrolysis) by Na^+/K^+-ATPase into the extracellular space. The enzyme molecules are confined to the basolateral parts of the cell membrane, facing the interstitium; Na^+ can, therefore, not escape back into tubular fluid.

All diuretics inhibit Na^+ reabsorption. Basically, either the inward or the outward transport of Na^+ can be affected.

Osmotic Diuretics (B)

Agents: mannitol, sorbitol. *Site of action:* mainly the proximal tubules. *Mode of action:* Since NaCl and H_2O are reabsorbed together in the proximal tubules, Na^+ concentration in the tubular fluid does not change despite the extensive reabsorption of Na^+ and H_2O. Body cells lack transport mechanisms for polyhydric alcohols such as mannitol (structure on p. 171) and sorbitol, which are thus prevented from penetrating cell membranes. Therefore, they need to be given by intravenous infusion. They also cannot be reabsorbed from the tubular fluid after glomerular filtration. These agents bind water osmotically and retain it in the tubular lumen. When Na ions are taken up into the tubule cell, water cannot follow in the usual amount. The fall in urine Na^+ concentration reduces Na^+ reabsorption, in part because the reduced concentration gradient towards the interior of tubule cells means a reduced driving force for Na^+ influx. The result of osmotic diuresis is a large volume of dilute urine.

Indications: prophylaxis of renal hypovolemic failure, mobilization of brain edema, and acute glaucoma.

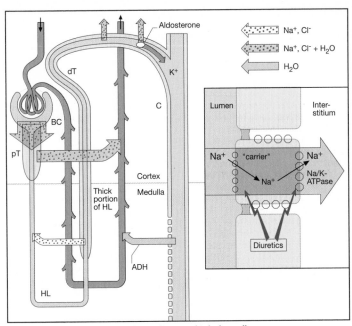

A. Kidney: NaCl reabsorption in nephron and tubular cell

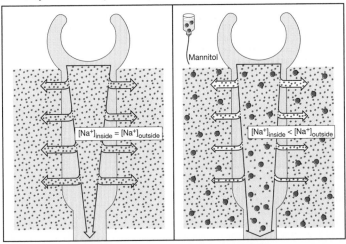

B. NaCl reabsorption in proximal tubule and effect of mannitol

Diuretics of the Sulfonamide Type

These drugs contain the sulfonamide group $-SO_2NH_2$. They are suitable for oral administration. In addition to being filtered at the glomerulus, they are subject to tubular secretion. Their concentration in urine is higher than in blood. They act on the luminal membrane of the tubule cells. Loop diuretics have the highest efficacy. Thiazides are most frequently used. Their forerunners, the carbonic anhydrase inhibitors, are now restricted to special indications.

Carbonic anhydrase (CAH) inhibitors, such as acetazolamide and sulthiame, act predominantly in the proximal tubules. CAH catalyzes CO_2 hydration/dehydration reactions:

$H^+ + HCO_3^- \leftrightarrow H_2CO_3 \leftrightarrow H_2O + CO_2$.

The enzyme is used in tubule cells to generate H^+, which is secreted into the tubular fluid in exchange for Na^+. There, H^+ captures HCO_3^-, leading to formation of CO_2 via the unstable carbonic acid. Membrane-permeable CO_2 is taken up into the tubule cell and used to regenerate H^+ and HCO_3^-. When the enzyme is inhibited, these reactions are slowed, so that less Na^+, HCO_3^- and water are reabsorbed from the fast-flowing tubular fluid. Loss of HCO_3^- leads to acidosis. The diuretic effectiveness of CAH inhibitors decreases with prolonged use. CAH is also involved in the production of ocular aqueous humor. Present *indications* for drugs in this class include: acute glaucoma, acute mountain sickness, and epilepsy. *Dorzolamide* can be applied topically to the eye to lower intraocular pressure in glaucoma.

Loop diuretics include furosemide (frusemide), piretanide, and bumetanide. With oral administration, a strong diuresis occurs within 1 h but persists for only about 4 h. The effect is rapid, intense, and brief (high-ceiling diuresis). The site of action of these agents is the thick portion of the ascending limb of Henle's loop, where they inhibit $Na^+/K^+/2Cl^-$ cotransport. As a result, these electrolytes, together with water, are excreted in larger amounts. Excretion of Ca^{2+} and Mg^{2+} also increases. Special *toxic effects* include: (reversible) hearing loss, enhanced sensitivity to renotoxic agents. *Indications:* pulmonary edema (added advantage of i.v. injection in left ventricular failure: immediate dilation of venous capacitance vessels → preload reduction); refractoriness to thiazide diuretics, e.g., in renal hypovolemic failure with creatinine clearance reduction (<30 mL/min); prophylaxis of acute renal hypovolemic failure; hypercalcemia. Ethacrynic acid is classed in this group although it is not a sulfonamide.

Thiazide diuretics (benzothiadiazines) include hydrochlorothiazide, benzthiazide, trichlormethiazide, and cyclothiazide. A long-acting analogue is chlorthalidone. These drugs affect the intermediate segment of the distal tubules, where they inhibit a Na^+/Cl^- cotransport. Thus, reabsorption of NaCl and water is inhibited. Renal excretion of Ca^{2+} decreases, that of Mg^{2+} increases. *Indications* are hypertension, cardiac failure, and mobilization of edema.

Unwanted effects of sulfonamide-type diuretics: (a) *hypokalemia* is a consequence of excessive K^+ loss in the terminal segments of the distal tubules where increased amounts of Na^+ are available for exchange with K^+; (b) hyperglycemia and glycosuria; (c) hyperuricemia—increase in serum urate levels may precipitate gout in predisposed patients. Sulfonamide diuretics compete with urate for the tubular organic anion secretory system.

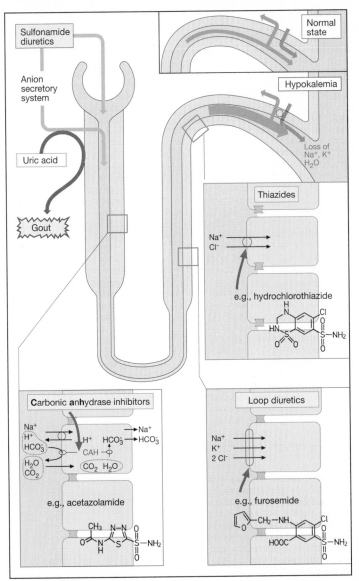

A. Diuretics of the sulfonamide type

Potassium-Sparing Diuretics (A)

These agents act in the distal portion of the distal tubule and the proximal part of the collecting ducts where Na^+ is reabsorbed in exchange for K^+ or H^+. Their diuretic effectiveness is relatively minor. In contrast to sulfonamide diuretics (p. 162), there is no increase in K^+ secretion; rather, there is a risk of hyperkalemia. These drugs are suitable for oral administration.

a) *Triamterene* and *amiloride*, in addition to glomerular filtration, undergo secretion in the proximal tubule. They act on the luminal membrane of tubule cells. Both inhibit the entry of Na^+, hence its exchange for K^+ and H^+. They are mostly used in combination with thiazide diuretics, e.g., hydrochlorothiazide, because the opposing effects on K^+ excretion cancel each other, while the effects on secretion of NaCl complement each other.

b) *Aldosterone antagonists.* The mineralocorticoid aldosterone promotes the reabsorption of Na^+ (Cl^- and H_2O follow) in exchange for K^+. Its hormonal effect on protein synthesis leads to augmentation of the reabsorptive capacity of tubule cells. *Spironolactone,* as well as its *metabolite canrenone,* are antagonists at the aldosterone receptor and attenuate the effect of the hormone. The diuretic effect of spironolactone develops fully only with continuous administration for several days. Two possible explanations are: (1) the conversion of spironolactone into and accumulation of the more slowly eliminated metabolite canrenone; (2) an inhibition of aldosterone-stimulated protein synthesis would become noticeable only if existing proteins had become nonfunctional and needed to be replaced by *de novo* synthesis. A particular *adverse effect* results from interference with gonadal hormones, as evidenced by the development of gynecomastia (enlargement of male breast). *Clinical uses* include conditions of increased aldosterone secretion, e.g., liver cirrhosis with ascites.

Antidiuretic Hormone (ADH) and Derivatives (B)

ADH, a nonapeptide, released from the posterior pituitary gland promotes reabsorption of water in the kidney. This response is mediated by vasopressin receptors of the V_2 subtype. ADH enhances the permeability of collecting duct epithelium for water (but not for electrolytes). As a result, water is drawn from urine into the hyperosmolar interstitium of the medulla. Nicotine augments (p. 110) and ethanol decreases ADH release. At concentrations above those required for antidiuresis, ADH stimulates smooth musculature, including that of blood vessels (**"vasopressin"**). The latter response is mediated by receptors of the V_1 subtype. Blood pressure rises; coronary vasoconstriction can precipitate angina pectoris. *Lypressin* (8-L-lysine vasopressin) acts like ADH. Other derivatives may display only one of the two actions.

Desmopressin is used for the therapy of diabetes insipidus (ADH deficiency), nocturnal enuresis, thrombasthemia (p. 148), and chronic hypotension (p. 314); it is given by injection or via the nasal mucosa (as "snuff").

Felypressin and *ornipressin* serve as adjunctive vasoconstrictors in infiltration local anesthesia (p. 206).

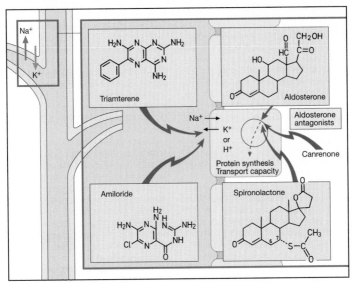

A. Potassium-sparing diuretics

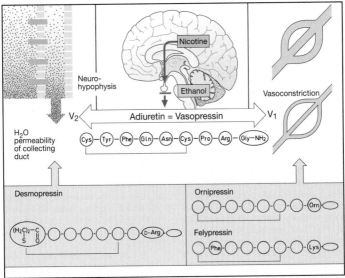

B. Antidiuretic hormone (ADH) and derivatives

Drugs for Gastric and Duodenal Ulcers

In the area of a gastric or duodenal peptic ulcer, the mucosa has been attacked by digestive juices to such an extent as to expose the subjacent connective tissue layer (submucosa). This self-digestion occurs when the equilibrium between the corrosive hydrochloric acid and acid-neutralizing mucus, which forms a protective cover on the mucosal surface, is shifted in favor of hydrochloric acid. Mucosal damage can be promoted by *Helicobacter pylori* bacteria that colonize the gastric mucus.

Drugs are employed with the following **therapeutic aims:** (1) to relieve pain; (2) to accelerate healing; and (3) to prevent ulcer recurrence. Therapeutic approaches are threefold: (a) to reduce aggressive forces by lowering H^+ output; (b) to increase protective forces by means of mucoprotectants; and (c) to eradicate *Helicobacter pylori*.

I. Drugs for Lowering Acid Concentration

Ia. Acid neutralization. H^+-binding groups such as CO_3^{2-}, HCO_3^- or OH^-, together with their counter ions, are contained in **antacid drugs**. Neutralization reactions occurring after intake of $CaCO_3$ and $NaHCO_3$, respectively, are shown in (**A**) at left. With nonabsorbable antacids, the counter ion is dissolved in the acidic gastric juice in the process of neutralization. Upon mixture with the alkaline pancreatic secretion in the duodenum, it is largely precipitated again by basic groups, e.g., as $CaCO_3$ or $AlPO_4$, and excreted in feces. Therefore, systemic absorption of counter ions or basic residues is minor. In the presence of renal insufficiency, however, absorption of even small amounts may cause an increase in plasma levels of counter ions (e.g., magnesium intoxication with paralysis and cardiac disturbances). Precipitation in the gut lumen is responsible for other side effects, such as reduced absorption of other drugs due to their adsorption to the surface of pre-

cipitated antacid or, phosphate depletion of the body with excessive intake of $Al(OH)_3$.

Na^+ ions remain in solution even in the presence of HCO_3^--rich pancreatic secretions and are subject to absorption, like HCO_3^-. Because of the uptake of Na^+, use of $NaHCO_3$ must be avoided in conditions requiring restriction of NaCl intake, such as hypertension, cardiac failure, and edema.

Since food has a buffering effect, antacids are taken between meals (e.g., 1 and 3 h after meals and at bedtime). Nonabsorbable antacids are preferred. Because $Mg(OH)_2$ produces a laxative effect (cause: osmotic action, p. 170, release of cholecystokinin by Mg^{2+}, or both) and $Al(OH)_3$ produces constipation (cause: astringent action of Al^{3+}, p. 178), these two antacids are frequently used in combination.

Ib. Inhibitors of acid production. Acting on their respective receptors, the transmitter acetylcholine, the hormone gastrin, and histamine released intramucosally stimulate the parietal cells of the gastric mucosa to increase output of HCl. Histamine comes from enterochromaffin-like (ECL) cells; its release is stimulated by the vagus nerve (via M_1 receptors) and hormonally by gastrin. The effects of acetylcholine and histamine can be abolished by orally applied antagonists that reach parietal cells via the blood.

The cholinoceptor antagonist **pirenzepine**, unlike atropine, prefers cholinoceptors of the M_1 type, does not penetrate into the CNS, and thus produces fewer atropine-like side effects (p. 104). The cholinoceptors on parietal cells probably belong to the M_3 subtype. Hence, pirenzepine may act by blocking M_1 receptors on ECL cells or submucosal neurons.

Histamine receptors on parietal cells belong to the H_2 type (p. 114) and are blocked by **H_2-antihistamines**. Because histamine plays a pivotal role in the activation of parietal cells, H_2-antihistamines also diminish responsivity to other stimulants, e.g., gastrin (in gas-

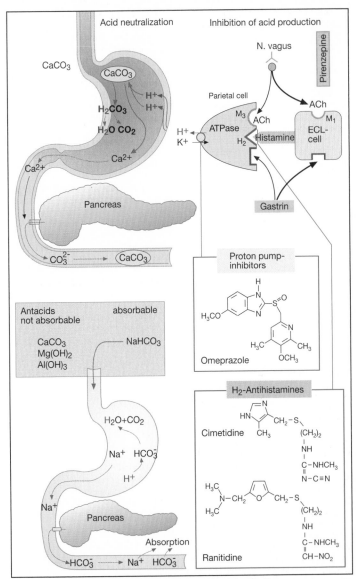

A. Drugs used to lower gastric acid concentration or production

trin-producing pancreatic tumors, Zollinger-Ellison syndrome). *Cimetidine,* the first H_2-antihistamine used therapeutically, only rarely produces side effects (CNS disturbances such as confusion; endocrine effects in the male, such as gynecomastia, decreased libido, impotence). Unlike cimetidine, its newer and more potent congeners, *ranitidine, nizatidine,* and *famotidine,* do not interfere with the hepatic biotransformation of other drugs.

Omeprazole (p. 167) can cause maximal inhibition of HCl secretion. Given orally in gastric juice-resistant capsules, it reaches parietal cells via the blood. In the acidic milieu of the mucosa, an active metabolite is formed and binds covalently to the ATP-driven proton pump (H^+/K^+ ATPase) that transports H^+ in exchange for K^+ into the gastric juice. *Lansoprazole* and *pantoprazole* produce analogous effects. The proton pump inhibitors are first-line drugs for the treatment of gastroesophageal reflux disease.

II. Protective Drugs

Sucralfate (A) contains numerous aluminum hydroxide residues. However, it is not an antacid because it fails to lower the overall acidity of gastric juice. After oral intake, sucralfate molecules undergo cross-linking in gastric juice, forming a paste that adheres to mucosal defects and exposed deeper layers. Here sucralfate intercepts H^+. Protected from acid, and also from pepsin, trypsin, and bile acids, the mucosal defect can heal more rapidly. Sucralfate is taken on an empty stomach (1 h before meals and at bedtime). It is well tolerated; however, released Al^{3+} ions can cause constipation.

Misoprostol (B) is a semisynthetic prostaglandin derivative with greater stability than natural prostaglandin, permitting absorption after oral administration. Like locally released prostaglandins, it promotes mucus production and inhibits acid secretion. Additional systemic effects (frequent diarrhea; risk of precipitating contractions of the gravid uterus) significantly restrict its therapeutic utility.

Carbenoxolone (B) is a derivative of glycyrrhetinic acid, which occurs in the sap of licorice root (succus liquiritiae). Carbenoxolone stimulates mucus production. At the same time, it has a mineralocorticoid-like action (due to inhibition of 11-β-hydroxysteroid dehydrogenase) that promotes renal reabsorption of NaCl and water. It may, therefore, exacerbate hypertension, congestive heart failure, or edemas. It is obsolete.

III. Eradication of *Helicobacter pylori* C.

This microorganism plays an important role in the pathogenesis of chronic gastritis and peptic ulcer disease. The combination of antibacterial drugs and omeprazole has proven effective. In case of intolerance to amoxicillin (p. 270) or clarithromycin (p. 276), metronidazole (p. 274) can be used as a substitute. Colloidal bismuth compounds are also effective; however, the problem of heavy-metal exposure compromises their long-term use.

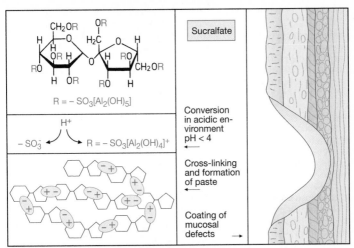

$R = - SO_3[Al_2(OH)_5]$

H^+

$- SO_3^- \quad \longleftrightarrow \quad R = - SO_3[Al_2(OH)_4]^+$

Sucralfate

Conversion in acidic environment pH < 4

Cross-linking and formation of paste

Coating of mucosal defects

A. Chemical structure and protective effect of sucralfate

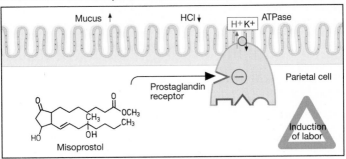

Mucus ↑   HCl ↓ $H^+ K^+$ ATPase

Prostaglandin receptor

Parietal cell

Misoprostol

Induction of labor

B. Chemical structure and protective effect of misoprostol

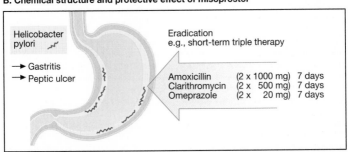

Helicobacter pylori

→ Gastritis
→ Peptic ulcer

Eradication e.g., short-term triple therapy

Amoxicillin	(2 x 1000 mg)	7 days
Clarithromycin	(2 x 500 mg)	7 days
Omeprazole	(2 x 20 mg)	7 days

C. Helicobacter eradication

Laxatives

Laxatives promote and facilitate bowel evacuation by acting locally to stimulate intestinal peristalsis, to soften bowel contents, or both.

1. Bulk laxatives. Distention of the intestinal wall by bowel contents stimulates propulsive movements of the gut musculature (peristalsis). Activation of intramural mechanoreceptors induces a neurally mediated ascending reflex contraction (red in **A**) and descending relaxation (blue) whereby the intraluminal bolus is moved in the anal direction.

Hydrophilic colloids or bulk gels (B) comprise insoluble and nonabsorbable carbohydrate substances that expand on taking up water in the bowel. *Vegetable fibers* in the diet act in this manner. They consist of the indigestible plant cell walls containing homoglycans that are resistant to digestive enzymes, e.g., *cellulose* ($1 \rightarrow 4\beta$-linked glucose molecules vs. $1 \rightarrow 4\alpha$ glucoside bond in starch, p. 153).

Bran, a grain milling waste product, and *linseed* (flaxseed) are both rich in cellulose. Other hydrophilic colloids derive from the seeds of *Plantago* species or *karaya gum.* Ingestion of hydrophilic gels for the prophylaxis of constipation usually entails a low risk of side effects. However, with low fluid intake in combination with a pathological bowel stenosis, mucilaginous viscous material could cause bowel occlusion (ileus).

Osmotically active laxatives (C) are soluble but nonabsorbable particles that retain water in the bowel by virtue of their osmotic action. The osmotic pressure (particle concentration) of bowel contents always corresponds to that of the extracellular space. The intestinal mucosa is unable to maintain a higher or lower osmotic pressure of the luminal contents. Therefore, absorption of molecules (e.g., glucose, NaCl) occurs isoosmotically, i.e., solute molecules are followed by a corresponding amount of water. Conversely, water remains in the bowel when molecules cannot be absorbed.

With *Epsom and Glauber's salts* ($MgSO_4$ and Na_2SO_4, respectively), the SO_4^{2-} anion is nonabsorbable and retains cations to maintain electroneutrality. Mg^{2+} ions are also believed to promote release from the duodenal mucosa of cholecystokinin/pancreozymin, a polypeptide that also stimulates peristalsis. These so-called saline cathartics elicit a watery bowel discharge 1–3 h after administration (preferably in isotonic solution). They are used to purge the bowel (e.g., before bowel surgery) or to hasten the elimination of ingested poisons. Glauber's salt (high Na^+ content) is contraindicated in hypertension, congestive heart failure, and edema. Epsom salt is contraindicated in renal failure (risk of Mg^{2+} intoxication).

Osmotic laxative effects are also produced by the *polyhydric alcohols, mannitol* and *sorbitol,* which unlike glucose cannot be transported through the intestinal mucosa, as well as by the nonhydrolyzable disaccharide, *lactulose.* Fermentation of lactulose by colon bacteria results in acidification of bowel contents and microfloral damage. Lactulose is used in hepatic failure in order to prevent bacterial production of ammonia and its subsequent absorption (absorbable $NH_3 \rightarrow$ nonabsorbable NH_4^+), so as to forestall hepatic coma.

2. Irritant laxatives—purgatives cathartics. Laxatives in this group exert an irritant action on the enteric mucosa (**A**). Consequently, less fluid is absorbed than is secreted. The increased filling of the bowel promotes peristalsis; excitation of sensory nerve endings elicits enteral hypermotility. According to the site of irritation, one distinguishes the small bowel irritant castor oil from the large bowel irritants anthraquinone and diphenolmethane derivatives (for details see p. 174).

Misuse of laxatives. It is a widely held belief that at least one bowel movement per day is essential for health; yet three bowel evacuations per week are quite normal. The desire for frequent bowel emptying probably stems from the time-honored, albeit

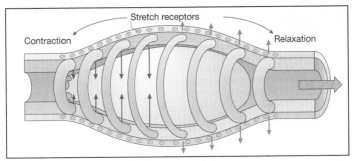

A. Stimulation of peristalsis by an intraluminal bolus

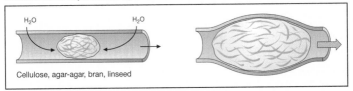

Cellulose, agar-agar, bran, linseed

B. Bulk laxatives

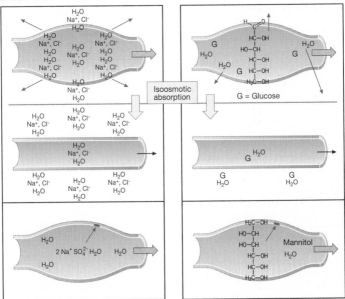

C. Osmotically active laxatives

mistaken, notion that absorption of colon contents is harmful. Thus, purging has long been part of standard therapeutic practice. Nowadays, it is known that intoxication from intestinal substances is impossible as long as the liver functions normally. Nonetheless, purgatives continue to be sold as remedies to "cleanse the blood" or to rid the body of "corrupt humors."

There can be no objection to the ingestion of bulk substances for the purpose of supplementing low-residue "modern diets." However, use of irritant purgatives or cathartics is not without hazards. Specifically, there is a risk of laxative dependence, i.e., the inability to do without them. Chronic intake of irritant purgatives disrupts the water and electrolyte balance of the body and can thus cause symptoms of illness (e.g., cardiac arrhythmias secondary to hypokalemia).

Causes of purgative dependence (B). The defecation reflex is triggered when the sigmoid colon and rectum are filled. A natural defecation empties the large bowel up to and including the descending colon. The interval between natural stool evacuations depends on the speed with which these colon segments are refilled. A large bowel irritant purgative clears out the entire colon. Accordingly, a longer period is needed until the next natural defecation can occur. Fearing constipation, the user becomes impatient and again resorts to the laxative, which then produces the desired effect as a result of emptying out the upper colonic segments. Therefore, a "compensatory pause" following cessation of laxative use must not give cause for concern (1).

In the colon, semifluid material entering from the small bowel is thickened by absorption of water and salts (from about 1000 to 150 mL/d). If, due to the action of an irritant purgative, the colon empties prematurely, an enteral loss of NaCl, KCl and water will be incurred. To forestall depletion of NaCl and water, the body responds with an increased release of aldosterone (p. 124), which stimulates their reabsorption in the kidney. The action of aldosterone is, however, associated with increased renal excretion of KCl. The enteral and renal K$^+$ loss add up to a K$^+$ depletion of the body, evidenced by a fall in serum K$^+$ concentration (hypokalemia). This condition is accompanied by a reduction in intestinal peristalsis (bowel atonia). The affected individual infers "constipation," again partakes of the purgative, and the vicious circle is closed (2).

Cholinogenic diarrhea results when bile acids fail to be absorbed in the ileum (e.g., after ileal resection) and enter the colon, where they cause enhanced secretion of electrolytes and water, leading to the discharge of fluid stools.

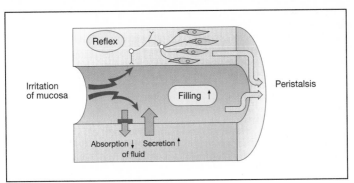

A. Stimulation of peristalsis by mucosal irritation

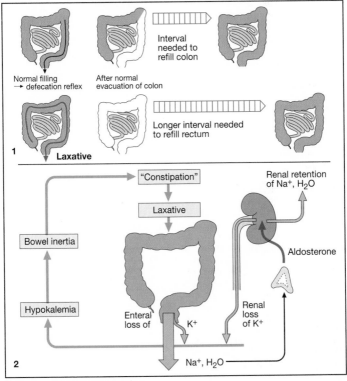

B. Causes of laxative habituation

174 Laxatives and Purgatives

2.a Small Bowel Irritant Purgative, Ricinoleic Acid

Castor oil comes from *Ricinus communis* (castor plants; Fig: sprig, panicle, seed); it is obtained from the first cold-pressing of the seed (shown in natural size). Oral administration of 10–30 mL of castor oil is followed within 0.5 to 3 h by discharge of a watery stool. Ricinoleic acid, but not the oil itself, is active. It arises as a result of the regular processes involved in fat digestion: the duodenal mucosa releases the enterohormone cholecystokinin/pancreozymin into the blood. The hormone elicits contraction of the gallbladder and discharge of bile acids via the bile duct, as well as release of lipase from the pancreas (intestinal peristalsis is also stimulated). Because of its massive effect, castor oil is hardly suitable for the treatment of ordinary constipation. It can be employed after oral ingestion of a toxin in order to hasten elimination and to reduce absorption of toxin from the gut. Castor oil is not indicated after the ingestion of lipophilic toxins likely to depend on bile acids for their absorption.

2.b Large Bowel Irritant Purgatives (p. 177 ff)

Anthraquinone derivatives (p. 176) are of plant origin. They occur in the leaves *(folia sennae)* or fruits *(fructus sennae)* of the *senna* plant, the bark of *Rhamnus frangulae* and *Rh. purshiana*, *(cortex frangulae, cascara sagrada)*, the roots of rhubarb *(rhizoma rhei)*, or the leaf extract from *Aloe* species (p. 176). The structural features of anthraquinone derivatives are illustrated by the prototype structure depicted on p. 177. Among other substituents, the anthraquinone nucleus contains hydroxyl groups, one of which is bound to a sugar (glucose, rhamnose). Following ingestion of galenical preparations or of the anthraquinone glycosides, discharge of soft stool occurs after a latency of 6 to 8 h. The anthraquinone glycosides themselves are inactive but are converted by colon bacteria to the active free aglycones.

Diphenolmethane derivatives (p. 177) were developed from *phenolphthalein*, an accidentally discovered laxative, use of which had been noted to result in rare but severe allergic reactions. *Bisacodyl* and *sodium picosulfate* are converted by gut bacteria into the active colon-irritant principle. Given by the enteral route, bisacodyl is subject to hydrolysis of acetyl residues, absorption, conjugation in liver to glucuronic acid (or also to sulfate, p. 38), and biliary secretion into the duodenum. Oral administration is followed after approx. 6 to 8 h by discharge of soft formed stool. When given by suppository, bisacodyl produces its effect within 1 h.

Indications for colon-irritant purgatives are the prevention of straining at stool following surgery, myocardial infarction, or stroke; and provision of relief in painful diseases of the anus, e.g., fissure, hemorrhoids.

Purgatives must not be given in abdominal complaints of unclear origin.

3. Lubricant laxatives. Liquid paraffin *(paraffinum subliquidum)* is almost nonabsorbable and makes feces softer and more easily passed. It interferes with the absorption of fat-soluble vitamins by trapping them. The few absorbed paraffin particles may induce formation of foreign-body granulomas in enteric lymph nodes (paraffinomas). Aspiration into the bronchial tract can result in lipoid pneumonia. Because of these adverse effects, its use is not advisable.

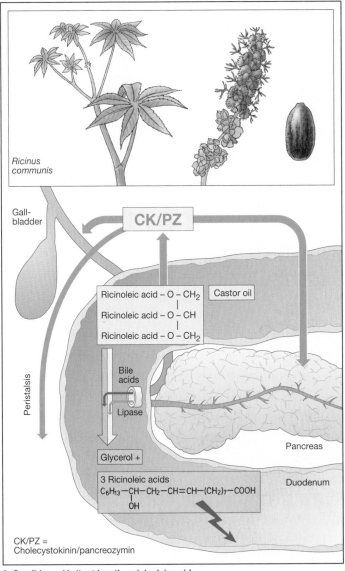

A. Small-bowel irritant laxative: ricinoleic acid

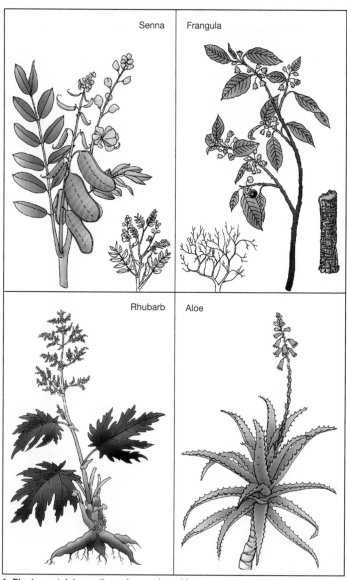

Senna

Frangula

Rhubarb

Aloe

A. Plants containing anthraquinone glycosides

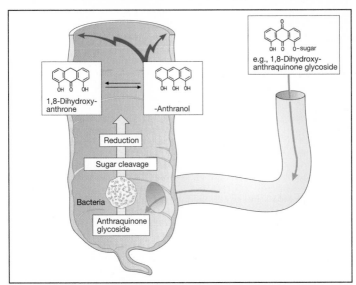

A. Large-bowel irritant laxatives: anthraquinone derivatives

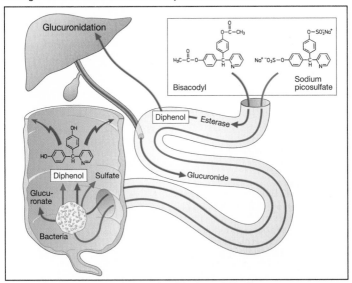

B. Large-bowel irritant laxatives: diphenylmethane derivatives

Antidiarrheal Agents

Causes of diarrhea (in red): Many bacteria (e.g., *Vibrio cholerae*) secrete **toxins** that inhibit the ability of mucosal enterocytes to absorb NaCl and water and, at the same time, stimulate mucosal secretory activity. **Bacteria** or **viruses** that invade the gut wall cause inflammation characterized by increased fluid secretion into the lumen. The enteric musculature reacts with increased peristalsis.

The **aims** of antidiarrheal **therapy** are to prevent: (1) dehydration and electrolyte depletion; and (2) excessively high stool frequency. **Different therapeutic approaches** (in green) listed are variously suited for these purposes.

Adsorbent powders are nonabsorbable materials with a large surface area. These bind diverse substances, including toxins, permitting them to be inactivated and eliminated. *Medicinal charcoal* possesses a particularly large surface because of the preserved cell structures. The recommended effective antidiarrheal dose is in the range of 4–8 g. Other adsorbents are kaolin (hydrated aluminum silicate) and chalk.

Oral rehydration solution (g/L of boiled water: NaCl 3.5, glucose 20, NaHCO$_3$ 2.5, KCl 1.5). Oral administration of glucose-containing salt solutions enables fluids to be absorbed because toxins do not impair the cotransport of Na$^+$ and glucose (as well as of H$_2$O) through the mucosal epithelium. In this manner, although frequent discharge of stool is not prevented, dehydration is successfully corrected.

Opioids. Activation of opioid receptors in the enteric nerve plexus results in inhibition of propulsive motor activity and enhancement of segmentation activity. This antidiarrheal effect was formerly induced by application of *opium tincture (paregoric)* containing *morphine*. Because of the CNS effects (sedation, respiratory depression, physical dependence), derivatives with peripheral actions have been developed. Whereas *diphenoxylate* can still produce clear CNS effects, *loperamide* does not affect brain functions at normal dosage. Loperamide is, therefore, the opioid antidiarrheal of first choice. The prolonged contact time of intestinal contents and mucosa may also improve absorption of fluid. With overdosage, there is a hazard of ileus. It is contraindicated in infants below age 2 y.

Antibacterial drugs. Use of these agents (e.g., cotrimoxazole, p. 272) is only rational when bacteria are the cause of diarrhea. This is rarely the case. It should be kept in mind that antibiotics also damage the intestinal flora which, in turn, can give rise to diarrhea.

Astringents such as tannic acid (home remedy: black tea) or metal salts precipitate surface proteins and are thought to help seal the mucosal epithelium. Protein denaturation must not include cellular proteins, for this would mean cell death. Although astringents induce constipation (cf. Al^{3+} salts, p. 166), a therapeutic effect in diarrhea is doubtful.

Demulcents, e.g., pectin (home remedy: grated apples) are carbohydrates that expand on absorbing water. They improve the consistency of bowel contents; beyond that they are devoid of any favorable effect.

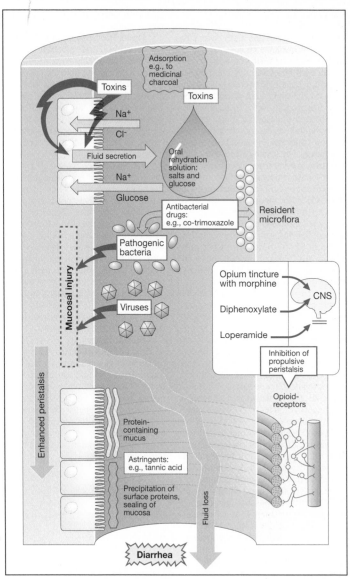

A. Antidiarrheals and their sites of action

Drugs for Dissolving Gallstones (A)

Following its secretion from liver into bile, water-insoluble cholesterol is held in solution in the form of micellar complexes with bile acids and phospholipids. When more cholesterol is secreted than can be emulsified, it precipitates and forms gallstones *(cholelithiasis)*. Precipitated cholesterol can be reincorporated into micelles, provided the cholesterol concentration in bile is below saturation. Thus, **cholesterol-containing stones** can be dissolved slowly. This effect can be achieved by long-term oral administration of **chenodeoxycholic acid** (CDCA) or **ursodeoxycholic acid** (UDCA). Both are physiologically occurring, stereoisomeric bile acids (position of the 7-hydroxy group being β in UDCA and α in CDCA). Normally, they represent a small proportion of the total amount of bile acid present in the body (circle diagram in *A*); however, this increases considerably with chronic administration because of *enterohepatic cycling*, p. 38). Bile acids undergo almost complete reabsorption in the ileum. Small losses via the feces are made up by *de novo* synthesis in the liver, keeping the *total amount of bile acids constant* (3–5 g). Exogenous supply removes the need for *de novo* synthesis of bile acids. The particular acid being supplied gains an increasingly larger share of the total store.

The altered composition of bile increases the capacity for cholesterol uptake. Thus, gallstones can be dissolved in the course of a 1- to 2 y treatment, provided that cholesterol stones are pure and not too large (<15 mm), gall bladder function is normal, liver disease is absent, and patients are of normal body weight. UCDA is more effective (daily dose, 8–10 mg) and better tolerated than is CDCA (15 mg/d; frequent diarrhea, elevation of liver enzymes in plasma). Stone formation may recur after cessation of successful therapy.

Compared with surgical treatment, drug therapy plays a subordinate role.

UCDA may also be useful in primary biliary cirrhosis.

Choleretics are supposed to stimulate production and secretion of dilute bile fluid. This principle has little therapeutic significance.

Cholekinetics stimulate the gallbladder to contract and empty, e.g., *egg yolk,* the osmotic laxative *MgSO₄,* the cholecystokinin-related *ceruletide* (given parenterally). Cholekinetics are employed to test gallbladder function for diagnostic purposes.

Pancreatic enzymes (B) from slaughtered animals are used to relieve excretory insufficiency of the pancreas (→ disrupted digestion of fats; steatorrhea, *inter alia*). Normally, secretion of pancreatic enzymes is activated by cholecystokinin/pancreozymin, the enterohormone that is released into blood from the duodenal mucosa upon contact with chyme. With oral administration of pancreatic enzymes, allowance must be made for their partial inactivation by gastric acid (the lipases, particularly). Therefore, they are administered in acid-resistant dosage forms.

Antiflatulents (carminatives) serve to alleviate *meteorism* (excessive accumulation of gas in the gastrointestinal tract). Aboral propulsion of intestinal contents is impeded when the latter are mixed with gas bubbles. Defoaming agents, such as *dimethicone* (dimethylpolysiloxane) and *simethicone,* in combination with charcoal, are given orally to promote separation of gaseous and semisolid contents.

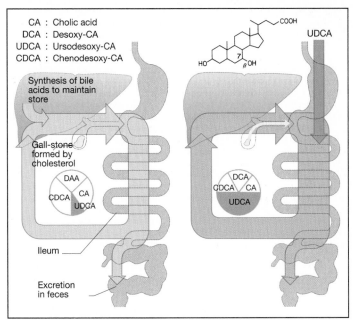

CA : Cholic acid
DCA : Desoxy-CA
UDCA : Ursodesoxy-CA
CDCA : Chenodesoxy-CA

UDCA

Synthesis of bile acids to maintain store

Gall-stone formed by cholesterol

DAA
CDCA   CA
UDCA

DCA
CDCA   CA
UDCA

Ileum

Excretion in feces

A. Gallstone dissolution

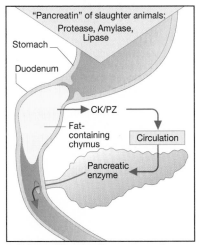

"Pancreatin" of slaughter animals:
Protease, Amylase, Lipase

Stomach

Duodenum

Fat-containing chymus

CK/PZ

Circulation

Pancreatic enzyme

B. Release of pancreatic enzymes and their replacement

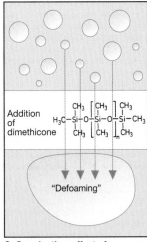

Addition of dimethicone

$H_3C-Si-O-\left[Si-O\right]_n Si-CH_3$ with CH_3 groups

"Defoaming"

C. Carminative effect of dimethicone

Drugs Affecting Motor Function

The smallest structural unit of skeletal musculature is the striated muscle fiber. It contracts in response to an impulse of its motor nerve. In executing motor programs, the brain sends impulses to the spinal cord. These converge on α-motoneurons in the anterior horn of the spinal medulla. Efferent axons course, bundled in motor nerves, to skeletal muscles. Simple reflex contractions to sensory stimuli, conveyed via the dorsal roots to the motoneurons, occur without participation of the brain. Neural circuits that propagate afferent impulses into the spinal cord contain inhibitory interneurons. These serve to prevent a possible overexcitation of motoneurons (or excessive muscle contractions) due to the constant barrage of sensory stimuli.

Neuromuscular transmission **(B)** of motor nerve impulses to the striated muscle fiber takes place at the motor endplate. The nerve impulse liberates acetylcholine (ACh) from the axon terminal. ACh binds to *nicotinic cholinoceptors* at the motor endplate. Activation of these receptors causes depolarization of the endplate, from which a propagated action potential (AP) is elicited in the surrounding sarcolemma. The AP triggers a release of Ca^{2+} from its storage organelles, the sarcoplasmic reticulum (SR), within the muscle fiber; the rise in Ca^{2+} concentration induces a contraction of the myofilaments (electromechanical coupling). Meanwhile, ACh is hydrolyzed by acetylcholinesterase (p. 100); excitation of the endplate subsides. If no AP follows, Ca^{2+} is taken up again by the SR and the myofilaments relax.

Clinically important drugs (with the exception of dantrolene) all interfere with neural control of the muscle cell **(A, B,** p. 183 ff.)

Centrally acting muscle relaxants (A) lower muscle tone by augmenting the activity of intraspinal inhibitory interneurons. They are used in the treatment of painful muscle spasms, e.g., in spinal disorders. *Benzodiazepines* enhance the effectiveness of the inhibitory transmitter GABA (p. 226) at $GABA_A$ receptors. *Baclofen* stimulates $GABA_B$ receptors. $α_2$-Adrenoceptor agonists such as *clonidine* and *tizanidine* probably act presynaptically to inhibit release of excitatory amino acid transmitters.

The **convulsant toxins,** *tetanus toxin* (cause of wound tetanus) and *strychnine* diminish the efficacy of interneuronal synaptic inhibition mediated by the amino acid glycine **(A)**. As a consequence of an unrestrained spread of nerve impulses in the spinal cord, motor convulsions develop. The involvement of respiratory muscle groups endangers life.

Botulinum toxin from *Clostridium botulinum* is the most potent poison known. The lethal dose in an adult is approx. 3×10^{-6} mg. The toxin blocks exocytosis of ACh in motor (and also parasympathetic) nerve endings. Death is caused by paralysis of respiratory muscles. Injected intramuscularly at minuscule dosage, *botulinum toxin type A* is used to treat blepharospasm, strabismus, achalasia of the lower esophageal sphincter, and spastic aphonia.

A pathological rise in *serum Mg^{2+}* levels also causes inhibition of ACh release, hence inhibition of neuromuscular transmission.

Dantrolene interferes with electromechanical coupling in the muscle cell by inhibiting Ca^{2+} release from the SR. It is used to treat painful muscle spasms attending spinal diseases and skeletal muscle disorders involving excessive release of Ca^{2+} (malignant hyperthermia).

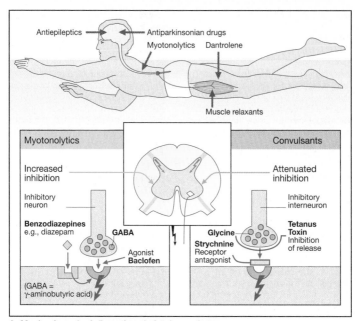

A. Mechanisms for influencing skeletal muscle tone

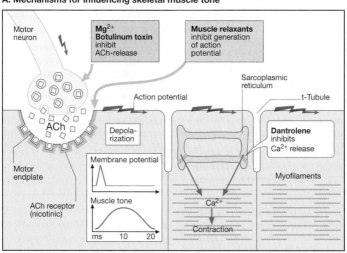

B. Inhibition of neuromuscular transmission and electromechanical coupling

Muscle Relaxants

Muscle relaxants cause a *flaccid paralysis of skeletal musculature* by binding to motor endplate cholinoceptors, thus blocking *neuromuscular transmission* (p. 182). According to whether receptor occupancy leads to a blockade or an excitation of the endplate, one distinguishes **nondepolarizing** from **depolarizing** muscle relaxants (p. 186). As adjuncts to general anesthetics, muscle relaxants help to ensure that surgical procedures are not disturbed by muscle contractions of the patient (p. 216).

Nondepolarizing muscle relaxants

Curare is the term for plant-derived arrow poisons of South American natives. When struck by a curare-tipped arrow, an animal suffers paralysis of skeletal musculature within a short time after the poison spreads through the body; death follows because respiratory muscles fail (respiratory paralysis). Killed game can be eaten without risk because absorption of the poison from the gastrointestinal tract is virtually nil. The curare ingredient of greatest medicinal importance is **d-tubocurarine.** This compound contains a quaternary nitrogen atom (N) and, at the opposite end of the molecule, a tertiary N that is protonated at physiological pH. These two positively charged N atoms are common to all other muscle relaxants. The fixed positive charge of the quaternary N accounts for the poor enteral absorbability.

d-Tubocurarine is given by i.v. injection (average dose approx. 10 mg). It binds to the endplate nicotinic cholinoceptors without exciting them, acting as a *competitive antagonist* towards ACh. By preventing the binding of released ACh, it blocks neuromuscular transmission. Muscular paralysis develops within about 4 min. *d*-Tubocurarine does not penetrate into the CNS. The patient would thus experience motor paralysis and inability to breathe, while remaining fully conscious but incapable of ex-

pressing anything. For this reason, care must be taken to eliminate consciousness by administration of an appropriate drug (general anesthesia) before using a muscle relaxant. The effect of a single dose lasts about 30 min.

The duration of the effect of *d*-tubocurarine can be shortened by administering an *acetylcholinesterase inhibitor,* such as *neostigmine* (p. 102). Inhibition of ACh breakdown causes the concentration of ACh released at the endplate to rise. Competitive "displacement" by ACh of *d*-tubocurarine from the receptor allows transmission to be restored.

Unwanted effects produced by *d*-tubocurarine result from a nonimmune-mediated release of histamine from mast cells, leading to bronchospasm, urticaria, and hypotension. More commonly, a fall in blood pressure can be attributed to ganglionic blockade by *d*-tubocurarine.

Pancuronium is a synthetic compound now frequently used and not likely to cause histamine release or ganglionic blockade. It is approx. 5-fold more potent than *d*-tubocurarine, with a somewhat longer duration of action. Increased heart rate and blood pressure are attributed to blockade of cardiac M_2-cholinoceptors, an effect not shared by newer pancuronium congeners such as **vecuronium** and **pipecuronium.**

Other nondepolarizing muscle relaxants include: **alcuronium,** derived from the alkaloid toxiferin; **rocuronium, gallamine, mivacurium,** and **atracurium.** The latter undergoes spontaneous cleavage and does not depend on hepatic or renal elimination.

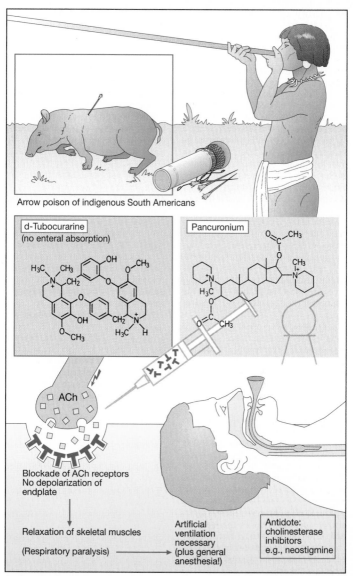

Arrow poison of indigenous South Americans

d-Tubocurarine
(no enteral absorption)

Pancuronium

ACh

Blockade of ACh receptors
No depolarization of
endplate

Relaxation of skeletal muscles

(Respiratory paralysis) ⟶

Artificial
ventilation
necessary
(plus general
anesthesia!)

Antidote:
cholinesterase
inhibitors
e.g., neostigmine

A. Non-depolarizing muscle relaxants

Depolarizing Muscle Relaxants

In this drug class, only **succinylcholine** (succinyldicholine, suxamethonium, **A**) is of clinical importance. Structurally, it can be described as a double ACh molecule. Like ACh, succinylcholine acts as agonist at endplate nicotinic cholinoceptors, yet it produces muscle relaxation. Unlike ACh, it is not hydrolyzed by acetylcholinesterase. However, it is a substrate of nonspecific plasma cholinesterase (serum cholinesterase, p. 100). Succinylcholine is degraded more slowly than is ACh and therefore remains in the synaptic cleft for several minutes, causing an endplate depolarization of corresponding duration. This depolarization initially triggers a propagated action potential (AP) in the surrounding muscle cell membrane, leading to contraction of the muscle fiber. After its i.v. injection, fine muscle twitches (fasciculations) can be observed. A new AP can be elicited near the endplate only if the membrane has been allowed to repolarize.

The AP is due to opening of voltage-gated Na-channel proteins, allowing Na^+ ions to flow through the sarcolemma and to cause depolarization. After a few milliseconds, the Na channels close automatically ("inactivation"), the membrane potential returns to resting levels, and the AP is terminated. As long as the membrane potential remains incompletely repolarized, renewed opening of Na channels, hence a new AP, is impossible. In the case of released ACh, rapid breakdown by ACh esterase allows repolarization of the endplate and hence a return of Na channel excitability in the adjacent sarcolemma. With succinylcholine, however, there is a persistent depolarization of the endplate and adjoining membrane regions. Because the Na channels remain inactivated, an AP cannot be triggered in the adjacent membrane.

Because most skeletal muscle fibers are innervated only by a single endplate, activation of such fibers, with lengths up to 30 cm, entails propagation of the AP through the entire cell. If the AP fails, the muscle fiber remains in a relaxed state.

The effect of a standard dose of succinylcholine lasts only about 10 min. It is often given at the start of anesthesia to facilitate intubation of the patient. As expected, cholinesterase inhibitors are unable to counteract the effect of succinylcholine. In the few patients with a genetic deficiency in pseudocholinesterase (= nonspecific cholinesterase), the succinylcholine effect is significantly prolonged.

Since persistent depolarization of endplates is associated with an efflux of K^+ ions, hyperkalemia can result (risk of cardiac arrhythmias).

Only in a few muscle types (e.g., extraocular muscle) are muscle fibers supplied with multiple endplates. Here succinylcholine causes depolarization distributed over the entire fiber, which responds with a contracture. Intraocular pressure rises, which must be taken into account during eye surgery.

In skeletal muscle fibers whose motor nerve has been severed, ACh receptors spread in a few days over the entire cell membrane. In this case, succinylcholine would evoke a persistent depolarization with contracture and hyperkalemia. These effects are likely to occur in polytraumatized patients undergoing follow-up surgery.

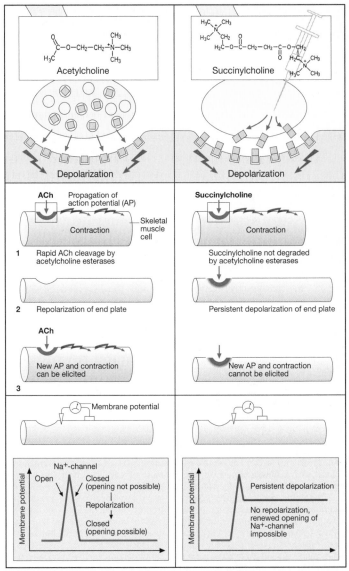

A. Action of the depolarizing muscle relaxant succinylcholine

Antiparkinsonian Drugs

Parkinson's disease (shaking palsy) and its syndromal forms are caused by a degeneration of **nigrostriatal** dopamine neurons. The resulting striatal dopamine deficiency leads to overactivity of cholinergic interneurons and imbalance of striopallidal output pathways, manifested by poverty of movement (akinesia), muscle stiffness (rigidity), tremor at rest, postural instability, and gait disturbance.

Pharmacotherapeutic measures are aimed at restoring dopaminergic function or suppressing cholinergic hyperactivity.

L-Dopa. Dopamine itself cannot penetrate the blood-brain barrier; however, its natural precursor, L-**d**ihydr**o**xy-**p**henyl**a**lanine (levodopa), is effective in replenishing striatal dopamine levels, because it is transported across the blood-brain barrier via an amino acid carrier and is subsequently decarboxylated by DOPA-decarboxylase, present in striatal tissue. Decarboxylation also takes place in peripheral organs where dopamine is not needed, likely causing undesirable effects (tachycardia, arrhythmias resulting from activation of β_1-adrenoceptors [p. 114], hypotension, and vomiting). Extracerebral production of dopamine can be prevented by inhibitors of DOPA-decarboxylase (carbidopa, benserazide) that do not penetrate the blood-brain barrier, leaving intracerebral decarboxylation unaffected. Excessive elevation of brain dopamine levels may lead to undesirable reactions, such as involuntary movements (dyskinesias) and mental disturbances.

Dopamine receptor agonists. Deficient dopaminergic transmission in the striatum can be compensated by ergot derivatives *(bromocriptine* [p. 114], *lisuride, cabergoline, and pergolide)* and nonergot compounds *(ropinirole, pramipexole)*. These agonists stimulate dopamine receptors (D_2, D_3, and D_1 subtypes), have lower clinical efficacy than levodopa, and share its main adverse effects.

Inhibitors of monoamine oxidase-B (MAO$_B$). This isoenzyme breaks down dopamine in the corpus striatum and can be selectively inhibited by *selegiline*. Inactivation of norepinephrine, epinephrine, and 5-HT via MAO$_A$ is unaffected. The antiparkinsonian effects of selegiline may result from decreased dopamine inactivation (enhanced levodopa response) or from neuroprotective mechanisms (decreased oxyradical formation or blocked bioactivation of an unknown neurotoxin).

Inhibitors of catechol-O-methyltransferase (COMT). L-Dopa and dopamine become inactivated by methylation. The responsible enzyme can be blocked by *entacapone*, allowing higher levels of L-dopa and dopamine to be achieved in corpus striatum.

Anticholinergics. Antagonists at muscarinic cholinoceptors, such as *benzatropine* and *biperiden* (p. 106), suppress striatal cholinergic overactivity and thereby relieve rigidity and tremor; however, akinesia is not reversed or is even exacerbated. Atropine-like peripheral side effects and impairment of cognitive function limit the tolerable dosage.

Amantadine. Early or mild parkinsonian manifestations may be temporarily relieved by amantadine. The underlying mechanism of action may involve, *inter alia,* blockade of ligand-gated ion channels of the glutamate/NMDA subtype, ultimately leading to a diminished release of acetylcholine.

Administration of levodopa plus carbidopa (or benserazide) remains the most effective treatment, but does not provide benefit beyond 3–5 y and is followed by gradual loss of symptom control, on-off fluctuations, and development of orobuccofacial and limb dyskinesias. These long-term drawbacks of levodopa therapy may be delayed by early monotherapy with dopamine receptor agonists. Treatment of advanced disease requires the combined administration of antiparkinsonian agents.

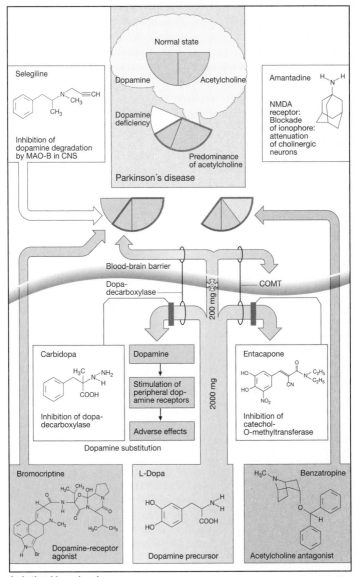

A. Antiparkinsonian drugs

Antiepileptics

Epilepsy is a chronic brain disease of diverse etiology; it is characterized by recurrent paroxysmal episodes of uncontrolled excitation of brain neurons. Involving larger or smaller parts of the brain, the electrical discharge is evident in the electroencephalogram (EEG) as synchronized rhythmic activity and manifests itself in motor, sensory, psychic, and vegetative (visceral) phenomena. Because both the affected brain region and the cause of abnormal excitability may differ, epileptic seizures can take many forms. From a pharmacotherapeutic viewpoint, these may be classified as:

- general vs. focal seizures;
- seizures with or without loss of consciousness;
- seizures with or without specific modes of precipitation.

The brief duration of a single epileptic fit makes acute drug treatment unfeasible. Instead, antiepileptics are used to *prevent* seizures and therefore need to be given chronically. Only in the case of *status epilepticus* (a succession of several tonic-clonic seizures) is acute anticonvulsant therapy indicated — usually with benzodiazepines given i.v. or, if needed, rectally.

The initiation of an epileptic attack involves "pacemaker" cells; these differ from other nerve cells in their unstable resting membrane potential, i.e., a depolarizing membrane current persists after the action potential terminates.

Therapeutic interventions aim to stabilize neuronal resting potential and, hence, to lower excitability. In specific forms of epilepsy, initially a single drug is tried to achieve control of seizures, valproate usually being the drug of first choice in generalized seizures, and carbamazepine being preferred for partial (focal), especially partial complex, seizures. Dosage is increased until seizures are no longer present or adverse effects become unacceptable. Only when monotherapy with different agents proves inadequate can changeover to a second-line drug or combined use ("add on") be recommended **(B)**, provided that the possible risk of pharmacokinetic interactions is taken into account (see below). The precise mode of action of antiepileptic drugs remains unknown. Some agents appear to lower neuronal excitability by several mechanisms of action. In principle, responsivity can be decreased by inhibiting excitatory or activating inhibitory neurons. Most excitatory nerve cells utilize glutamate and most inhibitory neurons utilize γ-aminobutyric acid (GABA) as their transmitter (p. 193A). Various drugs can lower seizure threshold, notably certain neuroleptics, the tuberculostatic isoniazid, and β-lactam antibiotics in high doses; they are, therefore, contraindicated in seizure disorders.

Glutamate receptors comprise three subtypes, of which the NMDA subtype has the greatest therapeutic importance. (**N**-methyl-**D**-aspartate is a synthetic selective agonist.) This receptor is a ligand-gated ion channel that, upon stimulation with glutamate, permits entry of both Na^+ and Ca^{2+} ions into the cell. The antiepileptics *lamotrigine, phenytoin,* and *phenobarbital* inhibit, among other things, the release of glutamate. *Felbamate* is a glutamate antagonist.

Benzodiazepines and *phenobarbital* augment activation of the $GABA_A$ receptor by physiologically released amounts of GABA **(B)** (see p. 226). Chloride influx is increased, counteracting depolarization. *Progabide* is a direct GABA-mimetic. *Tiagabin* blocks removal of GABA from the synaptic cleft by decreasing its re-uptake. *Vigabatrin* inhibits GABA catabolism. *Gabapentin* may augment the availability of glutamate as a precursor in GABA synthesis **(B)** and can also act as a K^+-channel opener.

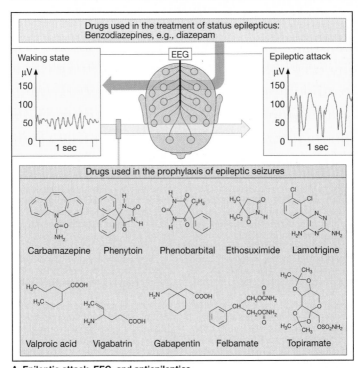

A. Epileptic attack, EEG, and antiepileptics

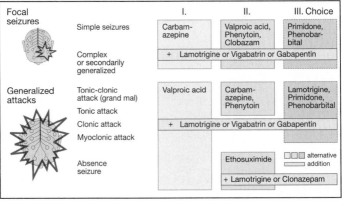

B. Indications for antiepileptics

Carbamazepine, valproate, and *phenytoin* enhance inactivation of voltage-gated sodium and calcium channels and limit the spread of electrical excitation by inhibiting sustained high-frequency firing of neurons.

Ethosuximide blocks a neuronal T-type Ca^{2+} channel **(A)** and represents a special class because it is effective only in absence seizures.

All antiepileptics are likely, albeit to different degrees, to produce adverse effects. *Sedation, difficulty in concentrating,* and *slowing of psychomotor drive* encumber practically all antiepileptic therapy. Moreover, cutaneous, hematological, and hepatic changes may necessitate a change in medication. Phenobarbital, primidone, and phenytoin may lead to *osteomalacia* (vitamin D prophylaxis) or *megaloblastic anemia* (folate prophylaxis). During treatment with phenytoin, *gingival hyperplasia* may develop in ca. 20% of patients.

Valproic acid (VPA) is gaining increasing acceptance as a first-line drug; it is less sedating than other anticonvulsants. Tremor, gastrointestinal upset, and weight gain are frequently observed; reversible hair loss is a rarer occurrence. Hepatotoxicity may be due to a toxic catabolite (4-en VPA).

Adverse reactions to **carbamazepine** include: nystagmus, ataxia, diplopia, particularly if the dosage is raised too fast. Gastrointestinal problems and skin rashes are frequent. It exerts an antidiuretic effect (sensitization of collecting ducts to vasopressin → water intoxication).

Carbamazepine is also used to treat trigeminal neuralgia and neuropathic pain.

Valproate, carbamazepine, and other anticonvulsants pose teratogenic risks. Despite this, treatment should continue during *pregnancy,* as the potential threat to the fetus by a seizure is greater. However, it is mandatory to administer the lowest dose affording safe and effective prophylaxis. Concurrent high-dose administration of folate may prevent neural tube developmental defects.

Carbamazepine, phenytoin, phenobarbital, and other anticonvulsants (except for gabapentin) induce hepatic enzymes responsible for drug biotransformation. *Combinations between anticonvulsants* or with other drugs may result in clinically **important interactions** (plasma level monitoring!).

For the often intractable **childhood epilepsies,** various other agents are used, including ACTH and the glucocorticoid, dexamethasone. Multiple (mixed) seizures associated with the slow spike-wave (Lennox–Gastaut) syndrome may respond to valproate, lamotrigine, and felbamate, the latter being restricted to drug-resistant seizures owing to its potentially fatal liver and bone marrow toxicity.

Benzodiazepines are the drugs of choice for status epilepticus (see above); however, development of tolerance renders them less suitable for long-term therapy. *Clonazepam* is used for myoclonic and atonic seizures. *Clobazam,* a 1,5-benzodiazepine exhibiting an increased anticonvulsant/sedative activity ratio, has a similar range of clinical uses. Personality changes and paradoxical excitement are potential side effects.

Clomethiazole can also be effective for controlling status epilepticus, but is used mainly to treat agitated states, especially alcoholic delirium tremens and associated seizures.

Topiramate, derived from D-fructose, has complex, long-lasting anticonvulsant actions that cooperate to limit the spread of seizure activity; it is effective in partial seizures and as an add-on in Lennox–Gastaut syndrome.

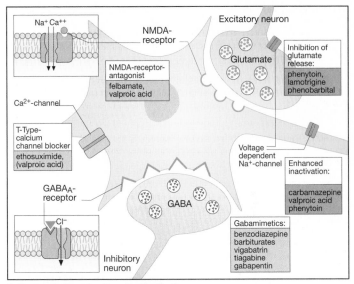

A. Neuronal sites of action of antiepileptics

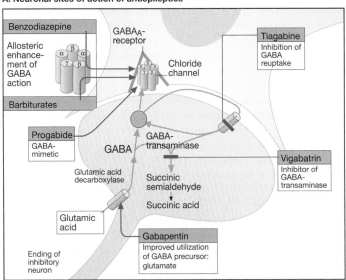

B. Sites of action of antiepileptics in GABAergic synapse

Pain Mechanisms and Pathways

Pain is a designation for a spectrum of sensations of highly divergent character and intensity ranging from unpleasant to intolerable. Pain stimuli are detected by physiological receptors (sensors, nociceptors) least differentiated morphologically, viz., free nerve endings. The body of the bipolar afferent first-order neuron lies in a dorsal root ganglion. Nociceptive impulses are conducted via unmyelinated (C-fibers, conduction velocity 0.2–2.0 m/s) and myelinated axons (Aδ-fibers, 5–30 m/s). The free endings of Aδ fibers respond to intense pressure or heat, those of C-fibers respond to chemical stimuli (H$^+$, K$^+$, histamine, bradykinin, etc.) arising from tissue trauma. Irrespective of whether chemical, mechanical, or thermal stimuli are involved, they become significantly more effective in the presence of prostaglandins (p. 196).

Chemical stimuli also underlie pain secondary to inflammation or ischemia (angina pectoris, myocardial infarction), or the intense pain that occurs during overdistention or spasmodic contraction of smooth muscle abdominal organs, and that may be maintained by local anoxemia developing in the area of spasm (visceral pain).

Aδ and C-fibers enter the spinal cord via the dorsal root, ascend in the dorsolateral funiculus, and then synapse on second-order neurons in the dorsal horn. The axons of the second-order neurons cross the midline and ascend to the brain as the anterolateral pathway or spinothalamic tract. Based on phylogenetic age, neo- and paleospinothalamic tracts are distinguished. Thalamic nuclei receiving neospinothalamic input project to circumscribed areas of the postcentral gyrus. Stimuli conveyed via this path are experienced as sharp, clearly localizable pain. The nuclear regions receiving paleospinothalamic input project to the postcentral gyrus as well as the frontal, limbic cortex and most likely represent the pathway subserving pain of a dull, aching, or burning character, i.e., pain that can be localized only poorly.

Impulse traffic in the neo- and paleospinothalamic pathways is subject to modulation by descending projections that originate from the reticular formation and terminate at second-order neurons, at their synapses with first-order neurons, or at spinal segmental interneurons **(descending antinociceptive system).** This system can inhibit impulse transmission from first- to second-order neurons via release of opiopeptides (enkephalins) or monoamines (norepinephrine, serotonin).

Pain sensation can be influenced or modified as follows:

- elimination of the cause of pain
- lowering of the **sensitivity of nociceptors** (antipyretic analgesics, local anesthetics)
- interrupting **nociceptive conduction** in sensory nerves (local anesthetics)
- suppression of **transmission of nociceptive impulses** in the spinal medulla (opioids)
- inhibition of **pain perception** (opioids, general anesthetics)
- altering **emotional responses** to pain, i.e., pain behavior (antidepressants as "co-analgesics," p. 230).

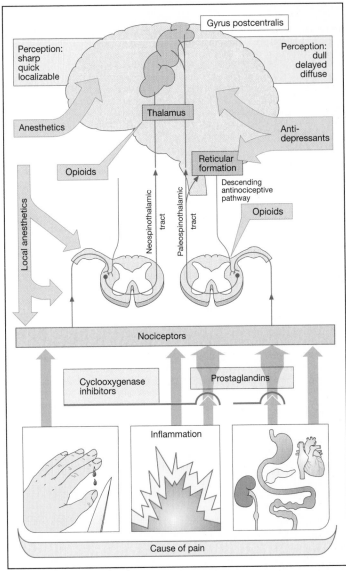

A. Pain mechanisms and pathways

Eicosanoids

Origin and metabolism. The eicosanoids, **prostaglandins, thromboxane, prostacyclin,** and **leukotrienes,** are formed in the organism from **arachidonic acid,** a C20 fatty acid with four double bonds (eicosatetraenoic acid). Arachidonic acid is a regular constituent of cell membrane phospholipids; it is released by phospholipase A_2 and forms the substrate of **cyclooxygenases** and **lipoxygenases.**

Synthesis of prostaglandins (PG), prostacyclin, and thromboxane proceeds via intermediary **cyclic endoperoxides.** In the case of PG, a cyclopentane ring forms in the acyl chain. The letters following PG (D, E, F, G, H, or I) indicate differences in substitution with hydroxyl or keto groups; the number subscripts refer to the number of double bonds, and the Greek letter designates the position of the hydroxyl group at C9 (the substance shown is $PGF_{2\alpha}$). PG are primarily inactivated by the enzyme 15-hydroxyprostaglandindehydrogenase. Inactivation in plasma is very rapid; during one passage through the lung, 90% of PG circulating in plasma are degraded. PG are **local mediators** that attain biologically effective concentrations only at their site of formation.

Biological effects. The individual PG (PGE, PGF, PGI = prostacyclin) possess different biological effects.

Nociceptors. PG increase sensitivity of sensory nerve fibers towards ordinary pain stimuli (p. 194), i.e., at a given stimulus strength there is an increased rate of evoked action potentials.

Thermoregulation. PG raise the set point of hypothalamic (preoptic) thermoregulatory neurons; body temperature increases (fever).

Vascular smooth muscle. PGE_2 and PGI_2 produce *arteriolar vasodilation;* $PGF_{2\alpha}$, venoconstriction.

Gastric secretion. PG promote the production of gastric *mucus* and reduce the formation of *gastric acid* (p. 160).

Menstruation. $PGF_{2\alpha}$ is believed to be responsible for the ischemic necrosis of the endometrium preceding menstruation. The relative proportions of individual PG are said to be altered in dysmenorrhea and excessive menstrual bleeding.

Uterine muscle. PG stimulate *labor contractions.*

Bronchial muscle. PGE_2 and PGI_2 induce *bronchodilation;* $PGF_{2\alpha}$ causes *constriction.*

Renal blood flow. When renal blood flow is lowered, vasodilating PG are released that act to restore blood flow.

Thromboxane A_2 and **prostacyclin** play a role in regulating the *aggregability of platelets* and *vascular diameter* (p. 150).

Leukotrienes increase capillary permeability and serve as chemotactic factors for neutrophil granulocytes. As "slow-reacting substances of anaphylaxis," they are involved in allergic reactions (p. 326); together with PG, they evoke the spectrum of characteristic inflammatory symptoms: redness, heat, swelling, and pain.

Therapeutic applications. PG derivatives are used to induce labor or to interrupt gestation (p. 126); in the therapy of peptic ulcer (p. 168), and in peripheral arterial disease.

PG are poorly tolerated if given systemically; in that case their effects cannot be confined to the intended site of action.

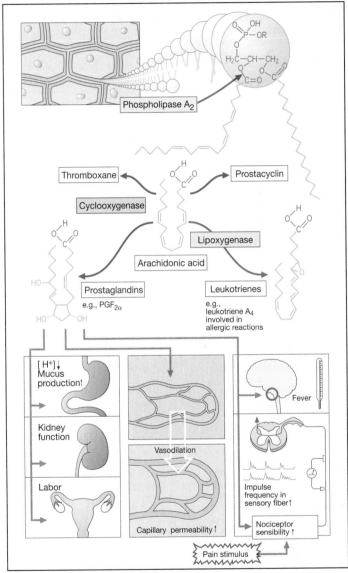

A. Origin and effects of prostaglandins

Antipyretic Analgesics

Acetaminophen, the amphiphilic acids acetylsalicylic acid (ASA), ibuprofen, and others, as well as some pyrazolone derivatives, such as aminopyrine and dipyrone, are grouped under the label **antipyretic analgesics** to distinguish them from opioid analgesics, because they share the ability to reduce fever.

Acetaminophen (paracetamol) has good analgesic efficacy in toothaches and headaches, but is of little use in inflammatory and visceral pain. Its mechanism of action remains unclear. It can be administered orally or in the form of rectal suppositories (single dose, 0.5–1.0 g). The effect develops after about 30 min and lasts for approx. 3 h. Acetaminophen undergoes conjugation to glucuronic acid or sulfate at the phenolic hydroxyl group, with subsequent renal elimination of the conjugate. At therapeutic dosage, a small fraction is oxidized to the highly reactive N-acetyl-p-benzoquinonimine, which is detoxified by coupling to glutathione. After ingestion of high doses (approx. 10 g), the glutathione reserves of the liver are depleted and the quinonimine reacts with constituents of liver cells. As a result, the cells are destroyed: liver necrosis. Liver damage can be avoided if the thiol group donor, N-acetylcysteine, is given intravenously within 6–8 h after ingestion of an excessive dose of acetaminophen. Whether chronic regular intake of acetaminophen leads to impaired renal function remains a matter of debate.

Acetylsalicylic acid (ASA) exerts an antiinflammatory effect, in addition to its analgesic and antipyretic actions. These can be attributed to inhibition of cyclooxygenase (p. 196). ASA can be given in tablet form, as effervescent powder, or injected systemically as lysinate (analgesic or antipyretic single dose, 0.5–1.0 g). ASA undergoes rapid ester hydrolysis, first in the gut and subsequently in the blood. The effect outlasts the presence of ASA in plasma ($t_{1/2}$ ~ 20 min), because cyclooxygenases are irreversibly inhibited due to covalent binding of the acetyl residue. Hence, the duration of the effect depends on the rate of enzyme resynthesis. Furthermore, salicylate may contribute to the effect. ASA irritates the gastric mucosa (direct acid effect and inhibition of cytoprotective PG synthesis, p. 200) and can precipitate bronchoconstriction ("aspirin asthma," pseudoallergy) due to inhibition of PGE_2 synthesis and overproduction of leukotrienes. Because ASA inhibits platelet aggregation and prolongs bleeding time (p. 150), it should not be used in patients with impaired blood coagulability. Caution is also needed in children and juveniles because of Reye's syndrome. The latter has been observed in association with febrile viral infections and ingestion of ASA; its prognosis is poor (liver and brain damage). Administration of ASA at the end of pregnancy may result in prolonged labor, bleeding tendency in mother and infant, and premature closure of the ductus arteriosus. Acidic nonsteroidal antiinflammatory drugs (**NSAIDS**; p. 200) are derived from ASA.

Among antipyretic analgesics, **dipyrone** (metamizole) displays the highest efficacy. It is also effective in visceral pain. Its mode of action is unclear, but probably differs from that of acetaminophen and ASA. It is rapidly absorbed when given via the oral or rectal route. Because of its water solubility, it is also available for injection. Its active metabolite, 4-aminophenazone, is eliminated from plasma with a $t_{1/2}$ of approx. 5 h. Dipyrone is associated with a low incidence of fatal agranulocytosis. In sensitized subjects, cardiovascular collapse can occur, especially after intravenous injection. Therefore, the drug should be restricted to the management of pain refractory to other analgesics. *Propyphenazone* presumably acts like metamizole both pharmacologically and toxicologically.

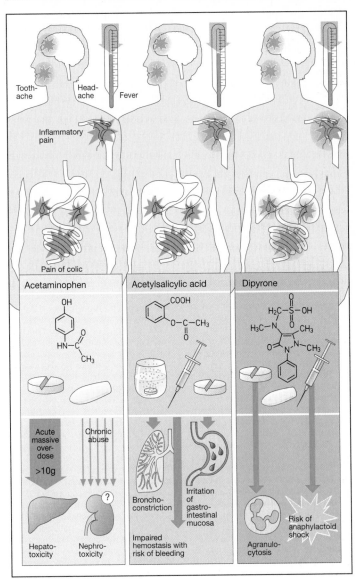

A. Antipyretic analgesics

Nonsteroidal Antiinflammatory (Antirheumatic) Agents

At relatively high dosage (> 4 g/d), **ASA** (p. 198) may exert antiinflammatory effects in rheumatic diseases (e.g., rheumatoid arthritis). In this dose range, central nervous signs of overdosage may occur, such as tinnitus, vertigo, drowsiness, etc. The search for better tolerated drugs led to the family of nonsteroidal antiinflammatory drugs (NSAIDs). Today, more than 30 substances are available, all of them sharing the organic acid nature of ASA. Structurally, they can be grouped into *carbonic acids* (e.g., diclofenac, ibuprofen, naproxene, indomethacin [p. 320]) or *enolic acids* (e.g., azapropazone, piroxicam, as well as the long-known but poorly tolerated phenylbutazone). Like ASA, these substances have analgesic, antipyretic, and antiinflammatory activity. In contrast to ASA, they *inhibit cyclooxygenase* in a *reversible* manner. Moreover, they are not suitable as inhibitors of platelet aggregation. Since their desired effects are similar, the choice between NSAIDs is dictated by their pharmacokinetic behavior and their adverse effects.

Salicylates additionally inhibit the transcription factor NF$_{KB}$, hence the expression of proinflammatory proteins. This effect is shared with glucocorticoids (p. 248) and ibuprofen, but not with some other NSAIDs.

Pharmacokinetics. NSAIDs are well absorbed enterally. They are highly bound to plasma proteins **(A)**. They are eliminated at different speeds: diclofenac ($t_{1/2} = 1-2$ h) and piroxicam ($t_{1/2} \sim 50$ h); thus, dosing intervals and risk of accumulation will vary. The elimination of *salicylate*, the rapidly formed metabolite of ASA, is notable for its dose dependence. Salicylate is effectively reabsorbed in the kidney, except at high urinary pH. A prerequisite for rapid renal elimination is a hepatic conjugation reaction (p. 38), mainly with glycine ($\rightarrow$ salicyluric acid) and glucuronic acid. At high dosage, the conjugation may become rate limiting. Elimination now increasingly depends on unchanged salicylate, which is excreted only slowly.

Group-specific **adverse effects** can be attributed to inhibition of cyclooxygenase **(B)**. The most frequent problem, *gastric mucosal injury* with risk of peptic ulceration, results from reduced synthesis of protective prostaglandins (PG), apart from a direct irritant effect. Gastropathy may be prevented by co-administration of the PG derivative, misoprostol (p. 168). In the intestinal tract, inhibition of PG synthesis would similarly be expected to lead to damage of the blood mucosa barrier and enteropathy. In predisposed patients, *asthma attacks* may occur, probably because of a lack of bronchodilating PG and increased production of leukotrienes. Because this response is not immune mediated, such "pseudoallergic" reactions are a potential hazard with all NSAIDs. PG also regulate renal blood flow as functional antagonists of angiotensin II and norepinephrine. If release of the latter two is increased (e.g., in hypovolemia), inhibition of PG production may result in *reduced renal blood flow and renal impairment.* Other unwanted effects are edema and a rise in blood pressure.

Moreover, drug-specific side effects deserve attention. These concern the CNS (e.g., indomethacin: drowsiness, headache, disorientation), the skin (piroxicam: photosensitization), or the blood (phenylbutazone: agranulocytosis).

Outlook: Cyclooxygenase (COX) has two isozymes: COX-1, a constitutive form present in stomach and kidney; and COX-2, which is induced in inflammatory cells in response to appropriate stimuli. Presently available NSAIDs inhibit both isozymes. The search for COX-2-selective agents (Celecoxib, Rofecoxib) is intensifying because, in theory, these ought to be tolerated better.

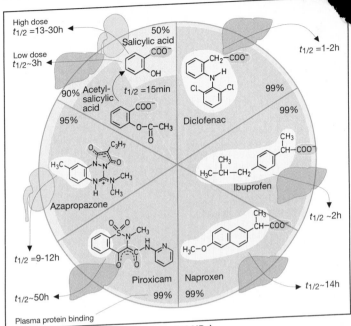

A. Nonsteroidal antiinflammatory drugs (NSAIDs)

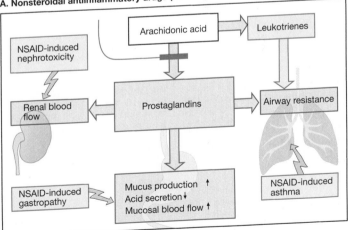

B. NSAIDs: group-specific adverse effects

...oregulation and Antipyretics

...ody core temperature in the human is about 37 °C and fluctuates within ± 1 °C during the 24 h cycle. In the resting state, the metabolic activity of vital organs contributes 60% (liver 25%, brain 20%, heart 8%, kidneys 7%) to total heat production. The absolute contribution to **heat production** from these organs changes little during physical activity, whereas muscle work, which contributes approx. 25% at rest, can generate up to 90% of heat production during strenuous exercise. The set point of the body temperature is programmed in the hypothalamic thermoregulatory center. The actual value is adjusted to the set point by means of various thermoregulatory mechanisms. Blood vessels supplying the skin penetrate the heat-insulating layer of subcutaneous adipose tissue and therefore permit controlled **heat exchange** with the environment as a function of vascular caliber and rate of blood flow. Cutaneous blood flow can range from ~ 0 to 30% of cardiac output, depending on requirements. **Heat conduction** via the blood from interior sites of production to the body surface provides a controllable mechanism for heat loss.

Heat dissipation can also be achieved by increased **production of sweat,** because evaporation of sweat on the skin surface consumes heat (**evaporative heat loss**). Shivering is a mechanism to **generate heat.** Autonomic neural regulation of cutaneous blood flow and sweat production permit homeostatic control of body temperature **(A).** The sympathetic system can either reduce heat loss via vasoconstriction or promote it by enhancing sweat production.

When sweating is inhibited due to poisoning with **anticholinergics** (e.g., atropine), cutaneous blood flow increases. If insufficient heat is dissipated through this route, overheating occurs **(hyperthermia).**

Thyroid hyperfunction poses a particular challenge to the thermoregulatory system, because the excessive secretion of thyroid hormones causes metabolic heat production to increase. In order to maintain body temperature at its physiological level, excess heat must be dissipated—the patients have a hot skin and are sweating.

The hypothalamic temperature controller **(B1)** can be inactivated by **neuroleptics** (p. 236), without impairment of other centers. Thus, it is possible to lower a patient's body temperature without activating counter-regulatory mechanisms (thermogenic shivering). This can be exploited in the treatment of severe febrile states (hyperpyrexia) or in open-chest surgery with cardiac by-pass, during which blood temperature is lowered to 10 °C by means of a heart-lung machine.

In higher doses, **ethanol** and **barbiturates** also depress the thermoregulatory center **(B1),** thereby permitting cooling of the body to the point of death, given a sufficiently low ambient temperature (freezing to death in drunkenness).

Pyrogens (e.g., bacterial matter) elevate—probably through mediation by prostaglandins (p. 196) and interleukin-1—the set point of the hypothalamic temperature controller **(B2).** The body responds by restricting heat loss (cutaneous vasoconstriction → chills) and by elevating heat production (shivering), in order to adjust to the new set point **(fever).** **Antipyretics** such as acetaminophen and ASA (p. 198) return the set point to its normal level **(B2)** and thus bring about a defervescence.

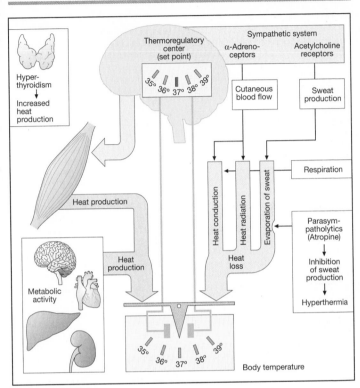

A. Thermoregulation

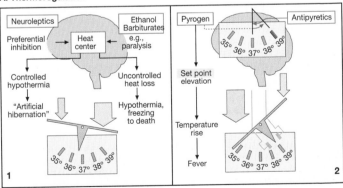

B. Disturbances of thermoregulation

Local Anesthetics

Local anesthetics reversibly inhibit impulse generation and propagation in nerves. In sensory nerves, such an effect is desired when painful procedures must be performed, e.g., surgical or dental operations.

Mechanism of action. Nerve impulse conduction occurs in the form of an action potential, a sudden reversal in resting transmembrane potential lasting less than 1 ms. The change in potential is triggered by an appropriate stimulus and involves a rapid influx of Na^+ into the interior of the nerve axon **(A).** This inward flow proceeds through a channel, a membrane pore protein, that, upon being opened (activated), permits rapid movement of Na^+ down a chemical gradient ($[Na^+]_{ext} \sim 150$ mM, $[Na^+]_{int} \sim 7$ mM). Local anesthetics are capable of inhibiting this rapid inward flux of Na^+; initiation and propagation of excitation are therefore blocked **(A).**

Most local anesthetics exist in part in the cationic amphiphilic form (cf. p. 208). This physicochemical property favors incorporation into membrane interphases, boundary regions between polar and apolar domains. These are found in phospholipid membranes and also in ion-channel proteins. Some evidence suggests that Na^+-channel blockade results from binding of local anesthetics to the channel protein. It appears certain that the site of action is reached from the cytosol, implying that the drug must first penetrate the cell membrane (p. 206).

Local anesthetic activity is also shown by uncharged substances, suggesting a binding site in apolar regions of the channel protein or the surrounding lipid membrane.

Mechanism-specific adverse effects. Since local anesthetics block Na^+ influx not only in sensory nerves but also in other excitable tissues, they are applied locally and measures are taken (p. 206) to impede their distribution into the body. Too rapid entry into the

circulation would lead to unwanted systemic reactions such as:

• *blockade of inhibitory CNS neurons,* manifested by restlessness and seizures (countermeasure: injection of a benzodiazepine, p. 226); general paralysis with respiratory arrest after higher concentrations.

• *blockade of cardiac impulse conduction,* as evidenced by impaired AV conduction or cardiac arrest (countermeasure: injection of epinephrine). Depression of excitatory processes in the heart, while undesired during local anesthesia, can be put to therapeutic use in cardiac arrhythmias (p. 134).

Forms of local anesthesia. Local anesthetics are applied via different routes, including infiltration of the tissue **(infiltration anesthesia)** or injection next to the nerve branch carrying fibers from the region to be anesthetized **(conduction anesthesia** of the nerve, **spinal anesthesia** of segmental dorsal roots), or by application to the surface of the skin or mucosa **(surface anesthesia).** In each case, the local anesthetic drug is required to diffuse to the nerves concerned from a depot placed in the tissue or on the skin.

High sensitivity of sensory nerves, low sensitivity of motor nerves. Impulse conduction in sensory nerves is inhibited at a concentration lower than that needed for motor fibers. This difference may be due to the higher impulse frequency and longer action potential duration in nociceptive, as opposed to motor, fibers.

Alternatively, it may be related to the thickness of sensory and motor nerves, as well as to the distance between nodes of Ranvier. In saltatory impulse conduction, only the nodal membrane is depolarized. Because depolarization can still occur after blockade of three or four nodal rings, the area exposed to a drug concentration sufficient to cause blockade must be larger for motor fibers (p. 205B).

This relationship explains why sensory stimuli that are conducted via

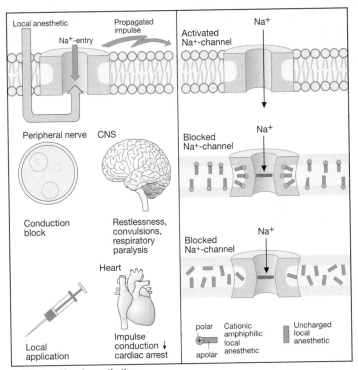

A. Effects of local anesthetics

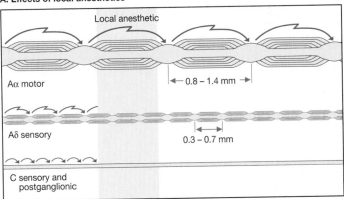

B. Inhibition of impulse conduction in different types of nerve fibers

myelinated Aδ-fibers are affected later and to a lesser degree than are stimuli conducted via unmyelinated C-fibers. Since autonomic postganglionic fibers lack a myelin sheath, they are particularly susceptible to blockade by local anesthetics. As a result, vasodilation ensues in the anesthetized region, because sympathetically driven vasomotor tone decreases. This local vasodilation is undesirable (see below).

Diffusion and Effect

During diffusion from the injection site (i.e., the interstitial space of connective tissue) to the axon of a sensory nerve, the local anesthetic must traverse the **perineurium.** The multilayered perineurium is formed by connective tissue cells linked by *zonulae occludentes* (p. 22) and therefore constitutes a closed lipophilic barrier.

Local anesthetics in clinical use are usually tertiary amines; at the pH of interstitial fluid, these exist partly as the neutral lipophilic base (symbolized by particles marked with two red dots) and partly as the protonated form, i.e., amphiphilic cation (symbolized by particles marked with one blue and one red dot). The uncharged form can penetrate the perineurium and enters the **endoneural space,** where a fraction of the drug molecules regains a positive charge in keeping with the local pH. The same process is repeated when the drug penetrates the axonal membrane (axolemma) into the **axoplasm,** from which it exerts its action on the sodium channel, and again when it diffuses out of the endoneural space through the unfenestrated endothelium of capillaries into the blood.

The concentration of local anesthetic at the site of action is, therefore, determined by the speed of penetration into the endoneurium and the speed of diffusion into the capillary blood. In order to ensure a sufficiently fast build-up of drug concentration at the site of action, there must be a correspondingly large concentration gradient between

drug depot in the connective tissue and the endoneural space. Injection of solutions of low concentration will fail to produce an effect; however, too high concentrations must also be avoided because of the danger of intoxication resulting from too rapid systemic absorption into the blood.

To ensure a reasonably long-lasting local effect with minimal systemic action, a **vasoconstrictor** (epinephrine, less frequently norepinephrine (p. 84) or a vasopressin derivative; p. 164) is often co-administered in an attempt to confine the drug to its site of action. As blood flow is diminished, diffusion from the endoneural space into the capillary blood decreases because the critical concentration gradient between endoneural space and blood quickly becomes small when inflow of drug-free blood is reduced. Addition of a vasoconstrictor, moreover, helps to create a relative ischemia in the surgical field. Potential disadvantages of catecholamine-type vasoconstrictors include reactive hyperemia following washout of the constrictor agent (p. 90) and cardiostimulation when epinephrine enters the systemic circulation. In lieu of epinephrine, the vasopressin analogue felypressin (p. 164, 165) can be used as an adjunctive vasoconstrictor (less pronounced reactive hyperemia, no arrhythmogenic action, but danger of coronary constriction). Vasoconstrictors must not be applied in local anesthesia involving the appendages (e.g., fingers, toes).

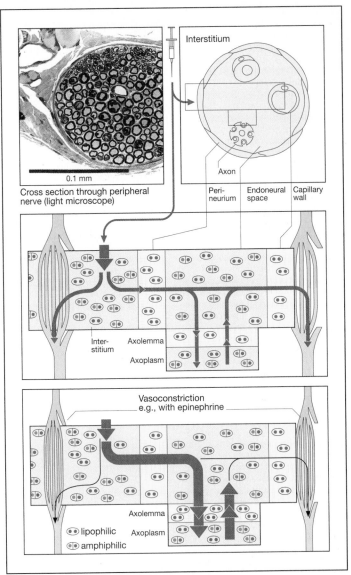

Interstitium

0.1 mm

Cross section through peripheral
nerve (light microscope)

Axon

Peri-
neurium

Endoneural
space

Capillary
wall

Inter-
stitium

Axolemma

Axoplasm

Vasoconstriction
e.g., with epinephrine

Axolemma

Axoplasm

lipophilic

amphiphilic

A. Disposition of local anesthetics in peripheral nerve tissue

Characteristics of chemical structure. Local anesthetics possess a uniform structure. Generally they are secondary or tertiary amines. The nitrogen is linked through an intermediary chain to a lipophilic moiety—most often an aromatic ring system.

The amine function means that local anesthetics exist either as the neutral amine or positively charged ammonium cation, depending upon their dissociation constant (pK_a value) and the actual pH value. The pK_a of typical local anesthetics lies between 7.5 and 9.0. The pk_a indicates the pH value at which 50% of molecules carry a proton. In its protonated form, the molecule possesses both a polar hydrophilic moiety (protonated nitrogen) and an apolar lipophilic moiety (ring system)—it is amphiphilic.

Graphic images of the procaine molecule reveal that the positive charge does not have a punctate localization at the N atom; rather it is distributed, as shown by the potential on the van der Waals' surface. The non-protonated form (right) possesses a negative partial charge in the region of the ester bond and at the amino group at the aromatic ring and is neutral to slightly positively charged (blue) elsewhere. In the protonated form (left), the positive charge is prominent and concentrated at the amino group of the side chain (dark blue).

Depending on the pK_a, 50 to 5% of the drug may be present at physiological pH in the uncharged lipophilic form. This fraction is important because it represents the lipid membrane-permeable form of the local anesthetic (p. 26), which must take on its cationic amphiphilic form in order to exert its action (p. 204).

Clinically used local anesthetics are either esters or amides. This structural element is unimportant for efficacy; even drugs containing a methylene bridge, such as chlorpromazine (p. 236) or imipramine (p. 230), would exert a local anesthetic effect with appropriate application. Ester-type local anesthetics are subject to inactivation by tissue esterases. This is advantageous because of the diminished danger of systemic intoxication. On the other hand, the high rate of bioinactivation and, therefore, shortened duration of action is a disadvantage.

Procaine cannot be used as a surface anesthetic because it is inactivated faster than it can penetrate the dermis or mucosa.

The amide type local anesthetic *lidocaine* is broken down primarily in the liver by oxidative N-dealkylation. This step can occur only to a restricted extent in *prilocaine* and *articaine* because both carry a substituent on the C-atom adjacent to the nitrogen group. Articaine possesses a carboxymethyl group on its thiophen ring. At this position, ester cleavage can occur, resulting in the formation of a polar -COO$^-$ group, loss of the amphiphilic character, and conversion to an inactive metabolite.

Benzocaine (ethoform) is a member of the group of local anesthetics lacking a nitrogen that can be protonated at physiological pH. It is used exclusively as a surface anesthetic.

Other agents employed for surface anesthesia include the uncharged *polidocanol* and the catamphiphilic *cocaine*, *tetracaine*, and *lidocaine*.

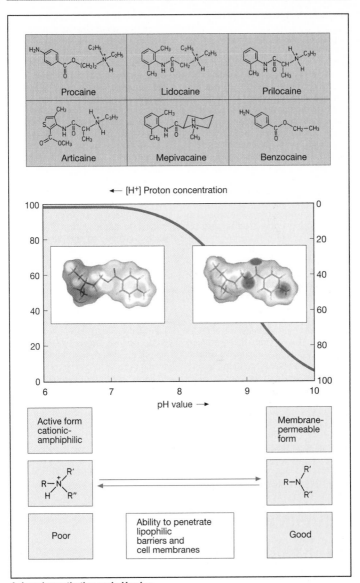

A. Local anesthetics and pH value

Opioid Analgesics—Morphine Type

Source of opioids. *Morphine* is an opium alkaloid (p. 4). Besides morphine, opium contains alkaloids devoid of analgesic activity, e.g., the spasmolytic papaverine, that are also classified as opium alkaloids. All semisynthetic derivatives (hydromorphone) and fully synthetic derivatives (pentazocine, pethidine = meperidine, l-methadone, and fentanyl) are collectively referred to as *opioids.* The high analgesic effectiveness of xenobiotic opioids derives from their affinity for receptors normally acted upon by endogenous opioids (enkephalins, β-endorphin, dynorphins; **A**). Opioid receptors occur in nerve cells. They are found in various brain regions and the spinal medulla, as well as in intramural nerve plexuses that regulate the motility of the alimentary and urogenital tracts. There are several types of opioid receptors, designated μ, δ, κ, that mediate the various opioid effects; all belong to the superfamily of G-protein-coupled receptors (p. 66).

Endogenous opioids are peptides that are cleaved from the precursors proenkephalin, pro-opiomelanocortin, and prodynorphin. All contain the amino acid sequence of the pentapeptides [Met]- or [Leu]-enkephalin (**A**). The effects of the opioids can be abolished by antagonists (e.g., naloxone; **A**), with the exception of buprenorphine.

Mode of action of opioids. Most neurons react to opioids with hyperpolarization, reflecting an increase in K^+ conductance. Ca^{2+} influx into nerve terminals during excitation is decreased, leading to a decreased release of excitatory transmitters and decreased synaptic activity (**A**). Depending on the cell population affected, this synaptic inhibition translates into a depressant or excitant effect (**B**).

Effects of opioids (B). The analgesic effect results from actions at the level of the spinal cord (inhibition of nociceptive impulse transmission) and the brain (attenuation of impulse spread, inhibition of pain perception). Attention and ability to concentrate are impaired. There is a **mood change,** the direction of which depends on the initial condition. Aside from the relief associated with the abatement of strong pain, there is a feeling of **detachment** (floating sensation) and sense of well-being **(euphoria),** particularly after intravenous injection and, hence, rapid build-up of drug levels in the brain. The desire to re-experience this state by renewed administration of drug may become overpowering: *development of psychological dependence.* The atttempt to quit repeated use of the drug results in withdrawal signs of both a physical (cardiovascular disturbances) and psychological (restlessness, anxiety, depression) nature. Opioids meet the criteria of "addictive" agents, namely, psychological and physiological dependence as well as a compulsion to increase the dose. For these reasons, prescription of opioids is subject to special rules (Controlled Substances Act, USA; Narcotic Control Act, Canada; etc). Regulations specify, among other things, maximum dosage (permissible single dose, daily maximal dose, maximal amount per single prescription). Prescriptions need to be issued on special forms the completion of which is rigorously monitored. Certain opioid analgesics, such as codeine and tramadol, may be prescribed in the usual manner, because of their lesser potential for abuse and development of dependence.

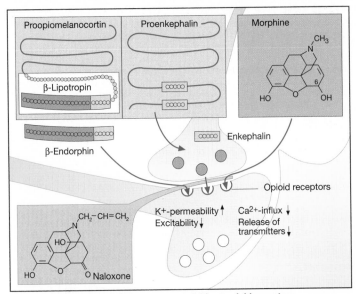

A. Action of endogenous and exogenous opioids at opioid receptors

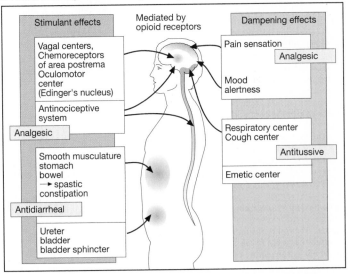

B. Effects of opioids

Differences between opioids regarding efficacy and potential for dependence probably reflect differing affinity and intrinsic activity profiles for the individual receptor subtypes. A given sustance does not necessarily behave as an agonist or antagonist at all receptor subtypes, but may act as an agonist at one subtype and as a partial agonist/antagonist or as a pure antagonist (p. 214) at another. The abuse potential is also determined by kinetic properties, because development of dependence is favored by rapid build-up of brain concentrations. With any of the high-efficacy opioid analgesics, overdosage is likely to result in *respiratory paralysis* (impaired sensitivity of medullary chemoreceptors to CO_2). The maximally possible extent of respiratory depression is thought to be less in partial agonist/antagonists at opioid receptors *(pentazocine, nalbuphine).*

The *cough-suppressant (antitussive)* effect produced by inhibition of the cough reflex is independent of the effects on nociception or respiration (antitussives: *codeine. noscapine*).

Stimulation of chemoreceptors in the area postrema (p. 330) results in *vomiting,* particularly after *first-time administration* or in the *ambulant* patient. The emetic effect disappears with repeated use because a direct inhibition of the emetic center then predominates, which overrides the stimulation of area postrema chemoreceptors.

Opioids elicit *pupillary narrowing (miosis)* by stimulating the parasympathetic portion (Edinger-Westphal nucleus) of the oculomotor nucleus.

Peripheral effects concern the *motility and tonus of gastrointestinal smooth muscle;* segmentation is enhanced, but propulsive peristalsis is inhibited. The tonus of sphincter muscles is raised markedly. In this fashion, morphine elicits the picture of spastic constipation. The antidiarrheic effect is used therapeutically (*loperamide,* p. 178). Gastric emptying is delayed (pyloric spasm) and drainage of bile and pancreatic juice is impeded, because the sphincter of Oddi contracts. Likewise, bladder function is affected; specifically *bladder emptying* is impaired due to increased tone of the vesicular sphincter.

Uses: The endogenous opioids (metenkephalin, leuenkephalin, β-endorphin) cannot be used therapeutically because, due to their peptide nature, they are either rapidly degraded or excluded from passage through the blood-brain barrier, thus preventing access to their sites of action even after parenteral administration **(A).**

Morphine can be given orally or parenterally, as well as epidurally or intrathecally in the spinal cord. The opioids heroin and fentanyl are highly lipophilic, allowing rapid entry into the CNS. Because of its high potency, fentanyl is suitable for transdermal delivery **(A).**

In **opiate abuse,** "smack" ("junk," "jazz," "stuff," "China white;" mostly heroin) is self administered by injection ("mainlining") so as to avoid first-pass metabolism and to achieve a faster rise in brain concentration. Evidently, psychic effects ("kick," "buzz," "rush") are especially intense with this route of administration. The user may also resort to other more unusual routes: opium can be smoked, and heroin can be taken as snuff **(B).**

Metabolism (C). Like other opioids bearing a hydroxyl group, morphine is conjugated to glucuronic acid and eliminated renally. Glucuronidation of the OH-group at position 6, unlike that at position 3, does not affect affinity. The extent to which the 6-glucuronide contributes to the analgesic action remains uncertain at present. At any rate, the activity of this polar metabolite needs to be taken into account in renal insufficiency (lower dosage or longer dosing interval).

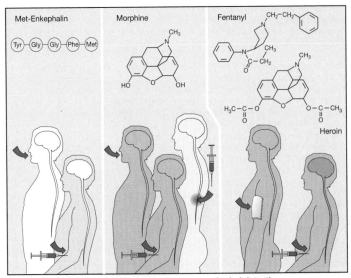

A. Bioavailability of opioids with different routes of administration

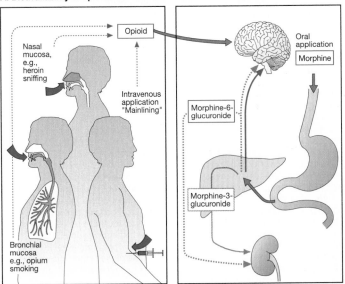

B. Application and rate of disposition

C. Metabolism of morphine

Tolerance. With repeated administration of opioids, their CNS effects can lose intensity (increased tolerance). In the course of therapy, progressively larger doses are needed to achieve the same degree of pain relief. Development of tolerance does not involve the peripheral effects, so that persistent constipation during prolonged use may force a discontinuation of analgesic therapy however urgently needed. Therefore, dietetic and pharmacological measures should be taken prophylactically to prevent constipation, whenever prolonged administration of opioid drugs is indicated.

Morphine antagonists and **partial agonists.** The effects of opioids can be abolished by the antagonists **naloxone** or **naltrexone (A),** irrespective of the receptor type involved. Given by itself, neither has any effect in normal subjects; however, in opioid-dependent subjects, both precipitate acute withdrawal signs. Because of its rapid presystemic elimination, naloxone is only suitable for parenteral use. Naltrexone is metabolically more stable and is given orally. Naloxone is effective as **antidote** in the treatment of opioid-induced respiratory paralysis. Since it is more rapidly eliminated than most opioids, repeated doses may be needed. Naltrexone may be used as an adjunct in withdrawal therapy.

Buprenorphine behaves like a partial agonist/antagonist at μ-receptors. Pentazocine is an antagonist at μ-receptors and an agonist at κ-receptors **(A).** Both are classified as "low-ceiling" opioids **(B),** because neither is capable of eliciting the maximal analgesic effect obtained with morphine or meperidine. The antagonist action of partial agonists may result in an initial decrease in effect of a full agonist during changeover to the latter. Intoxication with buprenorphine cannot be reversed with antagonists, because the drug dissociates only very slowly from the opioid receptors and competitive occupancy of the receptors cannot be achieved as fast as the clinical situation demands.

Opioids in chronic pain: In the management of chronic pain, opioid plasma concentration must be kept continuously in the effective range, because a fall below the critical level would cause the patient to experience pain. Fear of this situation would prompt intake of higher doses than necessary. Strictly speaking, the aim is a prophylactic analgesia.

Like other opioids (hydromorphone, meperidine, pentazocine, codeine), morphine is rapidly eliminated, limiting its duration of action to approx. 4 h. To maintain a steady analgesic effect, these drugs need to be given every 4 h. Frequent dosing, including at nighttime, is a major inconvenience for chronic pain patients. Raising the individual dose would permit the dosing interval to be lengthened; however, it would also lead to transient peaks above the therapeutically required plasma level with the attending risk of unwanted toxic effects and tolerance development. Preferred alternatives include the use of controlled-release preparations of morphine, a fentanyl adhesive patch, or a longer-acting opioid such as *l*-methadone. The kinetic properties of the latter, however, necessitate adjustment of dosage in the course of treatment, because low dosage during the first days of treatment fails to provide pain relief, whereas high dosage of the drug, if continued, will lead to accumulation into a toxic concentration range **(C).**

When the oral route is unavailable opioids may be administered by continuous infusion (pump) and when appropriate under control by the patient – advantage: constant therapeutic plasma level; disadvantage: indwelling catheter. When constipation becomes intolerable morphin can be applied near the spinal cord permitting strong analgesic effect at much lower total dosage.

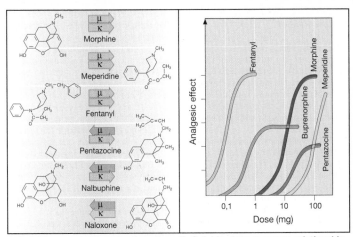

A. Opioids: μ- and κ-receptor ligands

B. Opioids: dose-response relationship

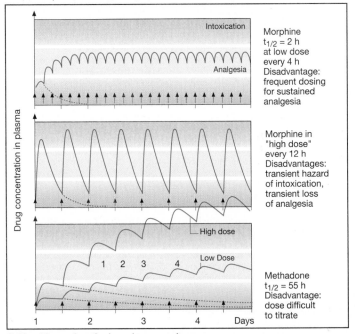

Morphine
t₁/₂ = 2 h
at low dose
every 4 h
Disadvantage:
frequent dosing
for sustained
analgesia

Morphine in
"high dose"
every 12 h
Disadvantages:
transient hazard
of intoxication,
transient loss
of analgesia

Methadone
t₁/₂ = 55 h
Disadvantage:
dose difficult
to titrate

C. Morphine and methadone dosage regimens

General Anesthesia and General Anesthetic Drugs

General anesthesia is a state of drug-induced reversible inhibition of central nervous function, during which surgical procedures can be carried out in the absence of consciousness, responsiveness to pain, defensive or involuntary movements, and significant autonomic reflex responses **(A)**.

The required level of anesthesia depends on the intensity of the pain-producing stimuli, i.e., the degree of nociceptive stimulation. The skilful anesthetist, therefore, dynamically adapts the plane of anesthesia to the demands of the surgical situation. Originally, anesthetization was achieved with a single anesthetic agent (e.g., diethylether—first successfully demonstrated in 1846 by W. T. G. Morton, Boston). To suppress defensive reflexes, such a "mono-anesthesia" necessitates a dosage in excess of that needed to cause unconsciousness, thereby increasing the risk of paralyzing vital functions, such as cardiovascular homeostasis **(B)**. Modern anesthesia employs a combination of different drugs to achieve the goals of surgical anesthesia **(balanced anesthesia)**. This approach reduces the hazards of anesthesia. In **C** are listed examples of drugs that are used concurrently or sequentially as anesthesia adjuncts. In the case of the inhalational anesthetics, the choice of adjuncts relates to the specific property to be exploited (see below). Muscle relaxants, opioid analgesics such as fentanyl, and the parasympatholytic atropine are discussed elsewhere in more detail.

Neuroleptanalgesia can be considered a special form of combination anesthesia, in which the short-acting **opioid analgesics** *fentanyl, alfentanil, remifentanil* is combined with the strongly sedating and affect-blunting **neuroleptic** *droperidol*. This procedure is used in high-risk patients (e.g., advanced age, liver damage).

Neuroleptanesthesia refers to the combined use of a short-acting analgesic, an injectable anesthetic, a short-acting muscle relaxant, and a low dose of a neuroleptic.

In **regional anesthesia** (spinal anesthesia) with a local anesthetic (p. 204), nociception is eliminated, while consciousness is preserved. This procedure, therefore, does not fall under the definition of general anesthesia.

According to their mode of application, **general anesthetics** in the restricted sense are divided into inhalational (gaseous, volatile) and injectable agents.

Inhalational anesthetics are administered in and, for the most part, eliminated via respired air. They serve to maintain anesthesia. Pertinent substances are considered on p. 218.

Injectable anesthetics (p. 220) are frequently employed for induction. Intravenous injection and rapid onset of action are clearly more agreeable to the patient than is breathing a stupefying gas. The effect of most injectable anesthetics is limited to a few minutes. This allows brief procedures to be carried out or to prepare the patient for inhalational anesthesia (intubation). Administration of the volatile anesthetic must then be titrated in such a manner as to counterbalance the waning effect of the injectable agent.

Increasing use is now being made of injectable, instead of inhalational, anesthetics during prolonged combined anesthesia (**t**otal **i**ntra**v**enous **a**nesthesia—TIVA).

"TIVA" has become feasible thanks to the introduction of agents with a suitably short duration of action, including the injectable anesthetics propofol and etomidate, the analgesics alfentanil und remifentanil, and the muscle relaxant mivacurium. These drugs are eliminated within minutes after being administered, irrespective of the duration of anesthesia.

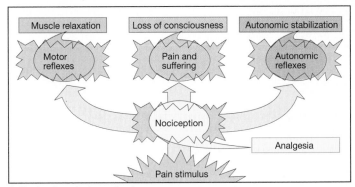

A. Goals of surgical anesthesia

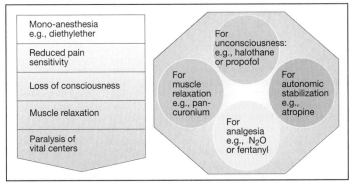

B. Traditional monoanesthesia vs. modern balanced anesthesia

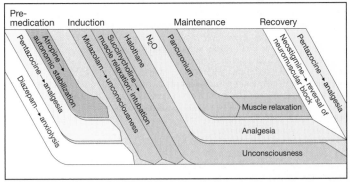

C. Regimen for balanced anesthesia

Inhalational Anesthetics

The **mechanism of action** of inhalational anesthetics is unknown. The diversity of chemical structures (inert gas xenon; hydrocarbons; halogenated hydrocarbons) possessing anesthetic activity appears to rule out involvement of specific receptors. According to one hypothesis, uptake into the hydrophobic interior of the plasmalemma of neurons results in inhibition of electrical excitability and impulse propagation in the brain. This concept would explain the *correlation between anesthetic potency and lipophilicity* of anesthetic drugs **(A).** However, an interaction with lipophilic domains of membrane proteins is also conceivable. Anesthetic potency can be expressed in terms of the **m**inimal **a**lveolar **c**oncentration **(MAC)** at which 50% of patients remain immobile following a defined painful stimulus (skin incision). Whereas the poorly lipophilic N_2O must be inhaled in high concentrations (>70% of inspired air has to be replaced), much smaller concentrations (<5%) are required in the case of the more lipophilic halothane.

The rates of onset and cessation of action vary widely between different inhalational anesthetics and also depend on the degree of lipophilicity. In the case of N_2O, there is rapid elimination from the body when the patient is ventilated with normal air. Due to the high partial pressure in blood, the driving force for transfer of the drug into expired air is large and, since tissue uptake is minor, the body can be quickly cleared of N_2O. In contrast, with halothane, partial pressure in blood is low and tissue uptake is high, resulting in a much slower elimination.

Given alone, N_2O (*nitrous oxide,* "laughing gas") is incapable of producing anesthesia of sufficient depth for surgery. It has good analgesic efficacy that can be exploited when it is used in conjunction with other anesthetics. As a gas, N_2O can be administered directly. Although it irreversibly oxidizes vitamin B_{12}, N_2O is not metabolized appre-

ciably and is cleared entirely by exhalation **(B).**

Halothane (boiling point [BP] 50 °C), *enflurane* (BP 56 °C), *isoflurane* (BP 48 °C), and the obsolete *methoxyflurane* (BP 104 °C) have to be vaporized by special devices. Part of the administered halothane is converted into hepatotoxic metabolites **(B).** Liver damage may result from halothane anesthesia. With a single exposure, the risk involved is unpredictable; however, there is a correlation with the frequency of exposure and the shortness of the interval between successive exposures.

Up to 70% of inhaled methoxyflurane is converted to metabolites that may cause nephrotoxicity, a problem that has led to the withdrawal of the drug.

Degradation products of enflurane or isoflurane (fraction biotransformed <2%) are of no concern.

Halothane exerts a pronounced hypotensive effect, to which a negative inotropic effect contributes. Enflurane and isoflurane cause less circulatory depression. Halothane sensitizes the myocardium to catecholamines (caution: serious tachyarrhythmias or ventricular fibrillation may accompany use of catecholamines as antihypotensives or tocolytics). This effect is much less pronounced with enflurane and isoflurane. Unlike halothane, enflurane and isoflurane have a muscle-relaxant effect that is additive with that of nondepolarizing neuromuscular blockers.

Desflurane is a close structural relative of isoflurane, but has low lipophilicity that permits rapid induction and recovery as well as good control of anesthetic depth.

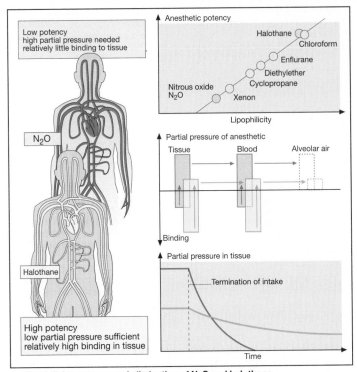

Anesthetic potency

Halothane
Chloroform
Enflurane
Diethylether
Cyclopropane
Nitrous oxide
N₂O
Xenon

Lipophilicity

Partial pressure of anesthetic

Tissue   Blood   Alveolar air

Binding

Partial pressure in tissue

Termination of intake

Time

Low potency
high partial pressure needed
relatively little binding to tissue

N₂O

Halothane

High potency
low partial pressure sufficient
relatively high binding in tissue

A. Lipophilicity, potency and elimination of N₂O and halothane

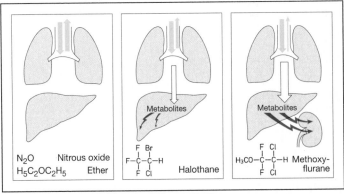

N_2O Nitrous oxide

$H_5C_2OC_2H_5$ Ether

Metabolites

$F-\overset{\displaystyle F}{\underset{\displaystyle F}{C}}-\overset{\displaystyle Br}{\underset{\displaystyle Cl}{C}}-H$ Halothane

Metabolites

$H_3CO-\overset{\displaystyle F}{\underset{\displaystyle F}{C}}-\overset{\displaystyle Cl}{\underset{\displaystyle Cl}{C}}-H$ Methoxy-flurane

B. Elimination routes of different volatile anesthetics

Injectable Anesthetics

Substances from different chemical classes suspend consciousness when given intravenously and can be used as injectable anesthetics (**B**). Unlike inhalational agents, most of these drugs affect consciousness only and are devoid of analgesic activity (exception: ketamine). The effect cannot be ascribed to nonselective binding to neuronal cell membranes, although this may hold for propofol.

Most injectable anesthetics are characterized by a short duration of action. The rapid cessation of action is largely due to **redistribution:** after intravenous injection, brain concentration climbs rapidly to anesthetic levels because of the high cerebral blood flow; the drug then distributes evenly in the body, i.e., concentration rises in the periphery, but falls in the brain—redistribution and cessation of anesthesia (**A**). Thus, the effect subsides before the drug has left the body. A second injection of the same dose, given immediately after recovery from the preceding dose, can therefore produce a more intense and longer effect. Usually, a single injection is administered. However, etomidate and propofol may be given by infusion over a longer time period to maintain unconsciousness.

Thiopental and *methohexital* belong to the barbiturates which, depending on dose, produce sedation, sleepiness, or anesthesia. Barbiturates lower the pain threshold and thereby facilitate defensive reflex movements; they also depress the respiratory center. Barbiturates are frequently used for induction of anesthesia.

Ketamine has analgesic activity that persists beyond the period of unconsciousness up to 1 h after injection. On regaining consciousness, the patient may experience a disconnection between outside reality and inner mental state *(dissociative anesthesia)*. Frequently there is memory loss for the duration of the recovery period; however, adults in particular complain about distressing dream-like experiences. These can be counteracted by administration of a benzodiazepine (e.g., midazolam). The CNS effects of ketamine arise, in part, from an interference with excitatory glutamatergic transmission via ligand-gated cation channels of the NMDA subtype, at which ketamine acts as a channel blocker. The non-natural excitatory amino acid **N-m**ethyl-**D**-**a**spartate is a selective agonist at this receptor. Release of catecholamines with a resultant increase in heart rate and blood pressure is another unrelated action of ketamine.

Propofol has a remarkably simple structure. Its effect has a rapid onset and decays quickly, being experienced by the patient as fairly pleasant. The intensity of the effect can be well controlled during prolonged administration.

Etomidate hardly affects the autonomic nervous system. Since it inhibits cortisol synthesis, it can be used in the treatment of adrenocortical overactivity (Cushing's disease).

Midazolam is a rapidly metabolized benzodiazepine (p. 228) that is used for induction of anesthesia. The longer-acting lorazepam is preferred as adjunct anesthetic in prolonged cardiac surgery with cardiopulmonary bypass; its amnesiogenic effect is pronounced.

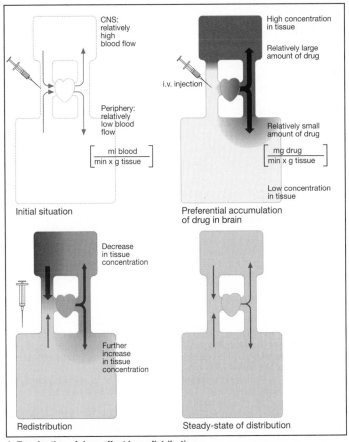

A. Termination of drug effect by redistribution

CNS: relatively high blood flow

Periphery: relatively low blood flow

$$\frac{ml\ blood}{min \times g\ tissue}$$

Initial situation

i.v. injection

High concentration in tissue

Relatively large amount of drug

Relatively small amount of drug

$$\frac{mg\ drug}{min \times g\ tissue}$$

Low concentration in tissue

Preferential accumulation of drug in brain

Decrease in tissue concentration

Further increase in tissue concentration

Redistribution

Steady-state of distribution

B. Intravenous anesthetics

Sodium thiopental

Sodium methohexital

Ketamine

Propofol

Etomidate

Midazolam

Soporifics, Hypnotics

During sleep, the brain generates a patterned rhythmic activity that can be monitored by means of the electroencephalogram (EEG). Internal sleep cycles recur 4 to 5 times per night, each cycle being interrupted by a **R**apid **E**ye **M**ovement (REM) sleep phase (**A**). The REM stage is characterized by EEG activity similar to that seen in the waking state, rapid eye movements, vivid dreams, and occasional twitches of individual muscle groups against a background of generalized atonia of skeletal musculature. Normally, the REM stage is entered only after a preceding non-REM cycle. Frequent interruption of sleep will, therefore, decrease the REM portion. Shortening of REM sleep (normally approx. 25% of total sleep duration) results in increased irritability and restlessness during the daytime. With undisturbed night rest, REM deficits are compensated by increased REM sleep on subsequent nights (**B**).

Hypnotics fall into different categories, including the **benzodiazepines** (e.g., triazolam, temazepam, clotiazepam, nitrazepam), **barbiturates** (e.g., hexobarbital, pentobarbital), chloral hydrate, and H$_1$-antihistamines with sedative activity (p. 114). Benzodiazepines act at specific receptors (p. 226). The site and mechanism of action of barbiturates, antihistamines, and chloral hydrate are incompletely understood.

All hypnotics shorten the time spent in the REM stages (**B**). With repeated ingestion of a hypnotic on several successive days, the proportion of time spent in REM vs. non-REM sleep returns to normal despite continued drug intake. Withdrawal of the hypnotic drug results in REM rebound, which tapers off only over many days (**B**). Since REM stages are associated with vivid dreaming, sleep with excessively long REM episodes is experienced as unrefreshing. Thus, the attempt to discontinue use of hypnotics may result in the impression that refreshing sleep calls for a hypnotic, probably promoting **hypnotic drug dependence.**

Depending on their blood levels, both benzodiazepines and barbiturates produce **calming** and **sedative** effects, the former group also being **anxiolytic.** At higher dosage, both groups **promote the onset** of sleep or **induce** it (**C**).

Unlike barbiturates, **benzodiazepine derivatives** administered orally lack a general anesthetic action; cerebral activity is not globally inhibited (respiratory paralysis is virtually impossible) and autonomic functions, such as blood pressure, heart rate, or body temperature, are unimpaired. Thus, benzodiazepines possess a therapeutic margin considerably wider than that of barbiturates.

Zolpidem (an imidazopyridine) and **zopiclone** (a cyclopyrrolone) are hypnotics that, despite their different chemical structure, possess agonist activity at the benzodiazepine receptor (p. 226).

Due to their narrower margin of safety (risk of misuse for suicide) and their potential to produce physical dependence, **barbiturates** are no longer or only rarely used as hypnotics. Dependence on them has all the characteristics of an addiction (p. 210).

Because of rapidly developing tolerance, **choral hydrate** is suitable only for short-term use.

Antihistamines are popular as **nonprescription** (over-the-counter) sleep remedies (e.g., diphenhydramine, doxylamine, p. 114), in which case their sedative side effect is used as the principal effect.

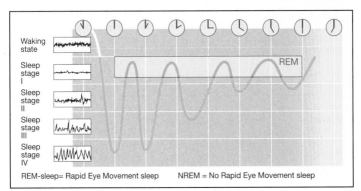

A. Succession of different sleep phases during night rest

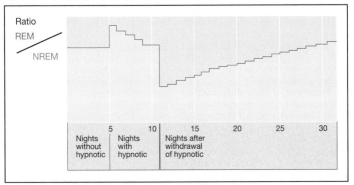

B. Effect of hypnotics on proportion of REM/NREM

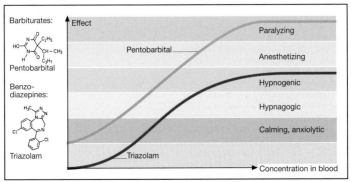

C. Concentration dependence of barbiturate and benzodiazepine effects

Sleep–Wake Cycle and Hypnotics

The physiological mechanisms regulating the sleep-wake rhythm are not completely known. There is evidence that histaminergic, cholinergic, glutamatergic, and adrenergic neurons are more active during waking than during the NREM sleep stage. Via their ascending thalamopetal projections, these neurons excite thalamocortical pathways and inhibit GABA-ergic neurons. During sleep, input from the brain stem decreases, giving rise to diminished thalamocortical activity and disinhibition of the GABA neurons **(A)**. The shift in balance between excitatory (red) and inhibitory (green) neuron groups underlies a circadian change in sleep propensity, causing it to remain low in the morning, to increase towards early afternoon (midday siesta), then to decline again, and finally to reach its peak before midnight **(B1)**.

Treatment of sleep disturbances. Pharmacotherapeutic measures are indicated only when causal therapy has failed. Causes of insomnia include emotional problems (grief, anxiety, "stress"), physical complaints (cough, pain), or the ingestion of stimulant substances (caffeine-containing beverages, sympathomimetics, theophylline, or certain antidepressants). As illustrated for emotional stress **(B2)**, these factors cause an imbalance in favor of excitatory influences. As a result, the interval between going to bed and falling asleep becomes longer, total sleep duration decreases, and sleep may be interrupted by several waking periods.

Depending on the type of insomnia, benzodiazepines (p. 226) with short or intermediate duration of action are indicated, e.g., triazolam and brotizolam ($t_{1/2} \sim 4$–6 h); lormetazepam or temazepam ($t_{1/2} \sim 10$–15 h). These drugs shorten the latency of falling asleep, lengthen total sleep duration, and reduce the frequency of nocturnal awakenings. They act by augmenting inhibitory activity. Even with the longer-acting benzodiazepines, the patient awakes after about 6–8 h of sleep, because in the morning excitatory activity exceeds the sum of physiological and pharmacological inhibition **(B3)**. The drug effect may, however, become unmasked at daytime when other sedating substances (e.g., ethanol) are ingested and the patient shows an unusually pronounced response due to a synergistic interaction (impaired ability to concentrate or react).

As the margin between excitatory and inhibitory activity decreases with age, there is an increasing tendency towards shortened daytime sleep periods and more frequent interruption of nocturnal sleep **(C)**.

Use of a hypnotic drug should not be extended beyond 4 wk, because tolerance may develop. The risk of a rebound decrease in sleep propensity after drug withdrawal may be avoided by tapering off the dose over 2 to 3 wk.

With any hypnotic, the risk of suicidal overdosage cannot be ignored. Since benzodiazepine intoxication may become life-threatening only when other central nervous depressants (ethanol) are taken simultaneously and can, moreover, be treated with specific benzodiazepine antagonists, the benzodiazepines should be given preference as sleep remedies over the all but obsolete barbiturates.

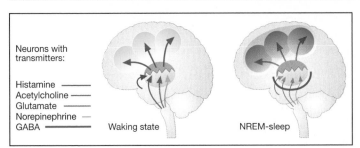

A. Transmitters: waking state and sleep

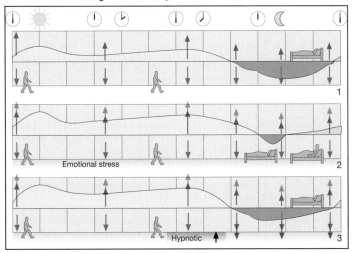

B. Wake-sleep pattern, stress, and hypnotic drug action

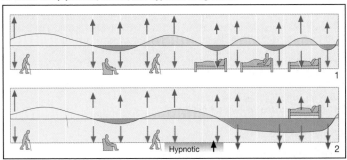

C. Changes of the arousal reaction in the elderly

Benzodiazepines

Benzodiazepines modify affective responses to sensory perceptions; specifically, they render a subject indifferent towards anxiogenic stimuli, i.e., **anxiolytic** action. Furthermore, benzodiazepines exert **sedating, anticonvulsant,** and **muscle-relaxant** (myotonolytic, p. 182) effects. All these actions result from augmenting the activity of **inhibitory neurons** and are mediated by specific **benzodiazepine receptors** that form an integral part of the GABA$_A$ receptor-chloride channel complex. The inhibitory transmitter GABA acts to open the membrane **chloride channels.** Increased chloride conductance of the neuronal membrane effectively short-circuits responses to depolarizing inputs. Benzodiazepine receptor agonists increase the affinity of GABA to its receptor. At a given concentration of GABA, binding to the receptors will, therefore, be increased, resulting in an augmented response. Excitability of the neurons is diminished.

Therapeutic indications for benzodiazepines include **anxiety states** associated with **neurotic, phobic, and depressive disorders,** or **myocardial infarction** (decrease in cardiac stimulation due to anxiety); **insomnia; preanesthetic** (preoperative) medication; **epileptic seizures;** and **hypertonia** of skeletal musculature (**spasticity,** rigidity).

Since GABA-ergic synapses are confined to neural tissues, specific inhibition of central nervous functions can be achieved; for instance, there is little change in blood pressure, heart rate, and body temperature. The therapeutic index of benzodiazepines, calculated with reference to the toxic dose producing respiratory depression, is greater than 100 and thus exceeds that of barbiturates and other sedative-hypnotics by more than tenfold. Benzodiazepine intoxication can be treated with a specific antidote (see below).

Since benzodiazepines depress responsivity to external stimuli, automotive driving skills and other tasks requiring precise sensorimotor coordination will be impaired.

Triazolam (t$_{1/2}$ of elimination ~1.5–5.5 h) is especially likely to impair memory (anterograde amnesia) and to cause rebound anxiety or insomnia and daytime confusion. The severity of these and other adverse reactions (e.g., rage, violent hostility, hallucinations), and their increased frequency in the elderly, has led to curtailed or suspended use of triazolam in some countries (UK).

Although benzodiazepines are well tolerated, the possibility of personality changes (nonchalance, paradoxical excitement) and the risk of physical dependence with chronic use must not be overlooked. Conceivably, benzodiazepine dependence results from a kind of habituation, the functional counterparts of which become manifest during abstinence as restlessness and anxiety; even seizures may occur. These symptoms reinforce chronic ingestion of benzodiazepines.

Benzodiazepine antagonists, such as flumazenil, possess affinity for benzodiazepine receptors, but they lack intrinsic activity. Flumazenil is an effective antidote in the treatment of benzodiazepine overdosage or can be used postoperatively to arouse patients sedated with a benzodiazepine.

Whereas benzodiazepines possessing agonist activity indirectly augment chloride permeability, **inverse agonists** exert an opposite action. These substances give rise to pronounced restlessness, excitement, anxiety, and convulsive seizures. There is, as yet, no therapeutic indication for their use.

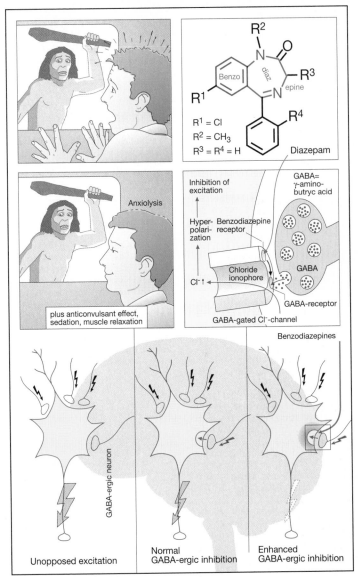

R¹ = Cl
R² = CH₃
R³ = R⁴ = H

$R^1 = Cl$
$R^2 = CH_3$
$R^3 = R^4 = H$

Diazepam

Inhibition of excitation

Hyper-polarization

Benzodiazepine receptor

Cl⁻ ↑

Chloride ionophore

GABA-gated Cl⁻-channel

GABA = γ-amino-butryc acid

GABA

GABA-receptor

plus anticonvulsant effect, sedation, muscle relaxation

Anxiolysis

Benzodiazepines

GABA-ergic neuron

Unopposed excitation

Normal GABA-ergic inhibition

Enhanced GABA-ergic inhibition

A. Action of benzodiazepines

228   Psychopharmacologicals

Pharmacokinetics of Benzodiazepines

All benzodiazepines exert their actions at specific receptors (p. 226). The choice between different agents is dictated by their speed, intensity, and duration of action. These, in turn, reflect physico-chemical and pharmacokinetic properties. Individual benzodiazepines remain in the body for very different lengths of time and are chiefly eliminated through biotransformation. Inactivation may entail a single chemical reaction or several steps (e.g., diazepam) before an inactive metabolite suitable for renal elimination is formed. Since the intermediary products may, in part, be pharmacologically active and, in part, be excreted more slowly than the parent substance, metabolites will accumulate with continued regular dosing and contribute significantly to the final effect.

Biotransformation begins either at substituents on the diazepine ring (*diazepam:* N-dealkylation at position 1; *midazolam:* hydroxylation of the methyl group on the imidazole ring) or at the diazepine ring itself. Hydroxylated midazolam is quickly eliminated following glucuronidation ($t_{1/2} \sim 2$ h). N-demethyldiazepam (nordazepam) is biologically active and undergoes hydroxylation at position 3 on the diazepine ring. The hydroxylated product (oxazepam) again is pharmacologically active. By virtue of their long half-lives, diazepam ($t_{1/2} \sim 32$ h) and, still more so, its metabolite, nordazepam ($t_{1/2}$ 50–90 h), are eliminated slowly and accumulate during repeated intake. Oxazepam undergoes conjugation to glucuronic acid via its hydroxyl group ($t_{1/2} = 8$ h) and renal excretion **(A)**.

The range of elimination half-lives for different benzodiazepines or their active metabolites is represented by the shaded areas **(B)**. Substances with a short half-life that are not converted to active metabolites can be used for induction or maintenance of sleep (light blue area in **B**). Substances with a long half-life are preferable for long-term anxiolytic treatment (light green area)

because they permit maintenance of steady plasma levels with single daily dosing. Midazolam enjoys use by the i.v. route in preanesthetic medication and anesthetic combination regimens.

Benzodiazepine Dependence

Prolonged regular use of benzodiazepines can lead to physical dependence. With the long-acting substances marketed initially, this problem was less obvious in comparison with other dependence-producing drugs because of the delayed appearance of withdrawal symptoms. The severity of the abstinence syndrome is inversely related to the elimination $t_{1/2}$, ranging from mild to moderate (restlessness, irritability, sensitivity to sound and light, insomnia, and tremulousness) to dramatic (depression, panic, delirium, grand mal seizures). Some of these symptoms pose diagnostic difficulties, being indistinguishable from the ones originally treated. Administration of a benzodiazepine antagonist would abruptly provoke abstinence signs. There are indications that substances with intermediate elimination half-lives are most frequently abused (violet area in **B**).

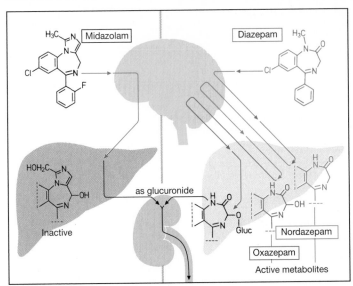

A. Biotransformation of benzodiazepines

B. Rate of elimination of benzodiazepines

Therapy of Manic-Depressive Illness

Manic-depressive illness connotes a psychotic disorder of affect that occurs episodically without external cause. In *endogenous depression* (melancholia), mood is persistently low. *Mania* refers to the opposite condition (p. 234). Patients may oscillate between these two extremes with interludes of normal mood. Depending on the type of disorder, mood swings may alternate between the two directions (bipolar depression, cyclothymia) or occur in only one direction (unipolar depression).

I. Endogenous Depression

In this condition, the patient experiences profound misery (beyond the observer's empathy) and feelings of severe guilt because of imaginary misconduct. The drive to act or move is inhibited. In addition, there are disturbances mostly of a somatic nature (insomnia, loss of appetite, constipation, palpitations, loss of libido, impotence, etc.). Although the patient may have suicidal thoughts, psychomotor retardation prevents suicidal impulses from being carried out. In **A,** endogenous depression is illustrated by the layers of somber colors; psychomotor drive, symbolized by a sine oscillation, is strongly reduced.

Therapeutic agents fall into two groups:

• **Thymoleptics,** possessing a pronounced ability to re-elevate depressed mood e.g., the tricyclic antidepressants;

• **Thymeretics,** having a predominant activating effect on psychomotor drive, e g., monoamine oxidase inhibitors.

It would be wrong to administer drive-enhancing drugs, such as amphetamines, to a patient with endogenous depression. Because this therapy fails to elevate mood but removes psychomotor inhibition **(A),** the danger of suicide increases.

Tricyclic antidepressants (TCA; prototype: **imipramine**) have had the longest and most extensive therapeutic use; however, in the past decade, they have been increasingly superseded by the serotonin-selective reuptake inhibitors (SSRI; prototype: fluoxetine).

The central seven-membered ring of the TCAs imposes a 120° angle between the two flanking aromatic rings, in contradistinction to the flat ring system present in phenothiazine type neuroleptics (p. 237). The side chain nitrogen is predominantly protonated at physiological pH.

The TCAs have affinity for both *receptors and transporters of monoamine transmitters* and behave as antagonists in both respects. Thus, the neuronal reuptake of norepinephrine (p. 82) and serotonin (p. 116) is inhibited, with a resultant increase in activity. Muscarinic acetylcholine receptors, α-adrenoceptors, and certain 5-HT and histamine(H_1) receptors are blocked. Interference with the dopamine system is relatively minor.

How interference with these transmitter/modulator substances translates into an antidepressant effect is still hypothetical. The clinical effect emerges only after prolonged intake, i.e., 2–3 wk, as evidenced by an elevation of mood and drive. However, the alteration in monoamine metabolism occurs as soon as therapy is started. Conceivably, adaptive processes (such as downregulation of cortical serotonin and β-adrenoceptors) are ultimately responsible. In healthy subjects, the TCAs do not improve mood (no euphoria).

Apart from the antidepressant effect, acute effects occur that are evident also in healthy individuals. These vary in degree among individual substances and thus provide a rationale for differentiated clinical use (p. 233), based upon the divergent patterns of interference with amine transmitters/modulators. **Amitriptyline** exerts anxiolytic, sedative and psychomotor dampening effects. These are useful in depressive patients who are anxious and agitated.

In contrast, **desipramine** produces psychomotor activation. **Imipramine**

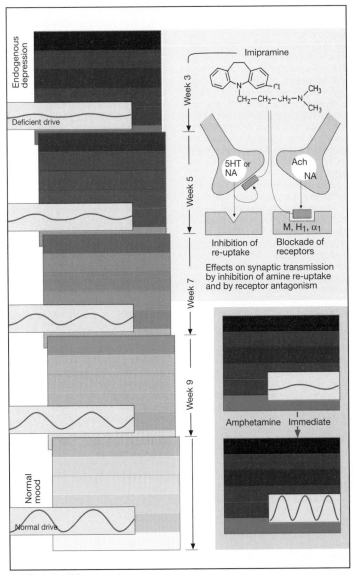

A. Effect of antidepressants

occupies an intermediate position. It should be noted that, in the organism, biotransformation of imipramine leads to desipramine (N-desmethylimipramine). Likewise, the desmethyl derivative of amitriptyline *(nortriptyline)* is less dampening.

In nondepressive patients whose complaints are of predominantly psychogenic origin, the anxiolytic-sedative effect may be useful in efforts to bring about a temporary "psychosomatic uncoupling." In this connection, clinical use as "co-analgesics" (p. 194) may be noted.

The **side effects** of tricyclic antidepressants are largely attributable to the ability of these compounds to bind to and block receptors for endogenous transmitter substances. These effects develop acutely. Antagonism at muscarinic cholinoceptors leads to *atropine-like* effects such as tachycardia, inhibition of exocrine glands, constipation, impaired micturition, and blurred vision.

Changes in adrenergic function are complex. Inhibition of neuronal catecholamine reuptake gives rise to superimposed indirect sympathomimetic stimulation. Patients are supersensitive to catecholamines (e.g., epinephrine in local anesthetic injections must be avoided). On the other hand, blockade of α_1-receptors may lead to orthostatic hypotension.

Due to their cationic amphiphilic nature, the TCA exert membrane-stabilizing effects that can lead to disturbances of cardiac impulse conduction with arrhythmias as well as decreases in myocardial contractility. All TCA lower the seizure threshold. Weight gain may result from a stimulant effect on appetite.

Maprotiline, a tetracyclic compound, largely resembles tricyclic agents in terms of its pharmacological and clinical actions. **Mianserine** also possesses a tetracyclic structure, but differs insofar as it increases intrasynaptic concentrations of norepinephrine by blocking presynaptic α_2-receptors, rather than reuptake. Moreover, it has less pronounced atropine-like activity.

Fluoxetine, along with sertraline, fluvoxamine, and paroxetine, belongs to the more recently developed group of SSRI. The clinical efficacy of SSRI is considered comparable to that of established antidepressants. Added advantages include: absence of cardiotoxicity, fewer autonomic nervous side effects, and relative safety with overdosage. Fluoxetine causes loss of appetite and weight reduction. Its main adverse effects include: overarousal, insomnia, tremor, akathisia, anxiety, and disturbances of sexual function.

Moclobemide is a new representative of the group of MAO inhibitors. Inhibition of intraneuronal degradation of serotonin and norepinephrine causes an increase in extracellular amine levels. A psychomotor stimulant *thymeretic* action is the predominant feature of MAO inhibitors. An older member of this group, **tranylcypromine,** causes irreversible inhibition of the two isozymes MAO_A and MAO_B. Therefore, presystemic elimination in the liver of biogenic amines, such as tyramine, which are ingested in food (e.g., aged cheese and Chianti), will be impaired. To avoid the danger of a hypertensive crisis, therapy with tranylcypromine or other nonselective MAO inhibitors calls for stringent dietary rules. With moclobemide, this hazard is much reduced because it inactivates only MAO_A and does so in a reversible manner.

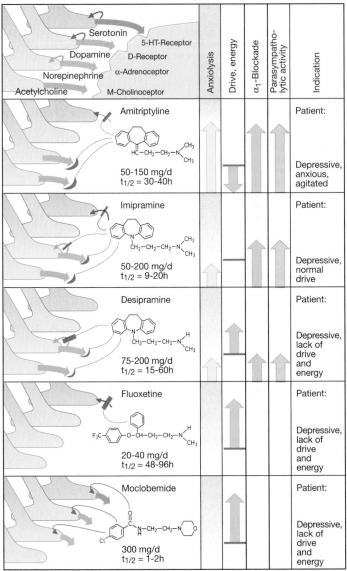

A. Antidepressants: activity profiles

II. Mania

The manic phase is characterized by ex-aggerated elation, flight of ideas, and a pathologically increased psychomotor drive. This is symbolically illustrated in **A** by a disjointed structure and aggressive color tones. The patients are over-confident, continuously active, show progressive incoherence of thought and loosening of associations, and act irresponsibly (financially, sexually etc.).

Lithium ions. Lithium salts (e.g., acetate, carbonate) are effective in controlling the **manic phase.** The effect becomes evident approx. 10 d after the start of therapy. The small therapeutic index necessitates frequent monitoring of Li^+ serum levels. Therapeutic levels should be kept between 0.8–1.0 mM in fasting morning blood samples. At higher values there is a risk of *adverse effects.* CNS symptoms include fine tremor, ataxia or seizures. Inhibition of the renal actions of vasopressin (p. 164) leads to polyuria and thirst. Thyroid function is impaired (p. 244), with compensatory development of (euthyroid) goiter.

The *mechanism of action* of Li ions remains to be fully elucidated. Chemically, lithium is the lightest of the alkali metals, which include such biologically important elements as sodium and potassium. Apart from interference with transmembrane cation fluxes (via ion channels and pumps), a lithium effect of major significance appears to be membrane depletion of phosphatidylinositol bisphosphates, the principal lipid substrate used by various receptors in transmembrane signalling (p. 66). Blockade of this important signal transduction pathway leads to impaired ability of neurons to respond to activation of membrane receptors for transmitters or other chemical signals. Another site of action of lithium may be GTP-binding proteins responsible for signal transduction initiated by formation of the agonist-receptor complex.

Rapid control of an acute attack of mania may require the use of a *neuroleptic* (see below).

Alternate treatments. Mood-sta-bilization and control of manic or hy-pomanic episodes in some subtypes of bipolar illness may also be achieved with the anticonvulsants valproate and carbamazepine, as well as with calcium channel blockers (e.g., verapamil, nifed-ipine, nimodipine). Effects are delayed and apparently unrelated to the mechanisms responsible for anticonvulsant and cardiovascular actions, respectively.

III. Prophylaxis

With continued treatment for 6 to 12 months, **lithium salts** prevent the recurrence of either manic or depressive states, effectively stabilizing mood at a normal level.

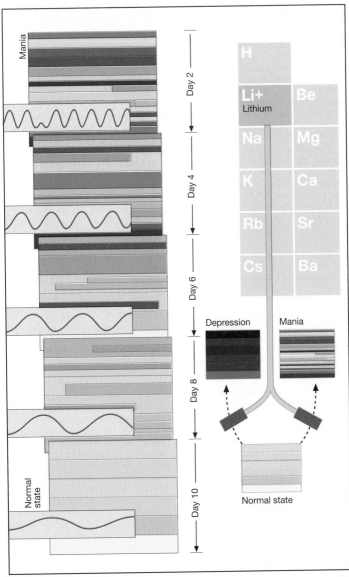

A. Effect of lithium salts in mania

Therapy of Schizophrenia

Schizophrenia is an endogenous psychosis of episodic character. Its chief symptoms reflect a thought disorder (i.e., distracted, incoherent, illogical thinking; impoverished intellectual content; blockage of ideation; abrupt breaking of a train of thought: claims of being subject to outside agencies that control the patient's thoughts), and a disturbance of affect (mood inappropriate to the situation) and of psychomotor drive. In addition, patients exhibit delusional paranoia (persecution mania) or hallucinations (fearfulness hearing of voices). Contrasting these "positive" symptoms, the so-called "negative" symptoms, viz., poverty of thought, social withdrawal, and anhedonia, assume added importance in determining the severity of the disease. The disruption and incoherence of ideation is symbolically represented at the top left **(A)** and the normal psychic state is illustrated as on p. 237 (bottom left).

Neuroleptics

After administration of a neuroleptic, there is at first only psychomotor dampening. Tormenting paranoid ideas and hallucinations lose their subjective importance **(A,** dimming of flashy colors); however, the psychotic processes still persist. In the course of weeks, psychic processes gradually normalize **(A)**; the psychotic episode wanes, although complete normalization often cannot be achieved because of the persistence of negative symptoms. Nonetheless, these changes are significant because the patient experiences relief from the torment of psychotic personality changes; care of the patient is made easier and return to a familiar community environment is accelerated.

The conventional (or classical) neuroleptics comprise two classes of compounds with distinctive chemical structures: 1. the **phenothiazines** derived from the antihistamine promethazine (prototype: chlorpromazine), including

their analogues (e.g., thioxanthenes); and 2. the **butyrophenones** (prototype: haloperidol). According to the chemical structure of the side chain, phenothiazines and thioxanthenes can be subdivided into aliphatic (chlorpromazine, triflupromazine, p. 239 and piperazine congeners (trifluperazine, fluphenazine, flupentixol, p. 239).

The antipsychotic effect is probably due to an *antagonistic action at dopamine receptors.* Aside from their main antipsychotic action, neuroleptics display additional actions owing to their antagonism at

- muscarinic acetylcholine receptors → atropine-like effects;
- α-adrenoceptors for norepinephrine → disturbances of blood pressure regulation;
- dopamine receptors in the nigrostriatal system → extrapyramidal motor disturbances; in the area postrema → antiemetic action (p. 330), and in the pituitary gland → increased secretion of prolactin (p. 242);
- histamine receptors in the cerebral cortex → possible cause of sedation.

These ancillary effects are also elicited in healthy subjects and vary in intensity among individual substances.

Other indications. Acutely, there is *sedation* with *anxiolysis* after neuroleptization has been started. This effect can be utilized for: *"psychosomatic uncoupling"* in disorders with a prominent psychogenic component; *neuroleptanalgesia* (p. 216) by means of the butyrophenone droperidol in combination with an opioid; *tranquilization* of overexcited, agitated patients; treatment of *delirium tremens* with haloperidol; as well as the control of *mania* (see p. 234).

It should be pointed out that neuroleptics do *not* exert an *anticonvulsant* action, on the contrary, they may lower seizure threshold.

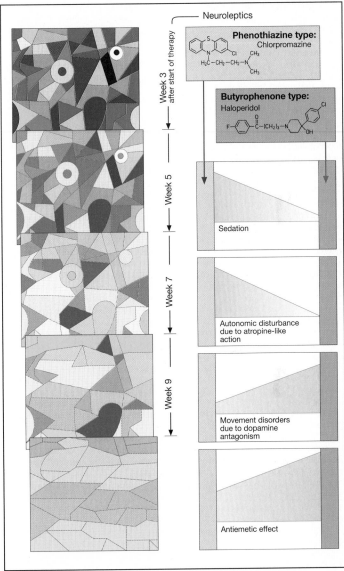

A. Effects of neuroleptics in schizophrenia

Because they *inhibit the thermoregulatory center,* neuroleptics can be employed for controlled hypothermia (p. 202).

Adverse Effects. Clinically most important and therapy-limiting are *extrapyramidal disturbances;* these result from dopamine receptor blockade. Acute dystonias occur immediately after neuroleptization and are manifested by motor impairments, particularly in the head, neck, and shoulder region. After several days to months, a *parkinsonian syndrome* (pseudoparkinsonism) or *akathisia* (motor restlessness) may develop. All these disturbances can be treated by administration of antiparkinson drugs of the anticholinergic type, such as biperiden (i.e., in acute dystonia). As a rule, these disturbances disappear after withdrawal of neuroleptic medication. *Tardive dyskinesia* may become evident after chronic neuroleptization for several years, particularly when the drug is discontinued. It is due to hypersensitivity of the dopamine receptor system and can be exacerbated by administration of anticholinergics.

Chronic use of neuroleptics can, on occasion, give rise to *hepatic damage* associated *with cholestasis.* A very rare, but dramatic, adverse effect is the *malignant neuroleptic syndrome* (skeletal muscle rigidity, hyperthermia, stupor) that can end fatally in the absence of intensive countermeasures (including treatment with dantrolene, p. 182).

Neuroleptic activity profiles. The marked differences in action spectra of the phenothiazines, their derivatives and analogues, which may partially resemble those of butyrophenones, are important in determining therapeutic uses of neuroleptics. Relevant parameters include: antipsychotic efficacy (symbolized by the arrow); the extent of sedation; and the ability to induce extrapyramidal adverse effects. The latter depends on relative differences in antagonism towards dopamine and acetylcholine, respectively (p. 188). Thus, the butyrophenones carry an increased risk of adverse motor reactions because

they lack anticholinergic activity and, hence, are prone to upset the balance between striatal cholinergic and dopaminergic activity.

Derivatives bearing a piperazine moiety (e.g., trifluperazine, fluphenazine) have greater antipsychotic potency than do drugs containing an aliphatic side chain (e.g., chlorpromazine, triflupromazine). However, their antipsychotic effects are qualitatively indistinguishable.

As structural analogues of the phenothiazines, *thioxanthenes* (e.g., chlorprothixene, flupentixol) possess a central nucleus in which the N atom is replaced by a carbon linked via a double bond to the side chain. Unlike the phenothiazines, they display an added *thymoleptic* activity.

Clozapine is the prototype of the so-called atypical neuroleptics, a group that combines a relative lack of extrapyramidal adverse effects with superior efficacy in alleviating negative symptoms. Newer members of this class include risperidone, olanzapine, and sertindole. Two distinguishing features of these atypical agents are a higher affinity for 5-HT$_2$ (or 5-HT$_6$) receptors than for dopamine D$_2$ receptors and relative selectivity for mesolimbic, as opposed to nigrostriatal, dopamine neurons. Clozapine also exhibits high affinity for dopamine receptors of the D$_4$ subtype, in addition to H$_1$ histamine and muscarinic acetylcholine receptors. Clozapine may cause dose–dependent seizures and agranulocytosis, necessitating close hematological monitoring. It is strongly sedating.

When esterified with a fatty acid, both fluphenazine and haloperidol can be applied intramuscularly as depot preparations.

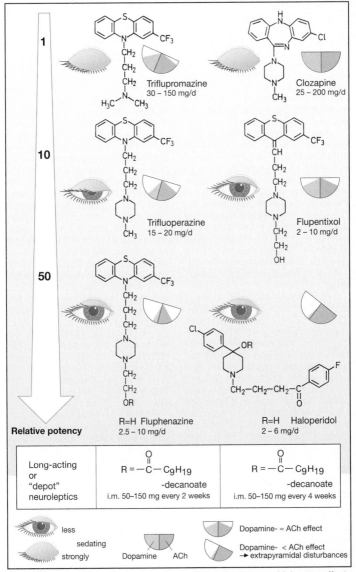

Relative potency

1	Triflupromazine 30 – 150 mg/d	Clozapine 25 – 200 mg/d
10	Trifluoperazine 15 – 20 mg/d	Flupentixol 2 – 10 mg/d
50	R=H Fluphenazine 2.5 – 10 mg/d	R=H Haloperidol 2 – 6 mg/d

| Long-acting or "depot" neuroleptics | $R = -\overset{O}{\overset{\|}{C}} - C_9H_{19}$ -decanoate i.m. 50–150 mg every 2 weeks | $R = -\overset{O}{\overset{\|}{C}} - C_9H_{19}$ -decanoate i.m. 50–150 mg every 4 weeks |

less sedating
strongly

Dopamine   ACh

Dopamine- ≈ ACh effect

Dopamine- < ACh effect
→ extrapyramidal disturbances

A. Neuroleptics: Antipsychotic potency, sedative, and extrapyramidal motor effects

Psychotomimetics
(Psychedelics, Hallucinogens)

Psychotomimetics are able to elicit psychic changes like those manifested in the course of a psychosis, such as **illusionary distortion of perception** and **hallucinations.** This experience may be of dreamlike character; its emotional or intellectual transposition appears inadequate to the outsider.

A psychotomimetic effect is pictorially recorded in the series of portraits drawn by an artist under the influence of lysergic acid diethylamide (LSD). As the intoxicated state waxes and wanes like waves, he reports seeing the face of the portrayed subject turn into a grimace, phosphoresce bluish-purple, and fluctuate in size as if viewed through a moving zoom lens, creating the illusion of abstruse changes in proportion and grotesque motion sequences. The diabolic caricature is perceived as threatening.

Illusions also affect the senses of hearing and smell; sounds (tones) are "experienced" as floating beams and visual impressions as odors ("synesthesia"). Intoxicated individuals see themselves temporarily from the outside and pass judgement on themselves and their condition. The boundary between self and the environment becomes blurred. An elating sense of being one with the other and the cosmos sets in. The sense of time is suspended; there is neither present nor past. Objects are seen that do not exist, and experiences felt that transcend explanation, hence the term "psychedelic" (Greek *delosis* = revelation) implying expansion of consciousness.

The contents of such illusions and hallucinations can occasionally become extremely threatening ("bad" or "bum trip"); the individual may feel provoked to turn violent or to commit suicide. Intoxication is followed by a phase of intense fatigue, feelings of shame, and humiliating emptiness.

The mechanism of the psychotogenic effect remains unclear. Some hallucinogens such as *LSD, psilocin, psilocybin* (from fungi), *bufotenin* (the cutaneous gland secretion of a toad), *mescaline* (from the Mexican cactuses Lophophora williamsii and L. diffusa; peyote) bear a structural resemblance to 5-HT (p. 116), and chemically synthesized amphetamine-derived hallucinogens (4-methyl-2,5-dimethoxyamphetamine; 3,4-dimethoxyamphetamine; 2,5-dimethoxy-4-ethyl amphetamine) are thought to interact with the agonist recognition site of the 5-HT$_{2A}$ receptor. Conversely, most of the psychotomimetic effects are annulled by *neuroleptics* having 5-HT$_{2A}$ antagonist activity (e.g. clozapine, risperidone). The structures of other agents such as *tetrahydrocannabinol* (from the hemp plant, *Cannabis sativa*— hashish, marihuana), *muscimol* (from the fly agaric, *Amanita muscaria*), or *phencyclidine* (formerly used as an injectable general anesthetic) do not reveal a similar connection. Hallucinations may also occur as adverse effects after intake of other substances, e.g., *scopolamine* and other centrally active parasympatholytics.

The popular psychostimulant, methylenedioxy-methamphetamine (MDMA, "ecstasy") acutely increases neuronal dopamine and norepinephrine release and causes a delayed and selective degeneration of forebrain 5-HT nerve terminals.

Although development of psychological dependence and permanent psychic damage cannot be considered established sequelae of chronic use of psychotomimetics, the manufacture and commercial distribution of these drugs are prohibited (Schedule I, Controlled Drugs).

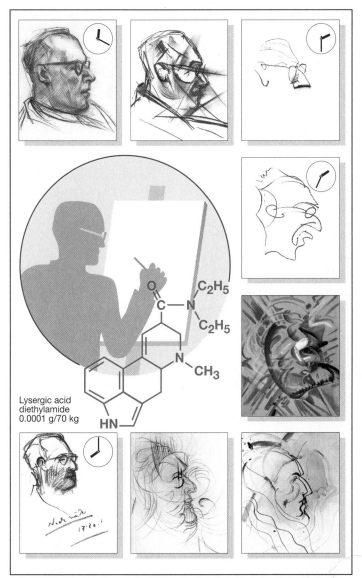

Lysergic acid
diethylamide
0.0001 g/70 kg

A. Psychotomimetic effect of LSD in a portrait artist

Hypothalamic and Hypophyseal Hormones

The endocrine system is controlled by the brain. **Nerve cells of the hypothalamus** synthesize and release messenger substances that regulate adenohypophyseal (AH) hormone release or are themselves secreted into the body as hormones. The latter comprise the so-called **neurohypophyseal (NH) hormones.**

The axonal processes of hypothalamic neurons project to the neurohypophysis, where they store the *nonapeptides vasopressin* (= *antidiuretic* hormone, ADH) and *oxytocin* and release them on demand into the blood. Therapeutically (ADH, p. 64, oxytocin, p. 126), these peptide hormones are given parenterally or via the nasal mucosa.

The **hypothalamic releasing hormones** are *peptides*. They reach their target cells in the AH lobe by way of a portal vascular route consisting of two serially connected capillary beds. The first of these lies in the hypophyseal stalk, the second corresponds to the capillary bed of the AH lobe. Here, the hypothalamic hormones diffuse from the blood to their target cells, whose activity they control. Hormones released from the AH cells enter the blood, in which they are distributed to peripheral organs **(1).**

Nomenclature of releasing hormones:

RH—releasing hormone; RIH—release inhibiting hormone.

GnRH: gonadotropin-RH = gonadorelin stimulates the release of FSH (follicle-stimulating hormone) and LH (luteinizing hormone).

TRH: thyrotropin-RH (protirelin) stimulates the release of TSH (thyroid stimulating hormone = thyrotropin).

CRH: corticotropin-RH stimulates the release of ACTH (adrenocorticotropic hormone = corticotropin).

GRH: growth hormone-RH (somatocrinin) stimulates the release of GH (growth hormone = STH, somatotropic hormone). **GRIH** somatostatin inhibits release of STH (and also other peptide hormones including insulin, glucagon, and gastrin).

PRH: prolactin-RH remains to be characterized or established. Both TRH and vasoactive intestinal peptide (VIP) are implicated.

PRIH inhibits the release of prolactin and could be identical with dopamine.

Hypothalamic releasing hormones are mostly administered (parenterally) for diagnostic reasons to test AH function.

Therapeutic control of AH cells. GnRH is used in *hypothalamic infertility in women* to stimulate FSH and LH secretion and to induce ovulation. For this purpose, it is necessary to mimic the physiologic intermittent "pulsatile" release (approx. every 90 min) by means of a programmed infusion pump.

Gonadorelin superagonists are GnRH analogues that bind with very high avidity to GnRH receptors of AH cells. As a result of the nonphysiologic uninterrupted receptor stimulation, initial augmentation of FSH and LH output is followed by a prolonged decrease. *Buserelin, leuprorelin, goserelin,* and *triptorelin* are used in patients with prostatic carcinoma to reduce production of testosterone, which promotes tumor growth. Testosterone levels fall as much as after extirpation of the testes **(2).**

The **dopamine D_2 agonists** bromocriptine and cabergoline (pp. 114, 188) inhibit prolactin-releasing AH cells (indications: suppression of lactation, prolactin-producing tumors). Excessive, but not normal, growth hormone release can also be inhibited (indication: acromegaly) **(3).**

Octreotide is a somatostatin analogue; it is used in the treatment of somatostatin-secreting pituitary tumors.

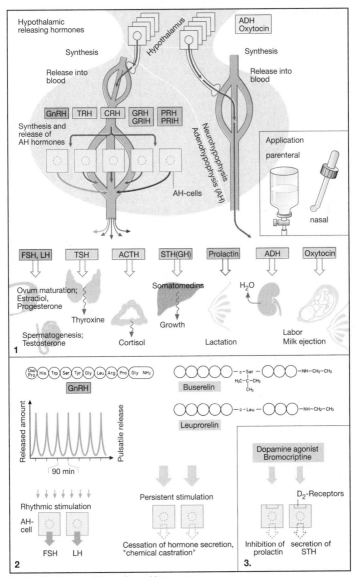

1

Hypothalamic releasing hormones

Synthesis

Release into blood

Hypothalamus

ADH
Oxytocin

Synthesis

Release into blood

GnRH | TRH | CRH | GRH GRIH | PRH PRIH

Synthesis and release of AH hormones

Neurohypophysis

Adenohypophysis (AH)

AH-cells

Application

parenteral

nasal

FSH, LH | TSH | ACTH | STH(GH) | Prolactin | ADH | Oxytocin

Ovum maturation; Estradiol, Progesterone

Somatomedins

H_2O

Thyroxine

Growth

Spermatogenesis; Testosterone

Cortisol

Lactation

Labor
Milk ejection

2

(Oxo Pro) His Trp Ser Tyr Gly Leu Arg Pro Gly NH_2

GnRH

Released amount

Pulsatile release

90 min

Buserelin

D-Ser — H_3C–C–CH_3 CH_3 — NH–CH_2–CH_3

Leuprorelin

D-Leu — NH–CH_2–CH_3

Dopamine agonist
Bromocriptine

D_2-Receptors

Rhythmic stimulation

AH-cell

FSH   LH

Persistent stimulation

Cessation of hormone secretion, "chemical castration"

3.

Inhibition of prolactin

secretion of STH

A. Hypothalamic and hypophyseal hormones

Thyroid Hormone Therapy

Thyroid hormones accelerate metabolism. Their release **(A)** is regulated by the hypophyseal glycoprotein TSH, whose release, in turn, is controlled by the hypothalamic tripeptide TRH. Secretion of TSH declines as the blood level of thyroid hormones rises; by means of this negative feedback mechanism, hormone production is "automatically" adjusted to demand.

The thyroid releases predominantly thyroxine (T_4). However, the active form appears to be triiodothyronine (T_3); T_4 is converted in part to T_3, receptor affinity in target organs being 10-fold higher for T_3. The effect of T_3 develops more rapidly and has a shorter duration than does that of T_4. Plasma elimination $t_{1/2}$ for T_4 is about 7 d; that for T_3, however, is only 1.5 d. Conversion of T_4 to T_3 releases iodide; 150 µg T_4 contains 100 µg of iodine.

For therapeutic purposes, T_4 is chosen, although T_3 is the active form and better absorbed from the gut. However, with T_4 administration, more constant blood levels can be achieved because degradation of T_4 is so slow. Since absorption of T_4 is maximal from an empty stomach, T_4 is taken about $1/2$ h before breakfast.

Replacement therapy of hypothyroidism. Whether primary, i.e., caused by thyroid disease, or secondary, i.e., resulting from TSH deficiency, hypothyroidism is treated by oral administration of T_4. Since too rapid activation of metabolism entails the hazard of cardiac overload (angina pectoris, myocardial infarction), therapy is usually started with low doses and gradually increased. The final maintenance dose required to restore a euthyroid state depends on individual needs (approx. 150 µg/d).

Thyroid suppression therapy of euthyroid goiter (B). The cause of goiter (struma) is usually a dietary deficiency of iodine. Due to an increased TSH action, the thyroid is activated to raise utilization of the little iodine available to a level at which hypothyroidism is averted. Therefore, the thyroid increases in size. In addition, intrathyroid depletion of iodine stimulates growth.

Because of the negative feedback regulation of thyroid function, thyroid activation can be inhibited by administration of T_4 doses equivalent to the endogenous daily output (approx. 150 µg/d). Deprived of stimulation, the inactive thyroid regresses in size.

If a euthyroid goiter has not persisted for too long, increasing iodine supply (potassium iodide tablets) can also be effective in reversing overgrowth of the gland.

In older patients with goiter due to iodine deficiency there is a risk of provoking hyperthyroidism by increasing iodine intake (p. 247): During chronic maximal stimulation, thyroid follicles can become independent of TSH stimulation ("autonomous tissue"). If the iodine supply is increased, thyroid hormone production increases while TSH secretion decreases due to feedback inhibition. The activity of autonomous tissue, however, persists at a high level; thyroxine is released in excess, resulting in iodine-induced hyperthyroidism.

Iodized salt prophylaxis. Goiter is endemic in regions where soils are deficient in iodine. Use of iodized table salt allows iodine requirements (150–300 µg/d) to be met and effectively prevents goiter.

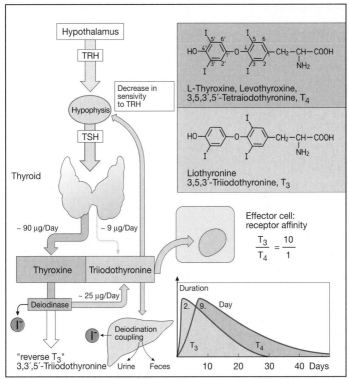

A. Thyroid hormones - release, effects, degradation

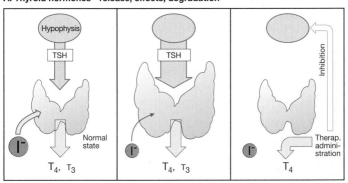

B. Endemic goiter and its treatment with thyroxine

Hyperthyroidism and Antithyroid Drugs

Thyroid overactivity in Graves' disease (**A**) results from formation of IgG antibodies that bind to and activate TSH receptors. Consequently, there is overproduction of hormone with cessation of TSH secretion. Graves' disease can abate spontaneously after 1–2 y. Therefore, initial therapy consists of reversible suppression of thyroid activity by means of antithyroid drugs. In other forms of hyperthyroidism, such as hormone-producing (morphologically benign) thyroid adenoma, the preferred therapeutic method is removal of tissue, either by surgery or administration of ^{131}iodine in sufficient dosage. Radioiodine is taken up into thyroid cells and destroys tissue within a sphere of a few millimeters by emitting β-(electron) particles during its radioactive decay.

Concerning iodine-induced hyperthyroidism, see p. 244 (**B**).

Antithyroid drugs inhibit thyroid function. Release of thyroid hormone (**C**) is preceded by a chain of events. A membrane transporter actively accumulates iodide in thyroid cells; this is followed by oxidation to iodine, iodination of tyrosine residues in thyroglobulin, conjugation of two diiodotyrosine groups, and formation of T_4 and T_3 moieties. These reactions are catalyzed by thyroid peroxidase, which is localized in the apical border of the follicular cell membrane. T_4-containing thyroglobulin is stored inside the thyroid follicles in the form of thyrocolloid. Upon endocytotic uptake, colloid undergoes lysosomal enzymatic hydrolysis, enabling thyroid hormone to be released as required. A "thyrostatic" effect can result from inhibition of synthesis or release. When synthesis is arrested, the antithyroid effect develops after a delay, as stored colloid continues to be utilized.

Antithyroid drugs for long-term therapy (C). Thiourea derivatives (thioureylenes, **thioamides**) inhibit peroxidase and, hence, hormone synthesis. In order to restore a euthyroid state, two therapeutic principles can be applied in Graves' disease: a) monotherapy with a thioamide with gradual dose reduction as the disease abates; b) administration of high doses of a thioamide with concurrent administration of thyroxine to offset diminished hormone synthesis. Adverse effects of thioamides are rare; however, the possibility of agranulocytosis has to be kept in mind.

Perchlorate, given orally as the sodium salt, inhibits the iodide pump. Adverse reactions include aplastic anemia. Compared with thioamides, its therapeutic importance is low but it is used as an adjunct in scintigraphic imaging of bone by means of technetate when accumulation in the thyroid gland has to be blocked.

Short-term thyroid suppression (C). Iodine in high dosage ($> 6000\ \mu g/d$) exerts a **transient** "thyrostatic" effect in hyperthyroid, but usually not in euthyroid, individuals. Since release is also blocked, the effect develops more rapidly than does that of thioamides.

Clinical applications include: preoperative suppression of thyroid secretion according to Plummer with *Lugol's* solution (5% iodine + 10% potassium iodide, 50–100 mg iodine/d for a maximum of 10 d). In thyrotoxic crisis, Lugol's solution is given together with thioamides and β-blockers. *Adverse effects:* allergies; *contraindications:* iodine-induced thyrotoxicosis.

Lithium ions inhibit thyroxine release. Lithium salts can be used instead of iodine for rapid thyroid suppression in iodine-induced thyrotoxicosis. Regarding administration of lithium in manic-depressive illness, see p. 234.

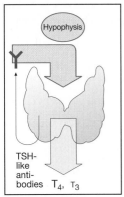
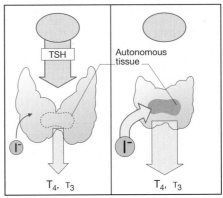

A. Graves' disease

B. Iodine hyperthyroidosis in endemic goiter

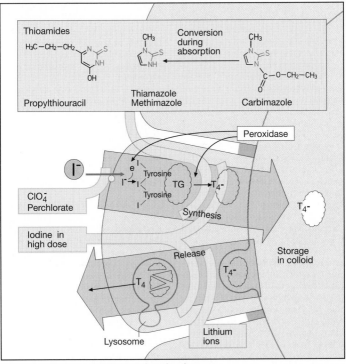

C. Antithyroid drugs and their modes of action

Glucocorticoid Therapy

I. Replacement therapy. The adrenal cortex (AC) produces the *glucocorticoid cortisol* (hydrocortisone) and the *mineralocorticoid aldosterone*. Both steroid hormones are vitally important in adaptation responses to stress situations, such as disease, trauma, or surgery. Cortisol secretion is stimulated by hypophyseal ACTH, aldosterone secretion by angiotensin II in particular (p. 124). In AC failure (*primary AC insuffiency:* Addison's disease), both *cortisol* and *aldosterone* must be replaced; when ACTH production is deficient *(secondary AC insufficiency), cortisol alone* needs to be replaced. Cortisol is effective when given orally (30 mg/d, 2/3 a.m., 1/3 p.m.). In stress situations, the dose is raised by 5- to 10-fold. Aldosterone is poorly effective via the oral route; instead, the mineralocorticoid fludrocortisone (0.1 mg/d) is given.

II. Pharmacodynamic therapy with glucocorticoids (A). In unphysiologically high concentrations, cortisol or other glucocorticoids suppress all phases (exudation, proliferation, scar formation) of the inflammatory reaction, i.e., the organism's defensive measures against foreign or noxious matter. This effect is mediated by multiple components, all of which involve alterations in gene transcription (p. 64). Glucocorticoids inhibit the expression of genes encoding for proinflammatory proteins (phospholipase-A2, cyclooxygenase 2, IL-2-receptor). The expression of these genes is stimulated by the transcription factor NF_{KB}. Binding to the glucocorticoid receptor complex prevents translocation af NF_{KB} to the nucleus. Conversely, glucocorticoids augment the expression of some anti-inflammatory proteins, e.g., lipocortin, which in turn inhibits phospholipase A2. Consequently, release of arachidonic acid is diminished, as is the formation of inflammatory mediators of the prostaglandin and leukotriene series (p. 196). At very high dosage, nongenomic effects may also contribute.

Desired effects. As *anti-allergics, immunosuppressants,* or *anti-inflammatory* drugs, glucocorticoids display excellent efficacy against "undesired" inflammatory reactions.

Unwanted effects. With *short-term use,* glucocorticoids are practically free of adverse effects, even at the highest dosage. **Long-term use** is likely to cause changes mimicking the signs of **Cushing's syndrome** (endogenous overproduction of cortisol). Sequelae of the anti-inflammatory action: lowered resistance to infection, delayed wound healing, impaired healing of peptic ulcers. Sequelae of exaggerated glucocorticoid action: a) increased gluconeogenesis and release of glucose; insulin-dependent conversion of glucose to triglycerides (adiposity mainly noticeable in the face, neck, and trunk); "steroid-diabetes" if insulin release is insufficient; b) increased protein catabolism with atrophy of skeletal musculature (thin extremities), osteoporosis, growth retardation in infants, skin atrophy. Sequelae of the intrinsically weak, but now manifest, mineralocorticoid action of cortisol: salt and fluid retention, hypertension, edema; KCl loss with danger of hypokalemia.

Measures for Attenuating or Preventing Drug-Induced Cushing's Syndrome

a) *Use of cortisol derivatives with less* (e.g., prednisolone) or *negligible mineralocorticoid activity* (e.g., triamcinolone, dexamethasone). Glucocorticoid activity of these congeners is more pronounced. Glucocorticoid, anti-inflammatory and feedback inhibitory (p. 250) actions on the hypophysis are correlated. An exclusively anti-inflammatory congener does not exist. The "glucocorticoid" related Cushingoid symptoms cannot be avoided. The table lists relative activity (potency) with reference to cortisol, whose mineralo- and glucocorticoid activities are assigned a value of 1.0. All listed glucocorticoids are effective orally.

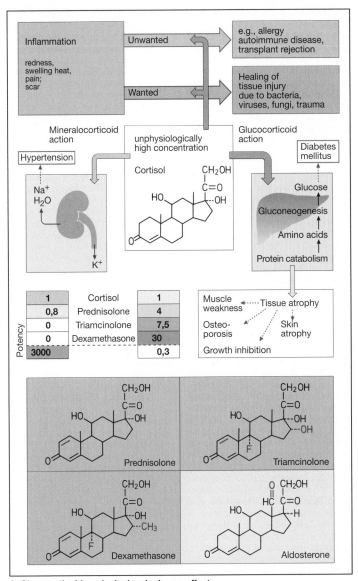

A. Glucocorticoids: principal and adverse effects

b) *Local application.* Typical adverse effects, however, also occur locally, e.g., skin atrophy or mucosal colonization with candidal fungi. To minimize systemic absorption after inhalation, derivatives should be used that have a high rate of presystemic elimination, such as beclomethasone dipropionate, flunisolide, budesonide, or fluticasone propionate (p. 14).

b) *Lowest dosage possible.* For long-term medication, a just sufficient dose should be given. However, in attempting to lower the dose to the minimal effective level, it is necessary to take into account that administration of exogenous glucocorticoids will suppress production of endogenous cortisol due to activation of an inhibitory feedback mechanism. In this manner, a very low dose could be "buffered," so that unphysiologically high glucocorticoid activity and the anti-inflammatory effect are both prevented.

Effect of glucocorticoid administration on adrenocortical cortisol production (A). Release of cortisol depends on stimulation by hypophyseal ACTH, which in turn is controlled by hypothalamic corticotropin-releasing hormone (CRH). In both the hypophysis and hypothalamus there are cortisol receptors through which cortisol can exert a feedback inhibition of ACTH or CRH release. By means of these cortisol "sensors," the regulatory centers can monitor whether the actual blood level of the hormone corresponds to the "set-point." If the blood level exceeds the set-point, ACTH output is decreased and, thus, also the cortisol production. In this way cortisol level is maintained within the required range. The regulatory centers respond to synthetic glucocorticoids as they do to cortisol. Administration of exogenous cortisol or any other glucocorticoid reduces the amount of endogenous cortisol needed to maintain homeostasis. Release of CRH and ACTH declines ("inhibition of higher centers by exogenous glucocorticoid") and, thus, cortisol secretion ("adrenocortical suppression"). After weeks of exposure to unphysio-

logically high glucocorticoid doses, the cortisol-producing portions of the adrenal cortex shrink ("adrenocortical atrophy"). Aldosterone-synthesizing capacity, however, remains unaffected. When glucocorticoid medication is suddenly withheld, the atrophic cortex is unable to produce sufficient cortisol and a potentially life-threatening cortisol deficiency may develop. Therefore, glucocorticoid therapy should always be tapered off by gradual reduction of the dosage.

Regimens for prevention of adrenocortical atrophy. Cortisol secretion is high in the early morning and low in the late evening (circadian rhythm). This fact implies that the regulatory centers continue to release CRH or ACTH in the face of high morning blood levels of cortisol; accordingly, sensitivity to feedback inhibition must be low in the morning, whereas the opposite holds true in the late evening.

a) *Circadian administration:* The daily dose of glucocorticoid is given in the morning. Endogenous cortisol production will have already begun, the regulatory centers being relatively insensitive to inhibition. In the early morning hours of the next day, CRF/-ACTH release and adrenocortical stimulation will resume.

b) *Alternate-day therapy:* Twice the daily dose is given on alternate mornings. On the "off" day, endogenous cortisol production is allowed to occur.

The disadvantage of either regimen is a recrudescence of disease symptoms during the glucocorticoid-free interval.

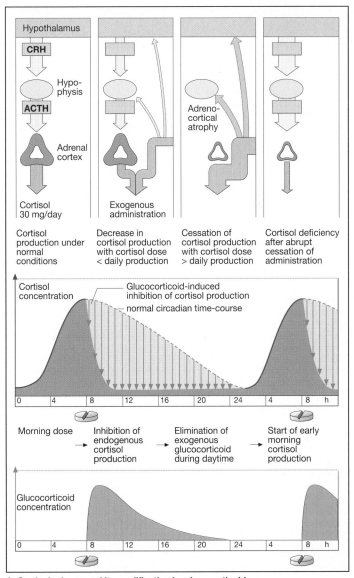

A. Cortisol release and its modification by glucocorticoids

Androgens, Anabolic Steroids, Antiandrogens

Androgens are masculinizing substances. The endogenous male gonadal hormone is the steroid **testosterone** from the interstitial Leydig cells of the testis. Testosterone secretion is stimulated by hypophyseal luteinizing hormone (LH), whose release is controlled by hypothalamic GnRH (gonadorelin, p. 242). Release of both hormones is subject to feedback inhibition by circulating testosterone. Reduction of testosterone to dihydrotestosterone occurs in most target organs; the latter possesses higher affinity for androgen receptors. Rapid intrahepatic degradation (plasma $t_{1/2} \sim$ 15 min) yields androsterone among other metabolites (17-ketosteroids) that are eliminated as conjugates in the urine. Because of rapid hepatic metabolism, testosterone is unsuitable for oral use. Although it is well absorbed, it undergoes virtually complete presystemic elimination.

Testosterone (T.) derivatives for clinical use. *T. esters for i.m. depot injection are T. propionate and T. heptanoate* (or *enanthate*). These are given in oily solution by deep intramuscular injection. Upon diffusion of the ester from the depot, esterases quickly split off the acyl residue, to yield free T. With increasing lipophilicity, esters will tend to remain in the depot, and the duration of action therefore lengthens. A *T. ester for oral use is the undecanoate.* Owing to the fatty acid nature of undecanoic acid, this ester is absorbed into the lymph, enabling it to bypass the liver and enter, via the thoracic duct, the general circulation. *17-a Methyltestosterone is* effective by the oral route due to its increased metabolic stability, but because of the hepatotoxicity of C17-alkylated androgens (cholestasis, tumors) its use should be avoided. Orally active *mesterolone* is 1α-methyl-dihydrotestosterone. Transdermal delivery systems for T. are also available.

Indications. For hormone replacement in deficiency of endogenous T. production and palliative treatment of breast cancer, T. esters for depot injection are optimally suited. Secondary sex characteristics and libido are maintained; however, fertility is not promoted. On the contrary, spermatogenesis may be suppressed because of feedback inhibition of hypothalamohypophyseal gonadotropin secretion.

Stimulation of spermatogenesis in gonadotropin (FSH, LH) deficiency can be achieved by injection of HMG and HCG. HMG or *human menopausal gonadotropin* is obtained from the urine of postmenopausal women and is rich in FSH activity. HCG, *human chorionic gonadotropin,* from the urine of pregnant women, acts like LH.

Anabolics are testosterone derivatives (e.g., clostebol, metenolone, nandrolone, stanozolol) that are used in debilitated patients, and misused by athletes, because of their protein anabolic effect. They act via stimulation of androgen receptors and, thus, also display androgenic actions (e.g., virilization in females, suppression of spermatogenesis).

The **antiandrogen cyproterone** acts as a competitive antagonist of T. In addition, it has progestin activity whereby it inhibits gonadotropin secretion (p. 254). **Indications:** in men, inhibition of sex drive in hypersexuality; prostatic cancer. In women: treatment of virilization, with potential utilization of the gestagenic contraceptive effect.

Flutamide, an androgen receptor antagonist possessing a different chemical structure, lacks progestin activity.

Finasteride inhibits 5α-reductase, the enzyme converting T. into dihydrotestosterone (DHT). Thus, the androgenic stimulus is reduced in those tissues in which DHT is the active species (e.g., prostate). T.-dependent tissues or functions are not or hardly affected (e.g., skeletal muscle, negative feedback inhibition of gonadotropin secretion, and libido). Finasteride can be used in benign prostate hyperplasia to shrink the gland and, possibly, to improve micturition.

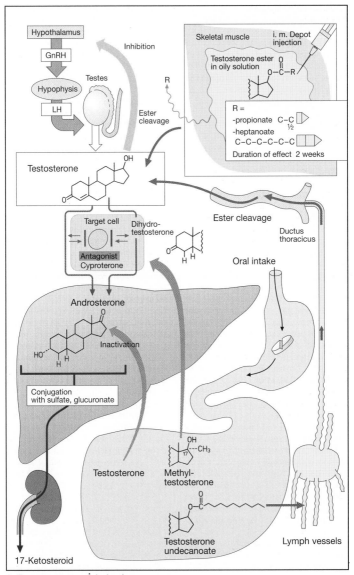

A. Testosterone and derivatives

Follicular Growth and Ovulation, Estrogen and Progestin Production

Follicular maturation and ovulation, as well as the associated production of female gonadal hormones, are controlled by the hypophyseal gonadotropins FSH (follicle-stimulating hormone) and LH (luteinizing hormone). In the first half of the menstrual cycle, FSH promotes growth and maturation of ovarian follicles that respond with accelerating synthesis of estradiol. Estradiol stimulates endometrial growth and increases the permeability of cervical mucus for sperm cells. When the estradiol blood level approaches a predetermined setpoint, FSH release is inhibited due to feedback action on the anterior hypophysis. Since follicle growth and estrogen production are correlated, hypophysis and hypothalamus can "monitor" the follicular phase of the ovarian cycle through their estrogen receptors. Within hours after ovulation, the tertiary follicle develops into the corpus luteum, which then also releases progesterone in response to LH. The former initiates the secretory phase of the endometrial cycle and lowers the permeability of cervical mucus. Nonruptured follicles continue to release estradiol under the influence of FSH. After 2 wk, production of progesterone and estradiol subsides, causing the secretory endometrial layer to be shed (menstruation).

The natural hormones are unsuitable for oral application because they are subject to presystemic hepatic elimination. Estradiol is converted via estrone to estriol; by conjugation, all three can be rendered water soluble and amenable to renal excretion. The major metabolite of progesterone is pregnandiol, which is also conjugated and eliminated renally.

Estrogen preparations. Depot preparations for i.m. injection are oily solutions of esters of estradiol (3- or 17-OH group). The hydrophobicity of the acyl moiety determines the rate of absorption, hence the duration of effect (p. 252). Released ester is hydrolyzed to yield free estradiol.

Orally used preparations. *Ethinylestradiol (EE)* is more stable metabolically, passes largely unchanged through the liver after oral intake and mimics estradiol at estrogen receptors. *Mestranol* itself is inactive; however, cleavage of the C-3 methoxy group again yields EE. In oral contraceptives, one of the two agents forms the estrogen component (p. 256). (Sulfate-)*conjugated estrogens* can be extracted from equine urine and are used for the prevention of postmenopausal osteoporosis and in the therapy of climacteric complaints. Because of their high polarity (sulfate, glucuronide), they would hardly appear suitable for this route of administration. For **transdermal delivery,** an adhesive patch is available that releases estradiol transcutaneously into the body.

Progestin preparations. Depot formulations for i.m. injection are *17-α-hydroxyprogesterone caproate* and *medroxyprogesterone acetate.* Preparations for oral use are derivatives of 17α-ethinyltestosterone = ethisterone (e.g., norethisterone, dimethisterone, lynestrenol, desogestrel, gestoden), or of 17α-hydroxyprogesterone acetate (e.g., chlormadinone acetate or cyproterone acetate). These agents are mainly used as the progestin component in oral contraceptives.

Indications for estrogens and progestins include: hormonal contraception (p. 256), hormone replacement, as in postmenopausal women for prophylaxis of osteoporosis; bleeding anomalies, menstrual complaints. Concerning adverse effects, see p. 256.

Estrogens with partial agonist activity (**raloxifene, tamoxifene**) are being investigated as agents used to replace estrogen in postmenopausal osteoporosis treatment, to lower plasma lipids, and as estrogen antagonists in the prevention of breast cancer. Raloxifen—in contrast to tamoxifen—is an antagonist at uterine estrogen receptors.

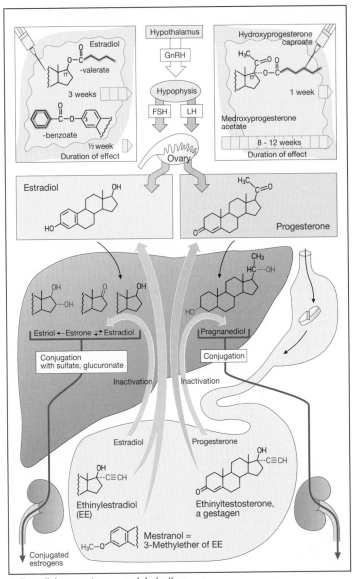

A. Estradiol, progesterone, and derivatives

Oral Contraceptives

Inhibitors of ovulation. Negative feedback control of gonadotropin release can be utilized to inhibit the ovarian cycle. **Administration of exogenous estrogens** (ethinylestradiol or mestranol) during the first half of the cycle permits **FSH production to be suppressed** (as it is by administration of progestins alone). Due to the reduced FSH stimulation of tertiary follicles, **maturation of follicles and, hence, ovulation are prevented.** In effect, the regulatory brain centers are deceived, as it were, by the elevated estrogen blood level, which signals normal follicular growth and a decreased requirement for FSH stimulation. If estrogens alone are given during the first half of the cycle, endometrial and cervical responses, as well as other functional changes, would occur in the normal fashion. By adding a progestin (p. 254) during the second half of the cycle, the secretory phase of the endometrium and associated effects can be elicited. Discontinuance of hormone administration would be followed by menstruation.

The physiological time course of estrogen-progesterone release is simulated in the so-called **biphasic (sequential) preparations (A).** In **monophasic preparations,** estrogen and progestin are taken concurrently. Early administration of progestin reinforces the inhibition of CNS regulatory mechanisms, prevents both normal endometrial growth and conditions for ovum implantation, and decreases penetrability of cervical mucus for sperm cells. The two latter effects also act to prevent conception. According to the staging of progestin administration, one distinguishes **(A):** one-, two-, and three-stage preparations. In all cases, "withdrawal-bleeding" occurs when hormone intake is discontinued (if necessary, by substituting dummy tablets).

Unwanted effects: An increased incidence of thrombosis and embolism is attributed to the estrogen component in particular. Hypertension, fluid retention, cholestasis, benign liver tumors, nausea, chest pain, etc. may occur. Apparently there is no increased overall risk of malignant tumors.

Minipill. Continuous low-dose administration of progestin alone can prevent conception. Ovulations are not suppressed regularly; the effect is then due to progestin-induced alterations in cervical and endometrial function. Because of the need for constant intake at the same time of day, a lower success rate, and relatively frequent bleeding anomalies, these preparations are now rarely employed.

"Morning-after" pill. This refers to administration of a high dose of estrogen and progestin, preferably within 12 to 24 h, but no later than 72 h after coitus. Menstrual bleeding ensues, which prevents implantation of the fertilized ovum (normally on the 7th day after fertilization, p. 74). Similarly, implantation can be inhibited by mifepristone, which is an antagonist at both progesterone and glucocorticoid receptors and which also offers a noninvasive means of inducing therapeutic abortion in early pregnancy.

Stimulation of ovulation. Gonadotropin secretion can be increased by *pulsatile delivery of GnRH* (p. 242). The *estrogen antagonists clomiphene* and *cyclofenil* block receptors mediating feedback inhibition of central neuroendocrine circuits and thereby disinhibit gonadotropin release. *Gonadotropins* can be given in the form of HMG and HCG (p. 252).

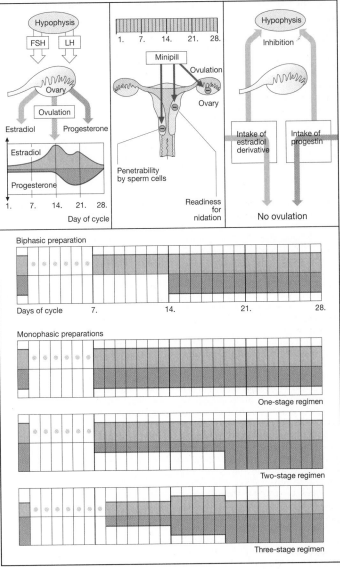

A. Oral contraceptives

Insulin Therapy

Insulin is synthesized in the B- (or β-) cells of the pancreatic islets of Langerhans. It is a protein (MW 5800) consisting of two peptide chains linked by two disulfide bridges; the A chain has 21 and the B chain 30 amino acids. Insulin is the "blood-sugar lowering" hormone. Upon ingestion of dietary carbohydrates, it is released into the blood and acts to prevent a significant rise in blood glucose concentration by promoting uptake of glucose in specific organs, viz., the heart, adipose tissue, and skeletal muscle, or its conversion to glycogen in the liver. It also increases lipogenesis and protein synthesis, while inhibiting lipolysis and release of free fatty acids.

Insulin is used in the **replacement therapy** of **diabetes mellitus** to supplement a deficient secretion of endogenous hormone.

Sources of therapeutic insulin preparations (A). Insulin can be obtained from pancreatic tissue of slaughtered animals. *Porcine insulin* differs from human insulin merely by one B chain amino acid, *bovine insulin* by two amino acids in the A chain and one in the B chain. With these slight differences, animal and human hormone display similar biological activity. Compared with human hormone, porcine insulin is barely antigenic and bovine insulin has a little higher antigenicity. *Human insulin* is produced by two methods: biosynthetically, by substituting threonine for the C-terminal alanine in the B chain of porcine insulin; or by gene technology involving insertion of the appropriate human DNA into *E. coli* bacteria.

Types of preparations (B). As a peptide, insulin is unsuitable for oral administration (destruction by gastrointestinal proteases) and thus needs to be given parenterally. Usually, insulin preparations are injected subcutaneously. The duration of action depends on the rate of absorption from the injection site.

Short-acting insulin is dispensed as a clear neutral **solution** known as **regular insulin.** In emergencies, such as hyperglycemic coma, it can be given intravenously (mostly by infusion because i.v. injections have too brief an action; plasma $t_{1/2}$ ~ 9 min). With the usual subcutaneous application, the effect is evident within 15 to 20 min, reaches a peak after approx. 3 h, and lasts for approx. 6 h. *Lispro insulin* has a faster onset and slightly shorter duration of action.

Insulin suspensions. When the hormone is injected as a suspension of insulin-containing particles, its dissolution and release in subcutaneous tissue are retarded (**rapid, intermediate,** and **slow insulins**). Suitable particles can be obtained by precipitation of apolar, poorly water-soluble complexes consisting of anionic insulin and cationic partners, e.g., the polycationic protein protamine or the compound aminoquinuride (Surfen). In the presence of zinc and acetate ions, insulin crystallizes; crystal size determines the rate of dissolution. Intermediate insulin preparations (NPH or isophane, lente or zinc insulin) act for 18 to 26 h, slow preparations (protamine zinc insulin, ultralente or extended zinc insulin) for up to 36 h.

Combination preparations contain insulin mixtures in solution and in suspension (e.g., *ultralente*); the plasma concentration-time curve represents the sum of the two components.

Unwanted effects. *Hypoglycemia* results from absolute or relative overdosage (see p. 260). *Allergic reactions* are rare—locally: redness at injection site, atrophy of adipose tissue (lipodystrophy); systemically: urticaria, skin rash, anaphylaxis. Insulin resistance can result from binding to inactivating antibodies. A possible local lipohypertrophy can be avoided by alternating injection sites.

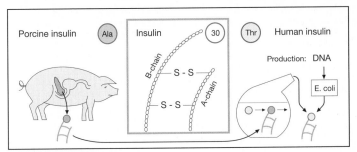

A. Insulin production

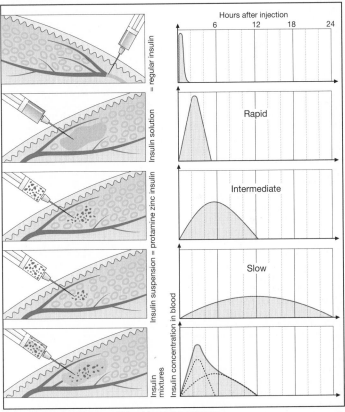

B. Insulin: preparations and blood level-time curves

Treatment of Insulin-Dependent Diabetes Mellitus

"Juvenile onset" (type I) diabetes mellitus is caused by the destruction of insulin-producing B cells in the pancreas, necessitating replacement of insulin (daily dose approx. 40 U, equivalent to approx. 1.6 mg).

Therapeutic objectives are: (1) prevention of life-threatening hyperglycemic (diabetic) coma; (2) prevention of diabetic sequelae (angiopathy with blindness, myocardial infarction, renal failure), with precise "titration" of the patient being essential to avoid even short-term spells of pathological hyperglycemia; (3) prevention of insulin overdosage leading to life-threatening hypoglycemic shock (CNS disturbance due to lack of glucose).

Therapeutic principles. In healthy subjects, the amount of insulin is "automatically" matched to carbohydrate intake, hence to blood glucose concentration. The critical secretory stimulus is the rise in plasma glucose level. Food intake and physical activity (increased glucose uptake into musculature, decreased insulin demand) are accompanied by corresponding changes in insulin secretion (**A**, left track).

In the diabetic, insulin could be administered as it is normally secreted; that is, injection of short-acting insulin before each main meal plus bedtime administration of a Lente preparation to avoid a nocturnal shortfall of insulin. This regimen requires a well-educated, cooperative, and competent patient. In other cases, a fixed-dosage schedule will be needed, e.g., morning and evening injections of a combination insulin in constant respective dosage (**A**). To avoid hypo- or hyperglycemias with this regimen, dietary carbohydrate (CH) intake must be synchronized with the time course of insulin absorption from the s.c. depot. Caloric intake is to be distributed (50% CH, 30% fat, 20% protein) in small meals over the day so as to achieve a steady CH supply—snacks, late night meal. Rapidly absorbable CH

(sweets, cakes) must be avoided (hyperglycemic−peaks) and replaced with slowly digestible ones.

Acarbose (an α-glucosidase inhibitor) delays intestinal formation of glucose from disaccharides.

Any change in eating and living habits can upset control of blood sugar: skipping a meal or unusual physical stress leads to hypoglycemia; increased CH intake provokes hyperglycemia.

Hypoglycemia is heralded by warning signs: tachycardia, unrest, tremor, pallor, profuse sweating. Some of these are due to the release of glucose-mobilizing epinephrine. *Countermeasures:* glucose administration, rapidly absorbed CH orally or 10–20 g glucose i.v. in case of unconsciousness; if necessary, injection of glucagon, the pancreatic hyperglycemic hormone.

Even with optimal control of blood sugar, s.c. administration of insulin cannot fully replicate the physiological situation. In healthy subjects, absorbed glucose and insulin released from the pancreas simultaneously reach the liver in high concentration, whereby effective presystemic elimination of both substances is achieved. In the diabetic, s.c. injected insulin is uniformly distributed in the body. Since insulin concentration in blood supplying the liver cannot rise, less glucose is extracted from portal blood. A significant amount of glucose enters extrahepatic tissues, where it has to be utilized.

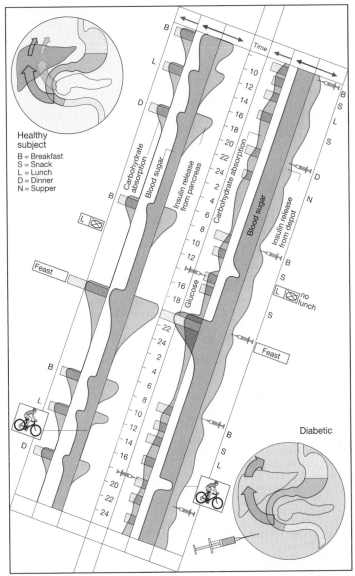

A. Control of blood sugar in healthy and diabetic subjects

Treatment of Maturity-Onset (Type II) Diabetes Mellitus

In overweight adults, a diabetic metabolic condition may develop (type II or *non-insulin-dependent diabetes*) when there is a relative insulin deficiency—enhanced demand cannot be met by a diminishing insulin secretion. The **cause of increased insulin requirement** is a loss of **insulin receptors** or an impairment of the signal cascade activated by the insulin receptor. Accordingly, insulin sensitivity of cells declines. This can be illustrated by comparing concentration-binding curves in cells from normal and obese individuals **(A)**. In the obese, the maximum binding possible (plateau of curve) is displaced downward, indicative of the reduction in receptor numbers. Also, at low insulin concentrations, there is less binding of insulin, compared with the control condition. For a given metabolic effect a certain number of receptors must be occupied. As shown by the binding curves (dashed lines), this can still be achieved with a reduced receptor number, although only at a higher concentration of insulin.

Development of adult diabetes (B). Compared with a normal subject, the obese subject requires a continually elevated output of insulin (orange curves) to avoid an excessive rise of blood glucose levels (green curves) during a glucose load. When the secretory capacity of the pancreas decreases, this is first noted as a rise in blood glucose during glucose loading (latent diabetes). Subsequently, not even the fasting blood level can be maintained (manifest, overt diabetes). A diabetic condition has developed, although insulin release is not lower than that in a healthy person (relative insulin deficiency).

Treatment. Caloric restriction to restore body weight to normal is associated with an increase in insulin receptor number or cellular responsiveness. The releasable amount of insulin is again adequate to maintain a normal metabolic rate.

Therapy of first choice is weight reduction, not administration of drugs! Should the diabetic condition fail to resolve, consideration should first be given to insulin replacement (p. 260). **Oral antidiabetics of the *sulfonylurea* type** increase the sensitivity of B-cells towards glucose, enabling them to increase release of insulin. These drugs probably promote depolarization of the β-cell membrane by closing off ATP-gated K^+ channels. Normally, these channels are closed when intracellular levels of glucose, hence of ATP, increase. This drug class includes tolbutamide (500–2000 mg/d) and glyburide (glibenclamide) (1.75–10.5 mg/d). In some patients, it is not possible to stimulate insulin secretion from the outset; in others, therapy fails later on. Matching dosage of the oral antidiabetic and caloric intake follows the same principles as apply to insulin. Hypoglycemia is the most important unwanted effect. Enhancement of the hypoglycemic effect can result from drug interactions: displacement of antidiabetic drug from plasma protein-binding sites by sulfonamides or acetylsalicylic acid.

Metformin, a biguanide derivative, can lower excessive blood glucose levels, provided that insulin is present. Metformin does not stimulate insulin release. Glucose release from the liver is decreased, while peripheral uptake is enhanced. The danger of hypoglycemia apparently is not increased. Frequent adverse effects include: anorexia, nausea, and diarrhea. Overproduction of lactic acid (lactate acidosis, lethality 50%) is a rare, potentially fatal reaction. Metformin is used in combination with sulfonylureas or by itself. It is contraindicated in renal insufficiency and should therefore be avoided in elderly patients.

Thiazolidinediones (**Glitazones:** rosiglitazone, pioglitazone) are insulin-sensitizing agents that augment tissue responsiveness by promoting the synthesis or the availability of plasmalemmal glucose transporters via activation of a transcription factor (peroxisome proliferator-activated receptor-γ).

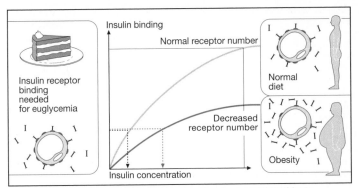

A. Insulin concentration and binding in normal and overweight subjects

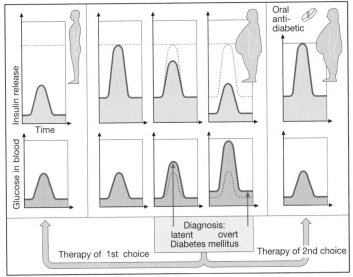

B. Development of maturity-onset diabetes

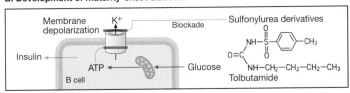

C. Action of oral antidiabetic drugs

Drugs for Maintaining Calcium Homeostasis

At rest, the intracellular concentration of free calcium ions (Ca^{2+}) is kept at 0.1 µM (see p. 128 for mechanisms involved). During excitation, a transient rise of up to 10 µM elicits contraction in muscle cells (electromechanical coupling) and secretion in glandular cells (electrosecretory coupling). The cellular content of Ca^{2+} is in equilibrium with the extracellular Ca^{2+} concentration (approx. 1000 µM), as is the plasma protein-bound fraction of calcium in blood. Ca^{2+} may crystallize with phosphate to form hydroxyapatite, the mineral of bone. Osteoclasts are phagocytes that mobilize Ca^{2+} by resorption of bone. Slight changes in extracellular Ca^{2+} concentration can alter organ function: thus, excitability of skeletal muscle increases markedly as Ca^{2+} is lowered (e.g., in hyperventilation tetany). Three hormones are available to the body for maintaining a constant extracellular Ca^{2+} concentration.

Vitamin D hormone is derived from *vitamin D (cholecalciferol).* Vitamin D can also be produced in the body; it is formed in the skin from dehydrocholesterol during irradiation with UV light. When there is lack of solar radiation, dietary intake becomes essential, cod liver oil being a rich source. Metabolically active vitamin D hormone results from two successive hydroxylations: in the liver at position 25 (→ calcifediol) and in the kidney at position 1 (→ calcitriol = vit. D hormone). 1-Hydroxylation depends on the level of calcium homeostasis and is stimulated by parathormone and a fall in plasma levels of Ca^{2+} or phosphate. Vit. D hormone promotes enteral absorption and renal reabsorption of Ca^{2+} and phosphate. As a result of the increased Ca^{2+} and phosphate concentration in blood, there is an increased tendency for these ions to be deposited in bone in the form of hydroxyapatite crystals. In vit. D deficiency, bone mineralization is inadequate (rickets, osteomalacia). **Therapeutic** use aims at *replacement.* Mostly, vit. D is given; in liver disease calcifediol may be indicated, in renal disease calcitriol. Effectiveness, as well as rate of onset and cessation of action, increase in the order vit. D. < 25-OH-vit. D < 1,25-di-OH-vit. D. **Overdosage** may induce hypercalcemia with deposits of calcium salts in tissues (particularly in kidney and blood vessels): calcinosis.

The polypeptide **parathormone** is released from the parathyroid glands when plasma Ca^{2+} level falls. It *stimulates osteoclasts* to increase bone resorption; in the kidneys, it promotes calcium reabsorption, while phosphate excretion is enhanced. As blood phosphate concentration diminishes, the tendency of calcium to precipitate as bone mineral decreases. By stimulating the formation of vit. D hormone, parathormone has an indirect effect on the enteral uptake of Ca^{2+} and phosphate. In parathormone deficiency, **vitamin D** can be used as a substitute that, unlike parathormone, is effective orally.

The polypeptide **calcitonin** is secreted by thyroid C-cells during imminent hypercalcemia. It lowers plasma Ca^{2+} levels by *inhibiting osteoclast activity.* Its uses include hypercalcemia and osteoporosis. Remarkably, calcitonin injection may produce a sustained *analgesic* effect that is not restricted to bone pain.

Hypercalcemia can be treated by (1) administering 0.9% NaCl solution plus furosemide (if necessary) → renal excretion ↑; (2) the osteoclast inhibitors calcitonin, plicamycin, or clodronate (a bisphosphonate) → bone calcium mobilization ↓; (3) the Ca^{2+} chelators EDTA sodium or sodium citrate; as well as (4) glucocorticoids.

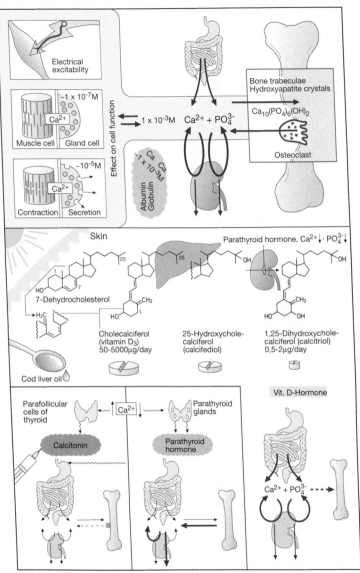

A. Calcium homeostasis of the body

Antibacterial Drugs

Drugs for Treating Bacterial Infections

When bacteria overcome the cutaneous or mucosal barriers and penetrate body tissues, a bacterial *infection* is present. Frequently the body succeeds in removing the invaders, without outward signs of disease, by mounting an immune response. If bacteria multiply faster than the body's defenses can destroy them, *infectious disease* develops with inflammatory signs, e.g., purulent wound infection or urinary tract infection. Appropriate treatment employs substances that injure bacteria and thereby prevent their further multiplication, without harming cells of the host organism (**1**).

Apropos nomenclature: **antibiotics** are produced by microorganisms (fungi, bacteria) and are directed "against life" at any phylogenetic level (prokaryotes, eukaryotes). **Chemotherapeutic agents** originate from chemical synthesis. This distinction has been lost in current usage.

Specific damage to bacteria is particularly practicable when a substance interferes with a metabolic process that occurs in bacterial but not in host cells. Clearly this applies to inhibitors of cell wall synthesis, because human and animal cells lack a cell wall. The **points of attack of antibacterial agents** are schematically illustrated in a grossly simplified bacterial cell, as depicted in (**2**).

In the following sections, polymyxins and tyrothricin are not considered further. These polypeptide antibiotics enhance cell membrane permeability. Due to their poor tolerability, they are prescribed in humans only for topical use.

The effect of antibacterial drugs can be observed *in vitro* (**3**). Bacteria multiply in a growth medium under control conditions. If the medium contains an antibacterial drug, two results can be discerned: 1. bacteria are killed—**bactericidal effect;** 2. bacteria survive, but do not multiply—**bacteriostatic effect.** Although variations may occur under therapeutic conditions, different drugs

can be classified according to their respective primary mode of action (color tone in **2** and **3**).

When bacterial growth remains unaffected by an antibacterial drug, bacterial **resistance** is present. This may occur because of certain metabolic characteristics that confer a natural insensitivity to the drug on a particular strain of bacteria *(natural resistance)*. Depending on whether a drug affects only a few or numerous types of bacteria, the terms **narrow-spectrum** (e.g., penicillin G) or **broad-spectrum** (e.g., tetracyclines) **antibiotic** are applied. Naturally susceptible bacterial strains can be transformed under the influence of antibacterial drugs into resistant ones *(acquired resistance)*, when a random genetic alteration (mutation) gives rise to a resistant bacterium. Under the influence of the drug, the susceptible bacteria die off, whereas the mutant multiplies unimpeded. The more frequently a given drug is applied, the more probable the emergence of resistant strains (e.g., hospital strains with multiple resistance)!

Resistance can also be acquired when DNA responsible for nonsusceptibility (so-called *resistance plasmid*) is passed on from other resistant bacteria by conjugation or transduction.

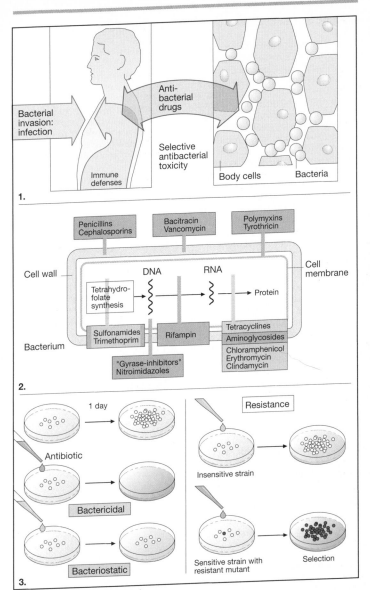

A. Principles of antibacterial therapy

Inhibitors of Cell Wall Synthesis

In most bacteria, a cell wall surrounds the cell like a rigid shell that protects against noxious outside influences and prevents rupture of the plasma membrane from a high internal osmotic pressure. The structural stability of the cell wall is due mainly to the **murein (peptidoglycan) lattice.** This consists of basic building blocks linked together to form a large macromolecule. Each basic unit contains the two linked aminosugars N-acetylglucosamine and N-acetylmuramyl acid; the latter bears a peptide chain. The building blocks are synthesized in the bacterium, transported outward through the cell membrane, and assembled as illustrated schematically. The enzyme transpeptidase cross-links the peptide chains of adjacent aminosugar chains.

Inhibitors of cell wall synthesis are suitable antibacterial agents, because animal and human cells lack a cell wall. They exert a **bactericidal** action on growing or multiplying germs. Members of this class include β-lactam antibiotics such as the *penicillins* and *cephalosporins*, in addition to *bacitracin* and *vancomycin.*

Penicillins (A). The parent substance of this group is **penicillin G (benzylpenicillin).** It is obtained from cultures of mold fungi, originally from *Penicillium notatum.* Penicillin G contains the basic structure common to all penicillins, **6-amino-penicillanic acid** (p. 271, 6-APA), comprised of a thiazolidine and a 4-membered β-**lactam ring.** 6-APA itself lacks antibacterial activity. Penicillins disrupt cell wall synthesis by inhibiting **transpeptidase.** When bacteria are in their growth and replication phase, penicillins are bactericidal; due to cell wall defects, the bacteria swell and burst.

Penicillins are generally well tolerated; with penicillin G, the **daily dose** can range from approx. 0.6 g i.m. (= 10^6 international units, 1 Mega I.U.) to 60 g by infusion. The most important **adverse effects** are due to *hypersensitivity* (incidence up to 5%), with manifestations ranging from skin eruptions to anaphylactic shock (in less than 0.05% of patients). Known penicillin allergy is a contraindication for these drugs. Because of an increased risk of sensitization, penicillins must not be used locally. *Neurotoxic effects,* mostly convulsions due to GABA antagonism, may occur if the brain is exposed to extremely high concentrations, e.g., after rapid i.v. injection of a large dose or intrathecal injection.

Penicillin G undergoes rapid renal **elimination** mainly in unchanged form (plasma $t_{1/2}$ ~ 0.5 h). The **duration of the effect can be prolonged** by:

1. *Use of higher doses,* enabling plasma levels to remain above the minimally effective antibacterial concentration;

2. *Combination with probenecid.* Renal elimination of penicillin occurs chiefly via the anion (acid)-secretory system of the proximal tubule (-COOH of 6-APA). The acid probenecid (p. 316) competes for this route and thus retards penicillin elimination;

3. *Intramuscular administration in depot form.* In its anionic form (-COO⁻) penicillin G forms poorly water-soluble salts with substances containing a positively charged amino group (procaine, p. 208; clemizole, an antihistamine; benzathine, dicationic). Depending on the substance, release of penicillin from the depot occurs over a variable interval.

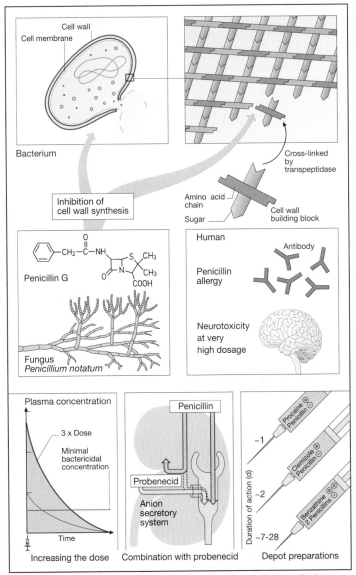

A. Penicillin G: structure and origin; mode of action of penicillins; methods for prolonging duration of action

Although very well tolerated, **penicillin G** has disadvantages **(A)** that limit its therapeutic usefulness: (1) It is inactivated by gastric acid, which cleaves the β-lactam ring, necessitating parenteral administration. (2) The β-lactam ring can also be opened by bacterial enzymes (β-lactamases); in particular, penicillinase, which can be produced by staphylococcal strains, renders them resistant to penicillin G. (3) The antibacterial spectrum is narrow; although it encompasses many gram-positive bacteria, gram-negative cocci, and spirochetes, many gram-negative pathogens are unaffected.

Derivatives with a different substituent on 6-APA possess **advantages (B):** (1) **Acid resistance** permits oral administration, provided that enteral absorption is possible. All derivatives shown in **(B)** can be given orally. *Penicillin V* (phenoxymethylpenicillin) exhibits antibacterial properties similar to those of penicillin G. (2) Due to their **penicillinase resistance,** *isoxazolylpenicillins (oxacillin dicloxacillin, flucloxacillin)* are suitable for the (oral) treatment of infections caused by penicillinase-producing staphylococci. (3) **Extended activity spectrum:** The aminopenicillin *amoxicillin* is active against many gram-negative organisms, e.g., coli bacteria or Salmonella typhi. It can be protected from destruction by penicillinase by combination with inhibitors of penicillinase *(clavulanic acid, sulbactam, tazobactam).*

The structurally close congener *ampicillin* (no 4-hydroxy group) has a similar activity spectrum. However, because it is poorly absorbed (<50%) and therefore causes more extensive damage to the gut microbial flora (side effect: diarrhea), it should be given only by injection.

A still broader spectrum (including Pseudomonas bacteria) is shown by *carboxypenicillins* (carbenicillin, ticarcillin) and acylaminopenicillins (mezlocillin, azlocillin, piperacillin). These substances are neither acid stable nor penicillinase resistant.

Cephalosporins (C). These β-lactam antibiotics are also fungal products and have bactericidal activity due to **inhibition of transpeptidase.** Their shared basic structure is 7-aminocephalosporanic acid, as exemplified by *cephalexin* (gray rectangle). Cephalosporins are acid stable, but many are poorly absorbed. Because they must be given parenterally, most—including those with high activity—are used only in clinical settings. A few, e.g., cephalexin, are suitable for oral use. Cephalosporins are penicillinase-resistant, but cephalosporinase-forming organisms do exist. Some derivatives are, however, also resistant to this β-lactamase. Cephalosporins are broad-spectrum antibacterials. Newer derivatives (e.g., cefotaxime, cefmenoxin, cefoperazone, ceftriaxone, ceftazidime, moxalactam) are also effective against pathogens resistant to various other antibacterials. Cephalosporins are mostly well tolerated. All can cause allergic reactions, some also renal injury, alcohol intolerance, and bleeding (vitamin K antagonism).

Other inhibitors of cell wall synthesis. Bacitracin and vancomycin interfere with the transport of peptidoglycans through the cytoplasmic membrane and are active only against gram-positive bacteria. **Bacitracin** is a polypeptide mixture, markedly nephrotoxic and used only topically. **Vancomycin** is a glycopeptide and the drug of choice for the (oral) treatment of bowel inflammations occurring as a complication of antibiotic therapy (pseudomembranous enterocolitis caused by *Clostridium difficile*). It is not absorbed.

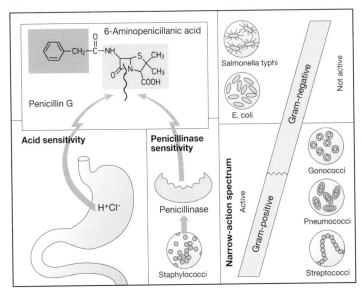

A. Disadvantages of penicillin G

	Acid	Penicillinase	Spectrum	Concentration needed to inhibit penicillin G-sensitive bacteria
Penicillin V	Resistant	Sensitive	Narrow	
Oxacillin	Resistant	Resistant	Narrow	
Amoxicillin	Resistant	Resistant	Broad	

B. Derivatives of penicillin G

Cefalexin	Resistant	Resistant, but sensitive to cephalosporinase	Broad	

C. Cephalosporin

Inhibitors of Tetrahydrofolate Synthesis

Tetrahydrofolic acid (THF) is a co-enzyme in the synthesis of purine bases and thymidine. These are constituents of DNA and RNA and required for cell growth and replication. Lack of THF leads to inhibition of cell proliferation. Formation of THF from dihydrofolate (DHF) is catalyzed by the enzyme dihydrofolate reductase. DHF is made from folic acid, a vitamin that cannot be synthesized in the body, but must be taken up from exogenous sources. Most bacteria do not have a requirement for folate, because they are capable of synthesizing folate, more precisely DHF, from precursors. Selective interference with bacterial biosynthesis of THF can be achieved with sulfonamides and trimethoprim.

Sulfonamides structurally resemble p-aminobenzoic acid (PABA), a precursor in bacterial DHF synthesis. As false substrates, sulfonamides competitively *inhibit* utilization of PABA, hence DHF *synthesis.* Because most bacteria cannot take up exogenous folate, they are depleted of DHF. Sulfonamides thus possess *bacteriostatic activity* against a *broad spectrum* of pathogens. Sulfonamides are produced by chemical synthesis. The basic structure is shown in **(A)**. Residue R determines the pharmacokinetic properties of a given sulfonamide. Most sulfonamides are well absorbed via the enteral route. They are metabolized to varying degrees and eliminated through the kidney. Rates of elimination, hence duration of effect, may vary widely. Some members are poorly absorbed from the gut and are thus suitable for the treatment of bacterial bowel infections. Adverse effects may include, among others, allergic reactions, sometimes with severe skin damage, displacement of other plasma protein-bound drugs or bilirubin in neonates (danger of kernicterus, hence contraindication for the last weeks of gestation and in the neonate). Because of the frequent emergence of resistant bacteria, sulfonamides are now rarely used. Introduced in 1935, they were the first broad-spectrum chemotherapeutics.

Trimethoprim inhibits bacterial DHF reductase, the human enzyme being significantly less sensitive than the bacterial one (rarely bone marrow depression). A 2,4-diaminopyrimidine, trimethoprim, has bacteriostatic activity against a broad spectrum of pathogens. It is used mostly as a component of co-trimoxazole.

Co-trimoxazole is a combination of *trimethoprim* and the sulfonamide *sulfamethoxazole.* Since THF synthesis is inhibited at two successive steps, the antibacterial effect of co-trimoxazole is better than that of the individual components. Resistant pathogens are infrequent; a bactericidal effect may occur. Adverse effects correspond to those of the components.

Although initially developed as an antirheumatic agent (p. 320), **sulfasalazine** (salazosulfapyridine) is used mainly in the treatment of inflammatory bowel disease (ulcerative colitis and terminal ileitis or Crohn's disease). Gut bacteria split this compound into the sulfonamide sulfapyridine and *mesalamine (5-aminosalicylic acid).* The latter is probably the anti-inflammatory agent (inhibition of synthesis of chemotactic signals for granulocytes, and of H_2O_2 formation in mucosa), but must be present on the gut mucosa in high concentrations. Coupling to the sulfonamide prevents premature absorption in upper small bowel segments. The cleaved-off sulfonamide can be absorbed and may produce typical adverse effects (see above).

Dapsone (p. 280) has several therapeutic uses: besides treatment of leprosy, it is used for prevention/prophylaxis of malaria, toxoplasmosis, and actinomycosis.

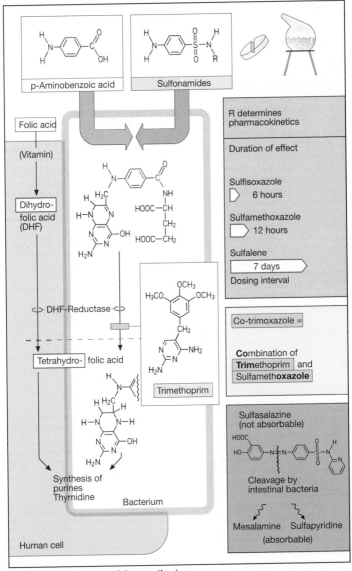

A. Inhibitors of tetrahydrofolate synthesis

Inhibitors of DNA Function

Deoxyribonucleic acid (DNA) serves as a template for the synthesis of nucleic acids. Ribonucleic acid (RNA) executes protein synthesis and thus permits cell growth. Synthesis of new DNA is a prerequisite for cell division. Substances that inhibit reading of genetic information at the DNA template damage the regulatory center of cell metabolism. The substances listed below are useful as antibacterial drugs because they do not affect human cells.

Gyrase inhibitors. The enzyme gyrase (topoisomerase II) permits the orderly accommodation of a ~1000 μm-long bacterial chromosome in a bacterial cell of ~1 μm. Within the chromosomal strand, double-stranded DNA has a double helical configuration. The former, in turn, is arranged in loops that are shortened by supercoiling. The gyrase catalyzes this operation, as illustrated, by opening, underwinding, and closing the DNA double strand such that the full loop need not be rotated.

Derivatives of 4-quinolone-3-carboxylic acid (green portion of ofloxacin formula) are inhibitors of bacterial gyrases. They appear to prevent specifically the resealing of opened strands and thereby act bactericidally. These agents are absorbed after oral ingestion. The older drug, *nalidixic acid,* affects exclusively gram-negative bacteria and attains effective concentrations only in urine; it is used as a urinary tract antiseptic. *Norfloxacin* has a broader spectrum. Ofloxacin, ciprofloxacin, enoxacin, and others, also yield systemically effective concentrations and are used for infections of internal organs.

Besides gastrointestinal problems and allergy, adverse effects particularly involve the CNS (confusion, hallucinations, seizures). Since they can damage epiphyseal chondrocytes and joint cartilages in laboratory animals, gyrase inhibitors should not be used during pregnancy, lactation, and periods of growth.

Azomycin (nitroimidazole) derivatives, such as **metronidazole,** damage DNA by complex formation or strand breakage. This occurs in obligate anaerobes, i.e., bacteria growing under O_2 exclusion. Under these conditions, conversion to reactive metabolites that attack DNA takes place (e.g., the hydroxylamine shown). The effect is bactericidal. A similar mechanism is involved in the antiprotozoal action on *Trichomonas vaginalis* (causative agent of vaginitis and urethritis) and *Entamoeba histolytica* (causative agent of large bowel inflammation, amebic dysentery, and hepatic abscesses). Metronidazole is well absorbed via the enteral route; it is also given i.v. or topically (vaginal insert). Because metronidazole is considered potentially mutagenic, carcinogenic, and teratogenic in the human, it should not be used longer than 10 d, if possible, and be avoided during pregnancy and lactation. *Timidazole* may be considered equivalent to metronidazole.

Rifampin inhibits the bacterial enzyme that catalyzes DNA template-directed RNA transcription, i.e., DNA-dependent RNA polymerase. Rifampin acts bactericidally against mycobacteria (M. tuberculosis, M. leprae), as well as many gram-positive and gram-negative bacteria. It is well absorbed after oral ingestion. Because resistance may develop with frequent usage, it is restricted to the treatment of tuberculosis and leprosy (p. 280).

Rifampin is contraindicated in the first trimester of gestation and during lactation.

Rifabutin resembles rifampin but may be effective in infections resistant to the latter.

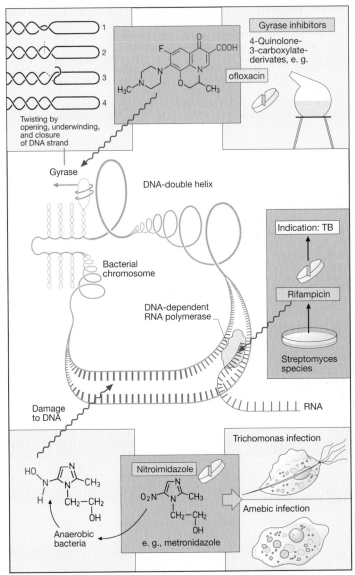

1
2
3
4

Twisting by opening, underwinding, and closure of DNA strand

Gyrase inhibitors

4-Quinolone-3-carboxylate-derivates, e. g.

ofloxacin

Gyrase

DNA-double helix

Bacterial chromosome

DNA-dependent RNA polymerase

Indication: TB

Rifampicin

Streptomyces species

Damage to DNA

RNA

Trichomonas infection

Nitroimidazole

Anaerobic bacteria

e. g., metronidazole

Amebic infection

A. Antibacterial drugs acting on DNA

Inhibitors of Protein Synthesis

Protein synthesis means translation into a peptide chain of a genetic message first copied (transcribed) into m-RNA (p. 274). Amino acid (AA) assembly occurs at the ribosome. Delivery of amino acids to m-RNA involves different transfer RNA molecules (t-RNA), each of which binds a specific AA. Each t-RNA bears an "anticodon" nucleobase triplet that is complementary to a particular m-RNA coding unit (codon, consisting of 3 nucleobases).

Incorporation of an AA normally involves the following steps **(A):**

1. The ribosome "focuses" two codons on m-RNA; one (at the left) has bound its t-RNA-AA complex, the AA having already been added to the peptide chain; the other (at the right) is ready to receive the next t-RNA-AA complex.

2. After the latter attaches, the AAs of the two adjacent complexes are linked by the action of the enzyme peptide synthetase (peptidyltransferase). Concurrently, AA and t-RNA of the left complex disengage.

3. The left t-RNA dissociates from m-RNA. The ribosome can advance along the m-RNA strand and focus on the next codon.

4. Consequently, the right t-RNA-AA complex shifts to the left, allowing the next complex to be bound at the right.

These individual steps are susceptible to inhibition by **antibiotics** of different groups. The examples shown originate primarily from Streptomyces bacteria, some of the aminoglycosides also being derived from Micromonospora bacteria.

1a. **Tetracyclines** inhibit the binding of t-RNA-AA complexes. Their action is bacteriostatic and affects a broad spectrum of pathogens.

1b. **Aminoglycosides** induce the binding of "wrong" t-RNA-AA complexes, resulting in synthesis of false proteins. Aminoglycosides are bactericidal. Their activity spectrum encompasses mainly gram-negative organisms. Streptomycin and kanamycin are used predominantly in the treatment of tuberculosis.

Note on spelling: -*mycin* designates origin from Streptomyces species; -*micin* (e.g., gentamicin) from Micromonospora species.

2. **Chloramphenicol** inhibits peptide synthetase. It has bacteriostatic activity against a broad spectrum of pathogens. The chemically simple molecule is now produced synthetically.

3. **Erythromycin** suppresses advancement of the ribosome. Its action is predominantly bacteriostatic and directed against gram-positve organisms. For oral administration, the acid-labile base (E) is dispensed as a salt (E. stearate) or an ester (e.g., E. succinate). Erythromycin is well tolerated. It is a suitable substitute in penicillin allergy or resistance. *Azithromycin, clarithromycin,* and *roxithromycin* are derivatives with greater acid stability and better bioavailability. The compounds mentioned are the most important members of the macrolide antibiotic group, which includes *josamycin* and *spiramycin.* An unrelated action of erythromycin is its mimicry of the gastrointestinal hormone motiline (↑ interprandial bowel motility).

Clindamycin has antibacterial activity similar to that of erythromycin. It exerts a bacteriostatic effect mainly on gram-positive aerobic, as well as on anaerobic pathogens. Clindamycin is a semisynthetic chloro analogue of lincomycin, which derives from a Streptomyces species. Taken orally, clindamycin is better absorbed than lincomycin, has greater antibacterial efficacy and is thus preferred. Both penetrate well into bone tissue.

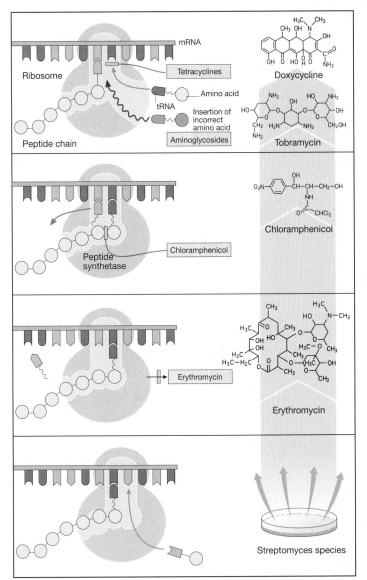

A. Protein synthesis and modes of action of antibacterial drugs

Tetracyclines are absorbed from the gastrointestinal tract to differing degrees, depending on the substance, absorption being nearly complete for *doxycycline* and *minocycline*. Intravenous injection is rarely needed (*rolitetracycline* is available only for i.v. administration). The most common unwanted effect is *gastrointestinal upset* (nausea, vomiting, diarrhea, etc.) due to (1) a direct mucosal irritant action of these substances and (2) damage to the natural bacterial gut flora (broad-spectrum antibiotics) allowing colonization by pathogenic organisms, including Candida fungi. Concurrent ingestion of antacids or milk would, however, be inappropriate because tetracyclines form insoluble *complexes* with *plurivalent cations* (e.g., Ca^{2+}, Mg^{2+}, Al^{3+}, $Fe^{2+/3+}$) resulting in their inactivation; that is, absorbability, antibacterial activity, and local irritant action are abolished. The ability to chelate Ca^{2+} accounts for the propensity of tetracyclines to accumulate in growing teeth and bones. As a result, there occurs an irreversible yellow-brown *discoloration of teeth* and a reversible *inhibition of bone growth.* Because of these adverse effects, tetracycline should not be given after the second month of pregnancy and not prescribed to children aged 8 y and under. Other adverse effects are increased *photosensitivity* of the skin and *hepatic damage,* mainly after i.v. administration.

The broad-spectrum antibiotic **chloramphenicol** is completely absorbed after oral ingestion. It undergoes even distribution in the body and readily crosses diffusion barriers such as the blood-brain barrier. Despite these advantageous properties, use of chloramphenicol is rarely indicated (e.g., in CNS infections) because of the danger of bone marrow damage. *Two types of bone marrow depression* can occur: (1) a dose-dependent, toxic, reversible form manifested during therapy and, (2) a frequently fatal form that may occur after a latency of weeks and is not dose dependent. Due to high tissue penetrability, the danger of bone marrow depression must also be taken into account after local use (e.g., eye drops).

Aminoglycoside antibiotics consist of glycoside-linked amino-sugars (cf. gentamicin $C_{1\alpha}$, a constituent of the gentamicin mixture). They contain numerous hydroxyl groups and amino groups that can bind protons. Hence, these compounds are highly polar, poorly membrane permeable, and not absorbed enterally. *Neomycin* and *paromomycin* are given orally to eradicate intestinal bacteria (prior to bowel surgery or for reducing NH_3 formation by gut bacteria in hepatic coma). Aminoglycosides for the treatment of serious infections must be injected (e.g., *gentamicin, tobramycin, amikacin, netilmicin, sisomycin*). In addition, local inlays of a gentamicin-releasing carrier can be used in infections of bone or soft tissues. Aminoglycosides gain access to the bacterial interior by the use of bacterial *transport systems.* In the kidney, they enter the cells of the proximal tubules via an uptake system for oligopeptides. Tubular cells are susceptible to damage (*nephrotoxicity,* mostly reversible). In the inner ear, sensory cells of the vestibular apparatus and Corti's organ may be injured (*ototoxicity,* in part irreversible).

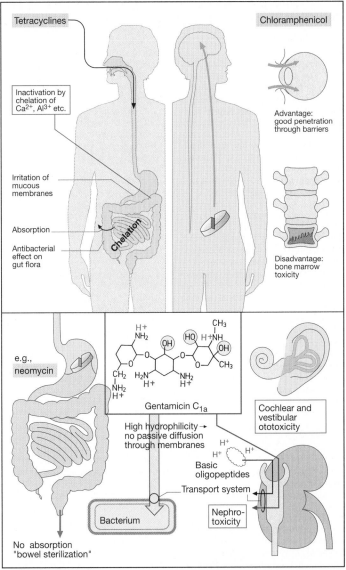

A. Aspects of the therapeutic use of tetracyclines, chloramphenicol, and aminoglycosides

Drugs for Treating Mycobacterial Infections

Mycobacteria are responsible for two diseases: tuberculosis, mostly caused by *M. tuberculosis,* and leprosy due to *M. leprae.* The therapeutic principle applicable to both is combined treatment with two or more drugs. Combination therapy prevents the emergence of resistant mycobacteria. Because the antibacterial effects of the individual substances are additive, correspondingly smaller doses are sufficient. Therefore, the risk of individual adverse effects is lowered. Most drugs are active against only one of the two diseases.

Antitubercular Drugs (1)

Drugs of choice are: isoniazid, rifampin, ethambutol, along with streptomycin and pyrazinamide. Less well tolerated, second-line agents include: *p*-aminosalicylic acid, cycloserine, viomycin, kanamycin, amikacin, capreomycin, ethionamide.

Isoniazid is bactericidal against growing *M. tuberculosis.* Its mechanism of action remains unclear. (In the bacterium it is converted to isonicotinic acid, which is membrane impermeable, hence likely to accumulate intracellularly.) Isoniazid is rapidly absorbed after oral administration. In the liver, it is inactivated by acetylation, the rate of which is genetically controlled and shows a characteristic distribution in different ethnic groups (fast vs. slow acetylators). Notable adverse effects are: peripheral neuropathy, optic neuritis preventable by administration of vitamin B_6 (pyridoxine); hepatitis, jaundice.

Rifampin. Source, antibacterial activity, and routes of administration are described on p. 274. Albeit mostly well tolerated, this drug may cause several adverse effects including hepatic damage, hypersensitivity with flu-like symptoms, disconcerting but harmless red/orange discoloration of body fluids, and enzyme induction (failure of oral contraceptives). Concerning rifabutin see p. 274.

Ethambutol. The cause of its specific antitubercular action is unknown. Ethambutol is given orally. It is generally well tolerated, but may cause dose-dependent damage to the optic nerve with disturbances of vision (red/green blindness, visual field defects).

Pyrazinamide exerts a bactericidal action by an unknown mechanism. It is given orally. Pyrazinamide may impair liver function; hyperuricemia results from inhibition of renal urate elimination.

Streptomycin must be given i.v. (pp. 278ff) like other aminoglycoside antibiotics. It damages the inner ear and the labyrinth. Its nephrotoxicity is comparatively minor.

Antileprotic Drugs (2)

Rifampin is frequently given in combination with one or both of the following agents:

Dapsone is a sulfone that, like sulfonamides, inhibits dihydrofolate synthesis (p. 272). It is bactericidal against susceptible strains of *M. leprae.* Dapsone is given orally. The most frequent adverse effect is methemoglobinemia with accelerated erythrocyte degradation (hemolysis).

Clofazimine is a dye with bactericidal activity against *M. leprae* and anti-inflammatory properties. It is given orally, but is incompletely absorbed. Because of its high lipophilicity, it accumulates in adipose and other tissues and leaves the body only rather slowly ($t_{1/2} \sim 70$ d). Red-brown skin pigmentation is an unwanted effect, particularly in fair-skinned patients.

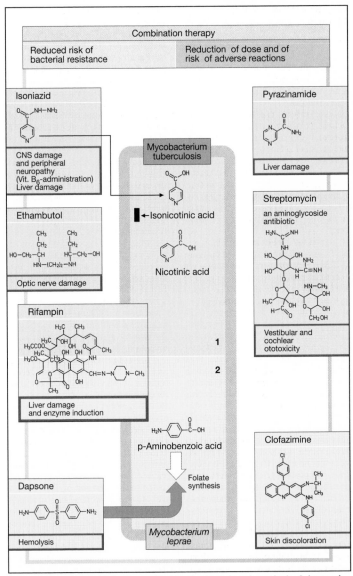

A. Drugs used to treat infections with mycobacteria (1. tuberculosis, 2. leprosy)

Drugs Used in the Treatment of Fungal Infections

Infections due to fungi are usually confined to the skin or mucous membranes: local or superficial mycosis. However, in immune deficiency states, internal organs may also be affected: systemic or deep mycosis.

Mycoses are most commonly due to *dermatophytes*, which affect the skin, hair, and nails following external infection. *Candida albicans*, a yeast organism normally found on body surfaces, may cause infections of mucous membranes, less frequently of the skin or internal organs when natural defenses are impaired (immunosuppression, or damage of microflora by broad-spectrum antibiotics).

Imidazole derivatives inhibit ergosterol synthesis. This steroid forms an integral constituent of cytoplasmic membranes of fungal cells, analogous to cholesterol in animal plasma membranes. Fungi exposed to imidazole derivatives stop growing (fungistatic effect) or die (fungicidal effect). The spectrum of affected fungi is very broad. Because they are poorly absorbed and poorly tolerated systemically, most imidazoles are suitable only for topical use (*clotrimazole, econazole oxiconazole, isoconazole, bifonazole,* etc.). Rarely, this use may result in contact dermatitis. *Miconazole* is given locally, or systemically by short-term infusion (despite its poor tolerability). Because it is well absorbed, *ketoconazole* is available for oral administration. Adverse effects are rare; however, the possibility of fatal liver damage should be noted. Remarkably, ketoconazole may inhibit steroidogenesis (gonadal and adrenocortical hormones). *Fluconazole* and *itraconazole* are newer, orally effective **triazole** derivatives. The topically active **allylamine** *naftidine* and the **morpholine** *amorolfine* also inhibit ergosterol synthesis, albeit at another step.

The **polyene antibiotics,** amphotericin B and nystatin, are of bacterial origin. They insert themselves into fungal cell membranes (probably next to ergosterol molecules) and cause formation of hydrophilic channels. The resultant increase in membrane permeability, e.g., to K^+ ions, accounts for the fungicidal effect. **Amphotericin B** is active against most organisms responsible for systemic mycoses. Because of its poor absorbability, it must be given by infusion, which is, however, poorly tolerated (chills, fever, CNS disturbances, impaired renal function, phlebitis at the infusion site). Applied topically to skin or mucous membranes, amphotericin B is useful in the treatment of candidal mycosis. Because of the low rate of enteral absorption, oral administration in intestinal candidiasis can be considered a topical treatment. *Nystatin* is used only for topical therapy.

Flucytosine is converted in candida fungi to 5-fluorouracil by the action of a specific cytosine deaminase. As an antimetabolite, this compound disrupts DNA and RNA synthesis (p. 298), resulting in a fungicidal effect. Given orally, flucytosine is rapidly absorbed. It is well tolerated and often combined with amphotericin B to allow dose reduction of the latter.

Griseofulvin originates from molds and has activity only against dermatophytes. Presumably, it acts as a spindle poison to inhibit fungal mitosis. Although targeted against local mycoses, griseofulvin must be used systemically. It is incorporated into newly formed keratin. "Impregnated" in this manner, keratin becomes unsuitable as a fungal nutrient. The time required for the eradication of dermatophytes corresponds to the renewal period of skin, hair, or nails. Griseofulvin may cause uncharacteristic adverse effects. The need for prolonged administration (several months), the incidence of side effects, and the availability of effective and safe alternatives have rendered griseofulvin therapeutically obsolete.

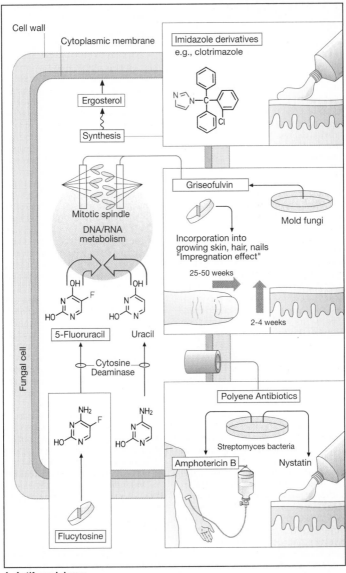

A. Antifungal drugs

Chemotherapy of Viral Infections

Viruses essentially consist of genetic material (nucleic acids, green strands in **(A)** and a capsular envelope made up of proteins (blue hexagons), often with a coat (gray ring) of a phospholipid (PL) bilayer with embedded proteins (small blue bars). They lack a metabolic system but depend on the infected cell for their growth and replication. Targeted therapeutic suppression of viral replication requires selective inhibition of those metabolic processes that specifically serve viral replication in infected cells. To date, this can be achieved only to a limited extent.

Viral replication as exemplified by Herpes simplex viruses (A): (1) The viral particle attaches to the host cell membrane *(adsorption)* by linking its capsular glycoproteins to specific structures of the cell membrane. (2) The viral coat fuses with the plasmalemma of the host cell and the nucleocapsid (nucleic acid plus capsule) enters the cell interior *(penetration)*. (3) The capsule opens ("uncoating") near the nuclear pores and viral DNA moves into the cell nucleus. The genetic material of the virus can now direct the cell's metabolic system. (4a) *Nucleic acid synthesis:* The genetic material (DNA in this instance) is replicated and RNA is produced for the purpose of *protein synthesis.* (4b) The proteins are used as "viral enzymes" catalyzing viral multiplication (e.g., DNA polymerase and thymidine kinase), as capsomers, or as coat components, or are incorporated into the host cell membrane. (5) Individual components are assembled into new virus particles *(maturation).* (6) Release of daughter viruses results in spread of virus inside and outside the organism. With herpes viruses, replication entails host cell destruction and development of disease symptoms.

Antiviral mechanisms (A). The organism can disrupt viral replication with the aid of cytotoxic T-lymphocytes that recognize and destroy virus-producing cells (viral surface proteins) or by means of antibodies that bind to and inactivate extracellular virus particles. Vaccinations are designed to activate **specific immune defenses.**

Interferons (IFN) are glycoproteins that, among other products, are released from virus-infected cells. In neighboring cells, interferon stimulates the production of "antiviral proteins." These inhibit the synthesis of viral proteins by (preferential) destruction of viral DNA or by suppressing its translation. Interferons are not directed against a specific virus, but have a broad spectrum of antiviral action that is, however, species-specific. Thus, interferon for use in humans must be obtained from cells of human origin, such as leukocytes (IFN-α), fibroblasts (IFN-β), or lymphocytes (IFN-γ). Interferons are also used to treat certain malignancies and autoimmune disorders (e.g., IFN-α for chronic hepatitis C and hairy cell leukemia; IFN-β for severe herpes virus infections and multiple sclerosis).

Virustatic antimetabolites are "false" DNA building blocks **(B)** or nucleosides. A nucleoside (e.g., thymidine) consists of a nucleobase (e.g., thymine) and the sugar deoxyribose. In antimetabolites, one of the components is defective. In the body, the abnormal nucleosides undergo bioactivation by attachment of three phosphate residues (p. 287).

Idoxuridine and congeners are incorporated into DNA with deleterious results. This also applies to the synthesis of human DNA. Therefore, idoxuridine and analogues are suitable only for topical use (e.g., in herpes simplex keratitis).

Vidarabine inhibits virally induced DNA polymerase more strongly than it does the endogenous enzyme. Its use is now limited to topical treatment of severe herpes simplex infection. Before the introduction of the better tolerated acyclovir, vidarabine played a major part in the treatment of herpes simplex encephalitis.

Among virustatic antimetabolites, **acyclovir (A)** has both specificity of the highest degree and optimal tolerability,

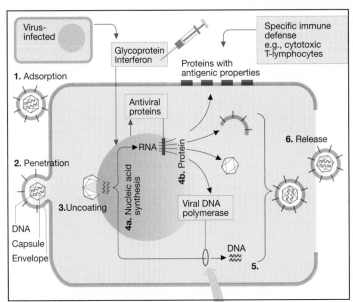

A. Virus multiplication and modes of action of antiviral agents

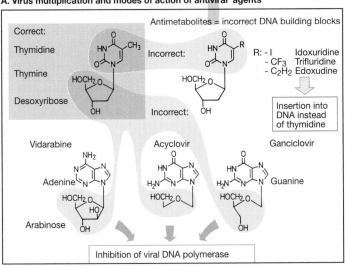

B. Chemical structure of virustatic antimetabolites

because it undergoes bioactivation only in infected cells, where it preferentially inhibits viral DNA synthesis. (1) A virally coded thymidine kinase (specific to H. simplex and varicella-zoster virus) performs the initial phosphorylation step; the remaining two phosphate residues are attached by cellular kinases. (2) The polar phosphate residues render acyclovir triphosphate membrane impermeable and cause it to accumulate in infected cells. (3) Acyclovir triphosphate is a preferred substrate of viral DNA polymerase; it inhibits enzyme activity and, following its incorporation into viral DNA, induces strand breakage because it lacks the 3'-OH group of deoxyribose that is required for the attachment of additional nucleotides. The high therapeutic value of acyclovir is evident in severe infections with H. simplex viruses (e.g., encephalitis, generalized infection) and varicella-zoster viruses (e.g., severe herpes zoster). In these cases, it can be given by i.v. infusion. Acyclovir may also be given orally despite its incomplete (15%–30%) enteral absorption. In addition, it has topical uses. Because host DNA synthesis remains unaffected, adverse effects do not include bone marrow depression. Acyclovir is eliminated unchanged in urine ($t_{1/2} \sim 2.5$ h).

Valacyclovir, the L-valyl ester of acyclovir, is a prodrug that can be administered orally in herpes zoster infections. Its absorption rate is approx. twice that of acyclovir. During passage through the intestinal wall and liver, the valine residue is cleaved by esterases, generating acyclovir.

Famcyclovir is an antiherpetic prodrug with good bioavailability when given orally. It is used in genital herpes and herpes zoster. Cleavage of two acetate groups from the "false sugar" and oxidation of the purine ring to guanine yields **penciclovir,** the active form. The latter differs from acyclovir with respect to its "false sugar" moiety, but mimics it pharmacologically. Bioactivation of penciclovir, like that of acyclovir, involves formation of the triphosphorylated antimetabolite via virally induced thymidine kinase.

Ganciclovir (structure on p. 285) is given by infusion in the treatment of severe infections with cytomegaloviruses (also belonging to the herpes group); these do not induce thymidine kinase, phosphorylation being initiated by a different viral enzyme. Ganciclovir is less well tolerated and, not infrequently, produces leukopenia and thrombopenia.

Foscarnet represents a diphosphate analogue.

As shown in (**A**), incorporation of **nucleotide** into a DNA strand entails cleavage of a **diphosphate residue.** Foscarnet (**B**) inhibits DNA polymerase by interacting with its binding site for the diphosphate group. *Indications:* systemic therapy of severe cytomegaly infection in AIDS patients; local therapy of herpes simplex infections.

Amantadine (C) specifically affects the replication of influenza A (RNA) viruses, the causative agent of true influenza. These viruses are endocytosed into the cell. Release of viral DNA requires protons from the acidic content of endosomes to penetrate the virus. Presumably, amantadine blocks a channel protein in the viral coat that permits influx of protons; thus, "uncoating" is prevented. Moreover, amantadine inhibits viral maturation. The drug is also used prophylactically and, if possible, must be taken *before* the outbreak of symptoms. It also is an antiparkinsonian (p. 188).

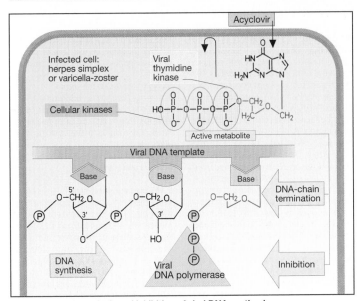

A. Activation of acyclovir and inhibition of viral DNA synthesis

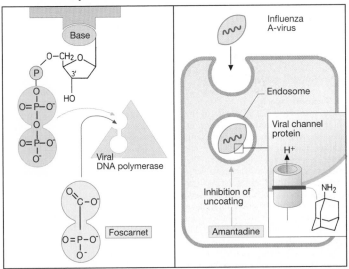

B. Inhibitor of DNA polymerase: Foscarnet

C. Prophylaxis for viral flu

Drugs for the Treatment of AIDS

Replication of the human immuno-deficiency virus (HIV), the causative agent of AIDS, is susceptible to targeted interventions, because several virus-specific metabolic steps occur in infected cells **(A).** Viral RNA must first be transcribed into DNA, a step catalyzed by viral "reverse transcriptase." Double-stranded DNA is incorporated into the host genome with the help of viral integrase. Under control by viral DNA, viral replication can then be initiated, with synthesis of viral RNA and proteins (including enzymes such as reverse transcriptase and integrase, and structural proteins such as the matrix protein lining the inside of the viral envelope). These proteins are assembled not individually but in the form of *polyproteins.* These precursor proteins carry an N-terminal fatty acid (myristoyl) residue that promotes their attachment to the interior face of the plasmalemma. As the virus particle buds off the host cell, it carries with it the affected membrane area as its envelope. During this process, a protease contained within the polyprotein cleaves the latter into individual, functionally active proteins.

I. Inhibitors of Reverse Transcriptase

IA. Nucleoside agents
These substances are analogues of thymine **(azidothymidine, stavudine),** adenine **(didanosine),** cytosine **(lamivudine, zalcitabine),** and guanine **(carbovir,** a metabolite of **abacavir**). They have in common an abnormal sugar moiety. Like the natural nucleosides, they undergo triphosphorylation, giving rise to nucleotides that both inhibit reverse transcriptase and cause strand breakage following incorporation into viral DNA.

The nucleoside inhibitors differ in terms of I) their ability to decrease circulating HIV load; 2) their pharmacokinetic properties (half life $\rightarrow$ dosing interval $\rightarrow$ compliance; organ distribution $\rightarrow$ passage through blood-brain-barrier); 3) the type of resistance-inducing mutations of the viral genome and the rate at which resistance develops; and 4) their adverse effects (bone marrow depression, neuropathy, pancreatitis).

IB. Non-nucleoside inhibitors
The non-nucleoside inhibitors of reverse transcriptase **(nevirapine, delavirdine, efavirenz)** are not phosphorylated. They bind to the enzyme with high selectivity and thus prevent it from adopting the active conformation. Inhibition is noncompetitive.

II. HIV protease inhibitors
Viral protease cleaves precursor proteins into proteins required for viral replication. The inhibitors of this protease **(saquinavir, ritonavir, indinavir,** and **nelfinavir**) represent abnormal proteins that possess high antiviral efficacy and are generally well tolerated in the short term. However, prolonged administration is associated with occasionally severe disturbances of lipid and carbohydrate metabolism. Biotransformation of these drugs involves cytochrome P_{450} (CYP 3A4) and is therefore subject to interaction with various other drugs inactivated via this route.

For the dual purpose of increasing the effectiveness of antiviral therapy and preventing the development of a therapy-limiting viral resistance, inhibitors of reverse transcriptase are combined with each other and/or with protease inhibitors.

Combination regimens are designed in accordance with substance-specific development of resistance and pharmacokinetic parameters (CNS penetrability, "neuroprotection," dosing frequency).

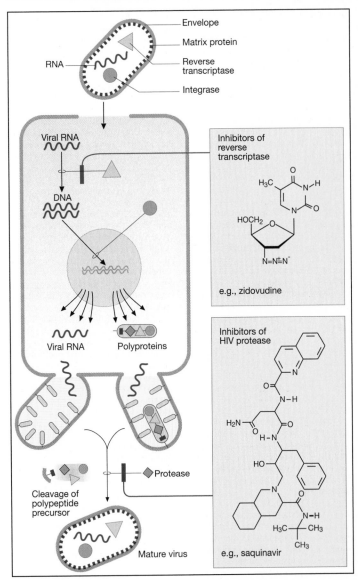

A. Antiretroviral drugs

290 Disinfectants

Disinfectants and Antiseptics

Disinfection denotes the inactivation or killing of pathogens (protozoa, bacteria, fungi, viruses) in the human environment. This can be achieved by chemical or physical means; the latter will not be discussed here. **Sterilization** refers to the killing of **all** germs, whether pathogenic, dormant, or nonpathogenic. **Antisepsis** refers to the *reduction* by chemical agents of germ numbers on skin and mucosal surfaces.

Agents for chemical disinfection ideally should cause *rapid, complete,* and *persistent* inactivation of all germs, but at the same time exhibit low toxicity (systemic toxicity, tissue irritancy, antigenicity) and be non-deleterious to inanimate materials. These requirements call for chemical properties that may exclude each other; therefore, compromises guided by the intended use have to be made.

Disinfectants come from various chemical classes, including oxidants, halogens or halogen-releasing agents, alcohols, aldehydes, organic acids, phenols, cationic surfactants (detergents) and formerly also heavy metals. The **basic mechanisms of action** involve denaturation of proteins, inhibition of enzymes, or a dehydration. Effects are dependent on concentration and contact time.

Activity spectrum. Disinfectants inactivate bacteria (gram-positive > gram-negative > mycobacteria), less effectively their sporal forms, and a few (e.g., formaldehyde) are virucidal.

Applications

Skin "disinfection." Reduction of germ counts prior to punctures or surgical procedures is desirable if the risk of wound infection is to be minimized. Useful agents include: alcohols (1- and 2-propanol; ethanol 60–90%; iodine-releasing agents like polyvinylpyrrolidone [povidone, PVP]-iodine as a depot form of the active principle iodine, instead of iodine tincture), cationic surfactants, and mixtures of these. Minimal contact times should be at least 15 s on skin areas with few sebaceous glands and at least 10 min on sebaceous gland-rich ones.

Mucosal disinfection: Germ counts can be reduced by PVP iodine or chlorhexidine (contact time 2 min), although not as effectively as on skin.

Wound disinfection can be achieved with hydrogen peroxide (0.3%–1% solution; short, foaming action on contact with blood and thus wound cleansing) or with potassium permanganate (0.0015% solution, slightly astringent), as well as PVP iodine, chlorhexidine, and biguanidines.

Hygienic and surgical hand disinfection: The former is required after a suspected contamination, the latter before surgical procedures. Alcohols, mixtures of alcohols and phenols, cationic surfactants, or acids are available for this purpose. Admixture of other agents prolongs duration of action and reduces flammability.

Disinfection of instruments: Instruments that cannot be heat- or steam-sterilized can be precleaned and then disinfected with aldehydes and detergents.

Surface (floor) disinfection employs aldehydes combined with cationic surfactants and oxidants or, more rarely, acidic or alkalizing agents.

Room disinfection: room air and surfaces can be disinfected by spraying or vaporizing of aldehydes, provided that germs are freely accessible.

Application sites	Examples	Active principles

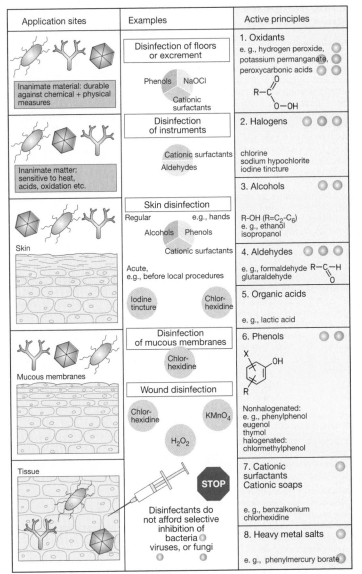

Inanimate material: durable against chemical + physical measures

Inanimate matter: sensitive to heat, acids, oxidation etc.

Skin

Mucous membranes

Tissue

Disinfection of floors or excrement

Phenols NaOCl

Cationic surfactants

Disinfection of instruments

Cationic surfactants

Aldehydes

Skin disinfection

Regular   e.g., hands

Alcohols Phenols

Cationic surfactants

Acute, e.g., before local procedures

Iodine tincture   Chlor-hexidine

Disinfection of mucous membranes

Chlor-hexidine

Wound disinfection

Chlor-hexidine   KMnO₄

H₂O₂

STOP

Disinfectants do not afford selective inhibition of bacteria viruses, or fungi

1. Oxidants

e. g., hydrogen peroxide, potassium permanganate, peroxycarbonic acids

$$R-C\begin{smallmatrix}O\\\\O-OH\end{smallmatrix}$$

2. Halogens

chlorine
sodium hypochlorite
iodine tincture

3. Alcohols

R-OH (R=C₂-C₆)
e. g., ethanol
isopropanol

4. Aldehydes

e.g., formaldehyde   R-C-H
glutaraldehyde   O

5. Organic acids

e. g., lactic acid

6. Phenols

X

OH

R

Nonhalogenated:
e. g., phenylphenol
eugenol
thymol
halogenated:
chlormethylphenol

7. Cationic surfactants Cationic soaps

e. g., benzalkonium chlorhexidine

8. Heavy metal salts

e. g., phenylmercury borate

A. Disinfectants

Drugs for Treating Endo- and Ectoparasitic Infestations

Adverse hygienic conditions favor human infestation with multicellular organisms (referred to here as parasites). Skin and hair are colonization sites for arthropod ectoparasites, such as insects (lice, fleas) and arachnids (mites). Against these, insecticidal or arachnicidal agents, respectively, can be used. Endoparasites invade the intestines or even internal organs, and are mostly members of the phyla of flatworms and roundworms. They are combated with anthelmintics.

Anthelmintics. As shown in the table, the newer agents *praziquantel* and *mebendazole* are adequate for the treatment of diverse worm diseases. They are generally well tolerated, as are the other agents listed.

Insecticides. Whereas fleas can be effectively dealt with by disinfection of clothes and living quarters, lice and mites require the topical application of insecticides to the infested subject.

Chlorphenothane (DDT) kills insects after absorption of a very small amount, e.g., via foot contact with sprayed surfaces (contact insecticide). The cause of death is nervous system damage and seizures. In humans DDT causes acute neurotoxicity only after absorption of very large amounts. DDT is chemically stable and degraded in the environment and body at extremely slow rates. As a highly lipophilic substance, it accumulates in fat tissues. Widespread use of DDT in pest control has led to its accumulation in food chains to alarming levels. For this reason its use has now been banned in many countries.

Lindane is the active γ-isomer of hexachlorocyclohexane. It also exerts a neurotoxic action on insects (as well as humans). Irritation of skin or mucous membranes may occur after topical use. Lindane is active also against intradermal mites (*Sarcoptes scabiei,* causative agent of scabies), besides lice and fleas. It is more readily degraded than DDT.

Permethrin, a synthetic pyrethroid, exhibits similar anti-ectoparasitic activity and may be the drug of choice due to its slower cutaneous absorption, fast hydrolytic inactivation, and rapid renal elimination.

Worms (helminths)	Anthelmintic drug of choice
Flatworms (platyhelminths) tape worms (cestodes) flukes (trematodes) e.g., Schistosoma species (bilharziasis)	praziquantel* praziquantel
Roundworms (nematodes) pinworm (*Enterobius vermicularis*) whipworm (*Trichuris trichiura*) *Ascaris lumbricoides* *Trichinella spiralis*** *Strongyloides stercoralis* Hookworm (*Necator americanus,* and *Ancylostoma duodenale*)	mebendazole or pyrantel pamoate mebendazole mebendazole or pyrantel pamoate mebendazole and thiabendazole thiabendazole mebendazole or pyrantel pamoate mebendazole or pyrantel pamoate

* not for ocular or spinal cord cysticercosis
** [thiabendazole: intestinal phase; mebendazole: tissue phase]

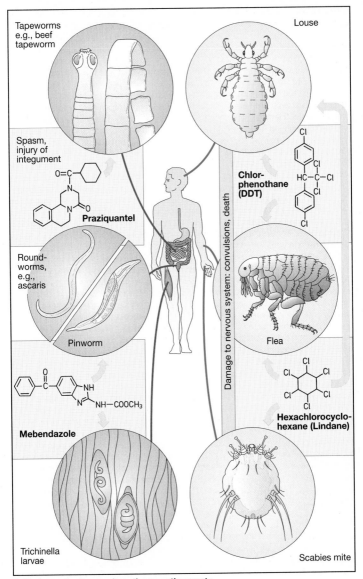

A. Endo- and ectoparasites: therapeutic agents

Antimalarials

The causative agents of malaria are plasmodia, unicellular organisms belonging to the order hemosporidia (class protozoa). The infective form, the sporozoite, is inoculated into skin capillaries when infected female Anopheles mosquitoes (A) suck blood from humans. The sporozoites invade liver parenchymal cells where they develop into primary tissue schizonts. After multiple fission, these schizonts produce numerous merozoites that enter the blood. The pre-erythrocytic stage is symptom free. In blood, the parasite enters erythrocytes (erythrocytic stage) where it again multiplies by schizogony, resulting in the formation of more merozoites. Rupture of the infected erythrocytes releases the merozoites and pyrogens. A fever attack ensues and more erythrocytes are infected. The generation period for the next crop of merozoites determines the interval between fever attacks. With *Plasmodium vivax* and *P. ovale,* there can be a parallel multiplication in the liver (paraerythrocytic stage). Moreover, some sporozoites may become dormant in the liver as "hypnozoites" before entering schizogony. When the sexual forms (gametocytes) are ingested by a feeding mosquito, they can initiate the sexual reproductive stage of the cycle that results in a new generation of transmittable sporozoites.

Different antimalarials selectively kill the parasite's different developmental forms. The mechanism of action is known for some of them: *pyrimethamine* and *dapsone* inhibit dihydrofolate reductase (p. 273), as does *chlorguanide (proguanil)* via its active metabolite. The sulfonamide *sulfadoxine* inhibits synthesis of dihydrofolic acid (p. 272). *Chloroquine* and *quinine* accumulate within the acidic vacuoles of blood schizonts and inhibit polymerization of heme, the latter substance being toxic for the schizonts.

Antimalarial drug choice takes into account tolerability and plasmodial resistance.

Tolerability. The first available antimalarial, quinine, has the smallest therapeutic margin. All newer agents are rather well tolerated.

Plasmodium (P.) falciparum, responsible for the most dangerous form of malaria, is particularly prone to develop **drug resistance.** The incidence of resistant strains rises with increasing frequency of drug use. Resistance has been reported for chloroquine and also for the combination pyrimethamine/sulfadoxine.

Drug choice for antimalarial chemoprophylaxis. In areas with a risk of malaria, continuous intake of antimalarials affords the best protection against the disease, although not against infection. *The drug of choice is chloroquine.* Because of its slow excretion (plasma $t_{1/2}$ = 3d and longer), a single weekly dose is sufficient. In areas with resistant *P. falciparum,* alternative regimens are chloroquine plus pyrimethamine/sulfadoxine (or proguanil, or doxycycline), the chloroquine analogue amodiaquine, as well as quinine or the better tolerated derivative mefloquine (blood-schizonticidal). Agents active against blood schizonts do not prevent the (symptom-free) hepatic infection, only the disease-causing infection of erythrocytes ("suppression therapy"). On return from an endemic malaria region, a 2 wk course of primaquine is adequate for eradication of the late hepatic stages *(P. vivax and P. ovale).*

Protection from mosquito bites (net, skin-covering clothes, etc.) is a very important prophylactic measure.

Antimalarial therapy employs the same agents and is based on the same principles. The blood-schizonticidal *halofantrine* is reserved for therapy only. The pyrimethamine-sulfadoxine combination may be used for initial self-treatment.

Drug resistance is accelerating in many endemic areas; malaria vaccines may hold the greatest hope for control of infection.

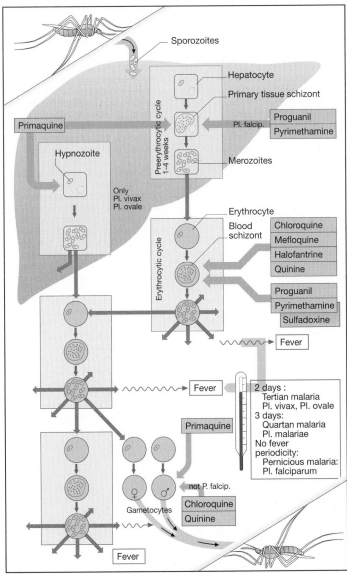

Sporozoites

Hepatocyte

Primary tissue schizont

Preerythrocytic cycle 1–4 weeks

Primaquine

Proguanil
Pyrimethamine

Pl. falcip.

Merozoites

Hypnozoite

Only
Pl. vivax
Pl. ovale

Erythrocyte

Blood schizont

Erythrocytic cycle

Chloroquine

Mefloquine

Halofantrine

Quinine

Proguanil

Pyrimethamine

Sulfadoxine

Fever

Fever

2 days :
Tertian malaria
Pl. vivax, Pl. ovale
3 days:
Quartan malaria
Pl. malariae
No fever
periodicity:
Pernicious malaria:
Pl. falciparum

Primaquine

not P. falcip.

Gametocytes

Chloroquine

Quinine

Fever

A. Malaria: stages of the plasmodial life cycle in the human;

Chemotherapy of Malignant Tumors

A tumor (neoplasm) consists of cells that proliferate independently of the body's inherent "building plan." A malignant tumor (cancer) is present when the tumor tissue destructively invades healthy surrounding tissue or when dislodged tumor cells form secondary tumors (metastases) in other organs. A cure requires the elimination of all malignant cells (curative therapy). When this is not possible, attempts can be made to slow tumor growth and thereby prolong the patient's life or improve quality of life (palliative therapy). Chemotherapy is faced with the problem that the malignant cells are endogenous and are not endowed with special metabolic properties.

Cytostatics (A) are cytotoxic substances that particularly affect proliferating or dividing cells. Rapidly dividing malignant cells are preferentially injured. Damage to mitotic processes not only retards tumor growth but may also initiate *apoptosis* (programmed cell death). Tissues with a low mitotic rate are largely unaffected; likewise, most healthy tissues. This, however, also applies to malignant tumors consisting of slowly dividing differentiated cells. Tissues that have a physiologically high mitotic rate are bound to be affected by cytostatic therapy. Thus, **typical adverse effects** occur:

Loss of hair results from injury to hair follicles; *gastrointestinal disturbances,* such as diarrhea, from inadequate replacement of enterocytes whose life span is limited to a few days; *nausea and vomiting* from stimulation of area postrema chemoreceptors (p. 330); and *lowered resistance to infection* from weakening of the immune system (p. 300). In addition, cytostatics cause *bone marrow depression.* Resupply of blood cells depends on the mitotic activity of bone marrow stem and daughter cells. When myeloid proliferation is arrested, the short-lived granulocytes are the first to be affected (neutropenia), then blood platelets (thrombopenia) and, finally,

the more long-lived erythrocytes (anemia). *Infertility* is caused by suppression of spermatogenesis or follicle maturation. Most cytostatics disrupt DNA metabolism. This entails the risk of a potential genomic alteration in healthy cells (*mutagenic* effect). Conceivably, the latter accounts for the occurrence of leukemias several years after cytostatic therapy (*carcinogenic* effect). Furthermore, congenital malformations are to be expected when cytostatics must be used during pregnancy (*teratogenic* effect).

Cytostatics possess different **mechanisms of action.**

Damage to the mitotic spindle (B). The contractile proteins of the spindle apparatus must draw apart the replicated chromosomes before the cell can divide. This process is prevented by the so-called *spindle poisons* (see also colchicine, p. 316) that arrest mitosis at metaphase by disrupting the assembly of microtubules into spindle threads. The vinca alkaloids, *vincristine* and *vinblastine* (from the periwinkle plant, *Vinca rosea*) exert such a cell-cycle-specific effect. Damage to the nervous system is a predicted adverse effect arising from injury to microtubule-operated axonal transport mechanisms.

Paclitaxel, from the bark of the pacific yew *(Taxus brevifolia),* inhibits disassembly of microtubules and induces atypical ones. *Docetaxel* is a semisynthetic derivative.

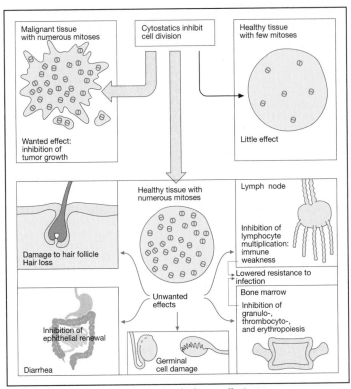

A. Chemotherapy of tumors: principal and adverse effects

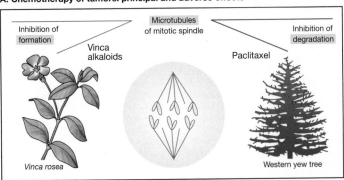

B. Cytostatics: inhibition of mitosis

Inhibition of DNA and RNA synthesis (A). Mitosis is preceded by replication of chromosomes (DNA synthesis) and increased protein synthesis (RNA synthesis). Existing DNA (gray) serves as a template for the synthesis of new (blue) DNA or RNA. *De novo* synthesis may be inhibited by:

Damage to the template (1). Alkylating cytostatics are reactive compounds that transfer alkyl residues into a covalent bond with DNA. For instance, *mechlorethamine (nitrogen mustard)* is able to cross-link double-stranded DNA on giving off its chlorine atoms. Correct reading of genetic information is thereby rendered impossible. Other alkylating agents are *chlorambucil, melphalan, thio-TEPA, cyclophosphamide* (p. 300, 320), *ifosfamide, lomustine,* and *busulfan.* Specific adverse reactions include irreversible pulmonary fibrosis due to busulfan and hemorrhagic cystitis caused by the cyclophosphamide metabolite acrolein (preventable by the uroprotectant mesna). *Cisplatin* binds to (but does not alkylate) DNA strands. **Cystostatic antibiotics** insert themselves into the DNA double strand; this may lead to strand breakage (e.g., with *bleomycin*). The *anthracycline antibiotics daunorubicin* and *adriamycin (doxorubicin)* may induce cardiomyopathy. Bleomycin can also cause pulmonary fibrosis.

The **epipodophyllotoxins,** *etoposide* and *teniposide*, interact with topoisomerase II, which functions to split, transpose, and reseal DNA strands (p. 274); these agents cause strand breakage by inhibiting resealing.

Inhibition of nucleobase synthesis (2). Tetrahydrofolic acid (THF) is required for the synthesis of both purine bases and thymidine. Formation of THF from folic acid involves dihydrofolate reductase (p. 272). The *folate analogues aminopterin* and *methotrexate* (amethopterin) inhibit enzyme activity as false substrates. As cellular stores of THF are depleted, synthesis of DNA and RNA building blocks ceases. The effect of these antimetabolites can be reversed by administration of folinic acid (5-formyl-THF, leucovorin, citrovorum factor).

Incorporation of false building blocks (3). Unnatural nucleobases (*6-mercaptopurine;* 5-fluorouracil) or nucleosides with incorrect sugars *(cytarabine)* act as antimetabolites. They inhibit DNA/RNA synthesis or lead to synthesis of missense nucleic acids.

6-Mercaptopurine results from biotransformation of the inactive precursor *azathioprine* (p. 37). The uricostatic *allopurinol* inhibits the degradation of 6-mercaptopurine such that co-administration of the two drugs permits dose reduction of the latter.

Frequently, the combination of cytostatics permits an improved therapeutic effect with fewer adverse reactions. Initial success can be followed by loss of effect because of the emergence of resistant tumor cells. **Mechanisms of resistance** are multifactorial:

Diminished cellular uptake may result from reduced synthesis of a transport protein that may be needed for membrane penetration (e.g., methotrexate).

Augmented drug extrusion: increased synthesis of the P-glycoprotein that extrudes drugs from the cell (e.g., anthracyclines, vinca alkaloids, epipodophyllotoxins, and paclitaxel) is responsible for multi-drug resistance (*mdr-1* gene amplification).

Diminished bioactivation of a prodrug, e.g., cytarabine, which requires intracellular phosphorylation to become cytotoxic.

Change in site of action: e.g., increased synthesis of dihydrofolate reductase may occur as a compensatory response to methotrexate.

Damage repair: DNA repair enzymes may become more efficient in repairing defects caused by cisplatin.

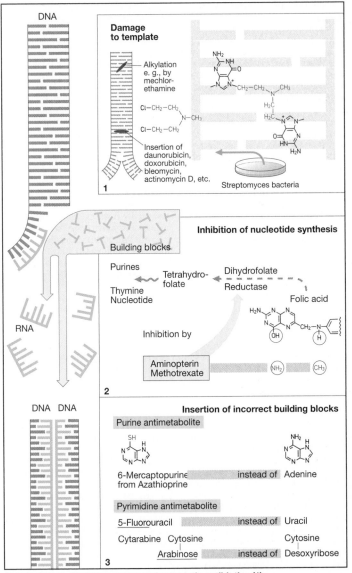

Damage to template

Alkylation e. g., by mechlorethamine

Insertion of daunorubicin, doxorubicin, bleomycin, actinomycin D, etc.

Streptomyces bacteria

1

Inhibition of nucleotide synthesis

Building blocks

Purines

Thymine Nucleotide

Tetrahydrofolate

Dihydrofolate Reductase

Folic acid

Inhibition by

Aminopterin Methotrexate

2

Insertion of incorrect building blocks

Purine antimetabolite

6-Mercaptopurine from Azathioprine — instead of — Adenine

Pyrimidine antimetabolite

5-Fluorouracil — instead of — Uracil

Cytarabine Cytosine — Cytosine

Arabinose — instead of — Desoxyribose

3

A. Cytostatics: alkylating agents and cytostatic antibiotics (1), inhibitors of tetrahydrofolate synthesis (2), antimetabolites (3)

Inhibition of Immune Responses

Both the prevention of *transplant rejection* and the treatment of *autoimmune disorders* call for a suppression of immune responses. However, immune suppression also entails weakened defenses against infectious pathogens and a long-term increase in the risk of neoplasms.

A specific **immune response** begins with the binding of antigen by lymphocytes carrying specific receptors with the appropriate antigen-binding site. B-lymphocytes "recognize" antigen surface structures by means of membrane receptors that resemble the antibodies formed subsequently. T-lymphocytes (and naive B-cells) require the antigen to be presented on the surface of macrophages or other cells in conjunction with the major histocompatibility complex (MHC); the latter permits recognition of antigenic structures by means of the T-cell receptor. T-helper cells carry adjacent CD-3 and CD-4 complexes, cytotoxic T-cells a CD-8 complex. The CD proteins assist in docking to the MHC. In addition to recognition of antigen, activation of lymphocytes requires stimulation by cytokines. Interleukin-1 is formed by macrophages, and various interleukins (IL), including IL-2, are made by T-helper cells. As antigen-specific lymphocytes proliferate, immune defenses are set into motion.

I. Interference with antigen recognition. Muromonab CD3 is a monoclonal antibody directed against mouse CD-3 that blocks antigen recognition by T-lymphocytes (use in graft rejection).

II. Inhibition of cytokine production or action. Glucocorticoids modulate the expression of numerous genes; thus, the production of IL-1 and IL-2 is inhibited, which explains the suppression of T-cell-dependent immune responses. Glucocorticoids are used in organ transplantations, autoimmune diseases, and allergic disorders. Systemic use carries the risk of iatrogenic Cushing's syndrome (p. 248).

Cyclosporin A is an antibiotic polypeptide from fungi and consists of 11, in part atypical, amino acids. Given orally, it is absorbed, albeit incompletely. In lymphocytes, it is bound by cyclophilin, a cytosolic receptor that inhibits the phosphatase calcineurin. The latter plays a key role in T-cell signal transduction. It contributes to the induction of cytokine production, including that of IL-2. The breakthroughs of modern transplantation medicine are largely attributable to the introduction of cyclosporin A. Prominent among its adverse effects are renal damage, hypertension, and hyperkalemia.

Tacrolimus, a macrolide, derives from a streptomyces species; pharmacologically it resembles cyclosporin A, but is more potent and efficacious.

The monoclonal antibodies daclizumab and basiliximab bind to the α-chain of the II-2 receptor of T-lymphocytes and thus prevent their activation, e.g., during transplant rejection.

III. Disruption of cell metabolism with inhibition of proliferation. At dosages below those needed to treat malignancies, some cytostatics are also employed for immunosuppression, e.g., azathioprine, methotrexate, and cyclophosphamide (p. 298). The antiproliferative effect is not specific for lymphocytes and involves both T- and B-cells.

Mycophenolate mofetil has a more specific effect on lymphocytes than on other cells. It inhibits inosine monophosphate dehydrogenase, which catalyzes purine synthesis in lymphocytes. It is used in acute tissue rejection responses.

IV. Anti-T-cell immune serum is obtained from animals immunized with human T-lymphocytes. The antibodies bind to and damage T-cells and can thus be used to attenuate tissue rejection.

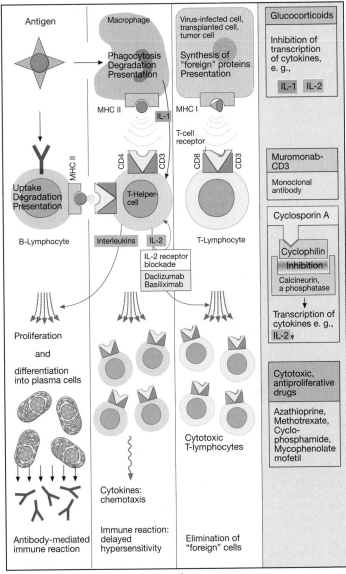

A. Immune reaction and immunosuppressives

Antidotes and treatment of poisonings

Drugs used to counteract drug overdosage are considered under the appropriate headings, e.g., physostigmine with atropine; naloxone with opioids; flumazenil with benzodiazepines; antibody (Fab fragments) with digitalis; and N-acetyl-cysteine with acetaminophen intoxication.

Chelating agents (A) serve as antidotes in poisoning with heavy metals. They act to complex and, thus, "inactivate" heavy metal ions. Chelates (from Greek: chele = claw [of crayfish]) represent complexes between a metal ion and molecules that carry several binding sites for the metal ion. Because of their high affinity, chelating agents "attract" metal ions present in the organism. The chelates are non-toxic, are excreted predominantly via the kidney, maintain a tight organometallic bond also in the concentrated, usually acidic, milieu of tubular urine and thus promote the elimination of metal ions.

Na_2Ca-EDTA is used to treat lead poisoning. This antidote cannot penetrate cell membranes and must be given parenterally. Because of its high binding affinity, the lead ion displaces Ca^{2+} from its bond. The lead-containing chelate is eliminated renally. Nephrotoxicity predominates among the unwanted effects. **Na_3Ca-Pentetate** is a complex of diethylenetriaminopentaacetic acid (DPTA) and serves as antidote in lead and other metal intoxications.

Dimercaprol (BAL, British Anti-Lewisite) was developed in World War II as an antidote against vesicant organic arsenicals (**B**). It is able to chelate various metal ions. Dimercaprol forms a liquid, rapidly decomposing substance that is given intramuscularly in an oily vehicle. A related compound, both in terms of structure and activity, is **dimercaptopropanesulfonic acid,** whose sodium salt is suitable for oral administration. Shivering, fever, and skin reactions are potential adverse effects.

Deferoxamine derives from the bacterium *Streptomyces pilosus.* The substance possesses a very high iron-binding capacity, but does not withdraw iron from hemoglobin or cytochromes. It is poorly absorbed enterally and must be given parenterally to cause increased excretion of iron. Oral administration is indicated only if enteral absorption of iron is to be curtailed. Unwanted effects include allergic reactions. It should be noted that blood letting is the most effective means of removing iron from the body; however, this method is unsuitable for treating conditions of iron overload associated with anemia.

D-penicillamine can promote the elimination of copper (e.g., in Wilson's disease) and of lead ions. It can be given orally. Two additional uses are cystinuria and rheumatoid arthritis. In the former, formation of cystine stones in the urinary tract is prevented because the drug can form a disulfide with cysteine that is readily soluble. In the latter, penicillamine can be used as a basal regimen (p. 320). The therapeutic effect may result in part from a reaction with aldehydes, whereby polymerization of collagen molecules into fibrils is inhibited. Unwanted effects are: cutaneous damage (diminished resistance to mechanical stress with a tendency to form blisters), nephrotoxicity, bone marrow depression, and taste disturbances.

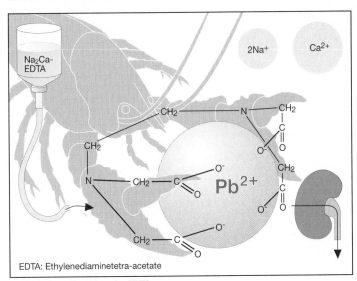

EDTA: Ethylenediaminetetra-acetate

A. Chelation of lead ions by EDTA

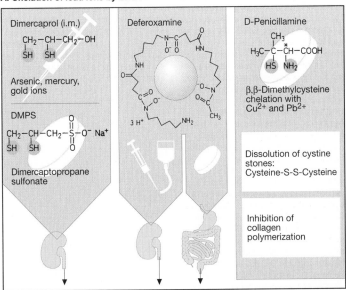

B. Chelators

Antidotes for cyanide poisoning

(A). Cyanide ions (CN⁻) enter the organism in the form of hydrocyanic acid (HCN); the latter can be inhaled, released from cyanide salts in the acidic stomach juice, or enzymatically liberated from bitter almonds in the gastrointestinal tract. The lethal dose of HCN can be as low as 50 mg. CN⁻ binds with high affinity to trivalent iron and thereby arrests utilization of oxygen via mitochondrial cytochrome oxidases of the respiratory chain. An internal asphyxiation *(histotoxic hypoxia)* ensues while erythrocytes remain charged with O_2 (venous blood colored bright red).

In small amounts, cyanide can be converted to the relatively nontoxic thiocyanate (SCN⁻) by hepatic "rhodanese" or sulfur transferase. As a therapeutic measure, thiosulfate can be given i.v. to promote formation of thiocyanate, which is eliminated in urine. However, this reaction is slow in onset. A more effective emergency treatment is the i.v. administration of the methemoglobin-forming agent 4-dimethylaminophenol, which rapidly generates trivalent from divalent iron in hemoglobin. Competition between methemoglobin and cytochrome oxidase for CN⁻ ions favors the formation of cyanmethemoglobin. Hydroxocobalamin is an alternative, very effective antidote because its central cobalt atom binds CN⁻ with high affinity to generate cyanocobalamin.

Tolonium chloride (Toluidin Blue). Brown-colored methemoglobin, containing tri- instead of divalent iron, is incapable of carrying O_2. Under normal conditions, methemoglobin is produced continuously, but reduced again with the help of glucose-6-phosphate dehydrogenase. Substances that promote formation of methemoglobin **(B)** may cause a lethal deficiency of O_2. Tolonium chloride is a redox dye that can be given i.v. to reduce methemoglobin.

Obidoxime is an antidote used to treat poisoning with insecticides of the organophosphate type (p. 102). Phosphorylation of acetylcholinesterase causes an irreversible inhibition of acetylcholine breakdown and hence flooding of the organism with the transmitter. Possible sequelae are exaggerated parasympathomimetic activity, blockade of ganglionic and neuromuscular transmission, and respiratory paralysis.

Therapeutic measures include: 1. administration of atropine in high dosage to shield muscarinic acetylcholine receptors; and 2. reactivation of acetylcholinesterase by obidoxime, which successively binds to the enzyme, captures the phosphate residue by a nucleophilic attack, and then dissociates from the active center to release the enzyme from inhibition.

Ferric Ferrocyanide ("Berlin Blue," B) is used to treat poisoning with thallium salts (e.g., in rat poison), the initial symptoms of which are gastrointestinal disturbances, followed by nerve and brain damage, as well as hair loss. Thallium ions present in the organism are secreted into the gut but undergo reabsorption. The insoluble, nonabsorbable colloidal Berlin Blue binds thallium ions. It is given orally to prevent absorption of acutely ingested thallium or to promote clearance from the organism by intercepting thallium that is secreted into the intestines.

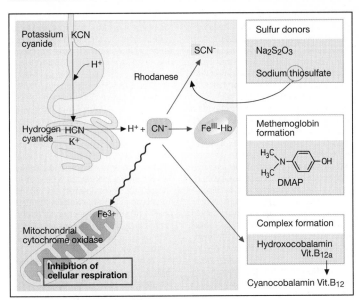

A. Cyanide poisoning and antidotes

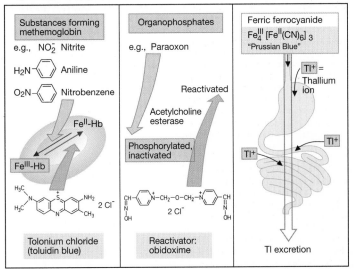

B. Poisons and antidotes

Angina Pectoris

An anginal pain attack signals a transient hypoxia of the myocardium. As a rule, the *oxygen deficit* results from inadequate myocardial blood flow due to narrowing of larger coronary arteries. The underlying causes are: most commonly, an atherosclerotic change of the vascular wall (*coronary sclerosis* with exertional angina); very infrequently, a spasmodic constriction of a morphologically healthy coronary artery (*coronary spasm* with angina at rest; variant angina); or more often, a coronary spasm occurring in an atherosclerotic vascular segment.

The goal of treatment is to prevent myocardial hypoxia either by raising blood flow *(oxygen supply)* or by lowering myocardial blood demand *(oxygen demand)* (**A**).

Factors determining oxygen supply. The force driving myocardial blood flow is the *pressure difference* between the coronary ostia *(aortic pressure)* and the opening of the coronary sinus *(right atrial pressure)*. Blood flow is opposed by *coronary flow resistance,* which includes three components. (1) Due to their large caliber, the *proximal coronary segments* do not normally contribute significantly to flow resistance. However, in coronary sclerosis or spasm, pathological obstruction of flow occurs here. Whereas the more common coronary sclerosis cannot be overcome pharmacologically, the less common coronary spasm can be relieved by appropriate vasodilators (nitrates, nifedipine). (2) The caliber of *arteriolar resistance vessels* controls blood flow through the coronary bed. Arteriolar caliber is determined by myocardial O_2 tension and local concentrations of metabolic products, and is "automatically" adjusted to the required blood flow (**B,** healthy subject). This *metabolic autoregulation* explains why anginal attacks in coronary sclerosis occur only during exercise (**B,** patient). At rest, the pathologically elevated flow resistance is compensated by a corresponding decrease in arteriolar resistance, ensuring adequate myocardial perfusion. During exercise, further dilation of arterioles is impossible. As a result, there is ischemia associated with pain. Pharmacological agents that act to dilate arterioles would thus be inappropriate because at rest they may divert blood from underperfused into healthy vascular regions on account of redundant arteriolar dilation. The resulting "steal effect" could provoke an anginal attack. (3) The intramyocardial pressure, i.e., systolic squeeze, compresses the capillary bed. Myocardial blood flow is halted during systole and occurs almost entirely during diastole. *Diastolic wall tension* ("preload") depends on ventricular volume and filling pressure. The organic nitrates reduce preload by decreasing venous return to the heart.

Factors determining oxygen demand. The heart muscle cell consumes the most energy to generate contractile force. O_2 demand rises with an increase in (1) *heart rate,* (2) *contraction velocity,* (3) *systolic wall tension* ("afterload"). The latter depends on ventricular volume and the systolic pressure needed to empty the ventricle. As peripheral resistance increases, aortic pressure rises, hence the resistance against which ventricular blood is ejected. O_2 demand is lowered by β-blockers and Ca-antagonists, as well as by nitrates (p. 308).

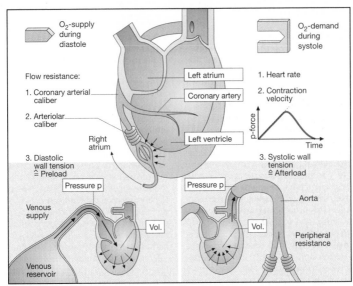

A. O₂ supply and demand of the myocardium

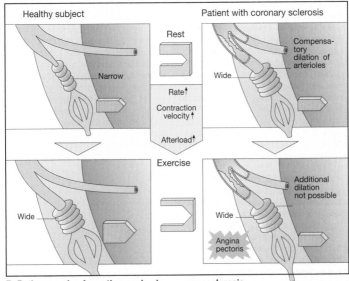

B. Pathogenesis of exertion angina in coronary sclerosis

Antianginal Drugs

Antianginal agents derive from three drug groups, the pharmacological properties of which have already been presented in more detail, viz., the organic nitrates (p. 120), the Ca^{2+} antagonists (p. 122), and the β-blockers (pp. 92ff).

Organic nitrates (A) increase blood flow, hence O_2 supply, because diastolic wall tension (preload) declines as venous return to the heart is diminished. Thus, the nitrates enable myocardial flow resistance to be reduced even in the presence of coronary sclerosis with angina pectoris. In angina due to coronary spasm, arterial dilation overcomes the vasospasm and restores myocardial perfusion to normal. O_2 demand falls because of the ensuing decrease in the two variables that determine systolic wall tension (afterload): ventricular filling volume and aortic blood pressure.

Calcium antagonists (B) decrease O_2 demand by lowering aortic pressure, one of the components contributing to afterload. The dihydropyridine *nifedipine* is devoid of a cardiodepressant effect, but may give rise to reflex tachycardia and an associated increase in O_2 demand. The catamphiphilic drugs *verapamil* and *diltiazem* are cardiodepressant. Reduced beat frequency and contractility contribute to a reduction in O_2 demand; however, AV-block and mechanical insufficiency can dangerously jeopardize heart function. In coronary spasm, calcium antagonists can induce spasmolysis and improve blood flow (p. 122).

β-Blockers (C) protect the heart against the O_2-wasting effect of sympathetic drive by inhibiting β-receptor-mediated increases in cardiac rate and speed of contraction.

Uses of antianginal drugs (D). For relief of the **acute anginal attack,** rapidly absorbed drugs devoid of cardiodepressant activity are preferred. The drug of choice is *nitroglycerin* (NTG, 0.8–2.4 mg sublingually; onset of action within 1 to 2 min; duration of effect ~30 min). Isosorbide dinitrate (ISDN)

can also be used (5–10 mg sublingually); compared with NTG, its action is somewhat delayed in onset but of longer duration. Finally, nifedipine may be useful in chronic stable, or in variant angina (5–20 mg, capsule to be bitten and the contents swallowed).

For sustained daytime **angina prophylaxis,** *nitrates* are of limited value because "nitrate pauses" of about 12 h are appropriate if nitrate tolerance is to be avoided. If attacks occur during the day, ISDN, or its metabolite *isosorbide mononitrate,* may be given in the morning and at noon (e.g., ISDN 40 mg in extended-release capsules). Because of hepatic presystemic elimination, NTG is not suitable for oral administration. Continuous delivery via a transdermal patch would also not seem advisable because of the potential development of tolerance. With *molsidomine,* there is less risk of a nitrate tolerance; however, due to its potential carcinogenicity, its clinical use is restricted.

The choice between *calcium antagonists* must take into account the differential effect of nifedipine versus verapamil or diltiazem on cardiac performance (see above). When β-*blockers* are given, the potential consequences of reducing cardiac contractility (withdrawal of sympathetic drive) must be kept in mind. Since vasodilating $β_2$-receptors are blocked, an increased risk of vasospasm cannot be ruled out. Therefore, monotherapy with β-blockers is recommended only in angina due to coronary sclerosis, but not in variant angina.

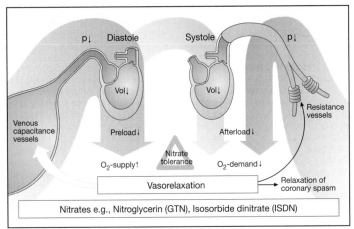

A. Effects of nitrates

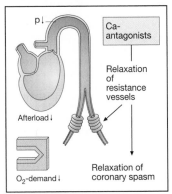

B. Effects of Ca-antagonists

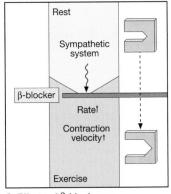

C. Effects of β-blockers

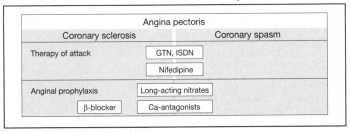

D. Clinical uses of antianginal drugs

Acute Myocardial Infarction

Myocardial infarction is caused by acute *thrombotic occlusion* of a coronary artery **(A)**. Therapeutic interventions aim to restore blood flow in the occluded vessel in order to reduce infarct size or to rescue ischemic myocardial tissue. In the area perfused by the affected vessel, inadequate supply of oxygen and glucose impairs the function of heart muscle: contractile force declines. In the great majority of cases, the left ventricle (anterior or posterior wall) is involved. The decreased work capacity of the infarcted myocardium leads to a reduction in stroke volume (SV) and hence cardiac output (CO). The fall in blood pressure (RR) triggers reflex activation of the sympathetic system. The resultant stimulation of cardiac β-adrenoceptors elicits an increase in both heart rate and force of systolic contraction, which, in conjunction with an α-adrenoceptor-mediated increase in peripheral resistance, leads to a compensatory rise in blood pressure. In ATP-depleted cells in the infarct border zone, resting membrane potential declines with a concomitant increase in excitability that may be further exacerbated by activation of β-adrenoceptors. Together, both processes promote the risk of fatal ventricular arrhythmias. As a consequence of local ischemia, extracellular concentrations of H^+ and K^+ rise in the affected region, leading to excitation of nociceptive nerve fibers. The resultant sensation of pain, typically experienced by the patient as annihilating, reinforces sympathetic activation.

The success of infarct therapy critically depends on the length of time between the onset of the attack and the start of treatment. Whereas some therapeutic measures are indicated only after the diagnosis is confirmed, others necessitate prior exclusion of contraindications or can be instituted only in specially equipped facilities. Without exception, however, prompt action is imperative. Thus, a staggered treatment schedule has proven useful.

The **antiplatelet agent, ASA,** is administered at the first suspected signs of infarction. Pain due to ischemia is treated predominantly with antianginal drugs (e.g., **nitrates**). In case this treatment fails (no effect within 30 min, administration of **morphine,** if needed in combination with an **antiemetic** to prevent morphine-induced vomiting, is indicated. If ECG signs of myocardial infarction are absent, the patient is stabilized by antianginal therapy (nitrates, β-blockers) and given ASA and heparin.

When the diagnosis has been confirmed by electrocardiography, attempts are started to dissolve the thrombus pharmacologically (thrombolytic therapy: **alteplase** or **streptokinase**) or to remove the obstruction by mechanical means (balloon dilation or angioplasty). **Heparin** is given to prevent a possible vascular reocclusion, i.e., to safeguard the patency of the affected vessel. Regardless of the outcome of thrombolytic therapy or balloon dilation, a β-**blocker** is administered to suppress imminent arrhythmias, unless it is contraindicated. Treatment of life-threatening ventricular arrhythmias calls for an antiarrhythmic of the class of Na^+-channel blockers, e.g., **lidocaine**. To improve long-term prognosis, use is made of a β-blocker (↓ incidence of reinfarction and acute cardiac mortality) and an **ACE inhibitor** (prevention of ventricular enlargement after myocardial infarction) **(A).**

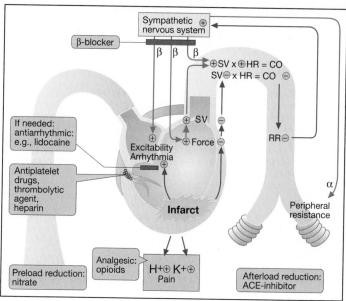

A. Drugs for the treatment of acute myocardial infarction

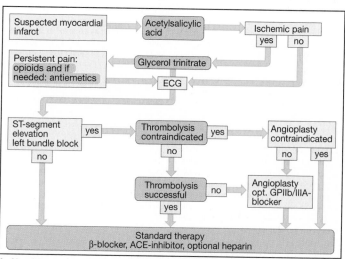

A. Algorithm for the treatment of acute myocardial infarction

Hypertension

Arterial hypertension (high blood pressure) generally does not impair the well-being of the affected individual; however, in the long term it leads to vascular damage and secondary complications (**A**). The aim of antihypertensive therapy is to prevent the latter and, thus, to prolong life expectancy.

Hypertension infrequently results from another disease, such as a catecholamine-secreting tumor (pheochromocytoma); in most cases the cause cannot be determined: **essential (primary) hypertension.** Antihypertensive drugs are indicated when blood pressure cannot be sufficiently controlled by means of **weight reduction** or a **low-salt diet.** In principle, lowering of either cardiac output or peripheral resistance may decrease blood pressure (cf. p. 306, 314, blood pressure determinants). The available drugs influence one or both of these determinants. The therapeutic utility of antihypertensives is determined by their efficacy and tolerability. The choice of a specific drug is determined on the basis of a benefit:risk assessment of the relevant drugs, in keeping with the patient's individual needs.

In instituting **single-drug therapy** (monotherapy), the following considerations apply: β-blockers (p. 92) are of value in the treatment of juvenile hypertension with tachycardia and high cardiac output; however, in patients disposed to bronchospasm, even β_1-selective blockers are contraindicated. Thiazide diuretics (p. 162) are potentially well suited in hypertension associated with congestive heart failure; however, they would be unsuitable in hypokalemic states. When hypertension is accompanied by angina pectoris, the preferred choice would be a β-blocker or calcium antagonist (p. 122) rather than a diuretic. As for the calcium antagonists, it should be noted that verapamil, unlike nifedipine, possesses cardiodepressant activity. α-Blockers may be of particular benefit in patients with benign prostatic hyperplasia and im-paired micturition. At present, only β-blockers and diuretics have undergone large-scale clinical trials, which have shown that reduction in blood pressure is associated with decreased morbidity and mortality due to stroke and congestive heart failure.

In **multidrug therapy,** it is necessary to consider which agents rationally complement each other. A β-blocker (bradycardia, cardiodepression due to sympathetic blockade) can be effectively combined with nifedipine (reflex tachycardia), but obviously not with verapamil (bradycardia, cardiodepression). Monotherapy with ACE inhibitors (p. 124) produces an adequate reduction of blood pressure in 50% of patients; the response rate is increased to 90% by combination with a (thiazide) diuretic. When vasodilators such as dihydralazine or minoxidil (p. 118) are given, β-blockers would serve to prevent reflex tachycardia, and diuretics to counteract fluid retention.

Abrupt termination of continuous treatment can be followed by rebound hypertension (particularly with short $t_{1/2}$ β-blockers).

Drugs for the control of hypertensive crises include nifedipine (capsule, to be chewed and swallowed), nitroglycerin (sublingually), clonidine (p.o. or i.v., p. 96), dihydralazine (i.v.), diazoxide (i.v.), fenoldopam (by infusion, p. 114) and sodium nitroprusside (p. 120, by infusion). The nonselective α-blocker phentolamine (p. 90) is indicated only in pheochromocytoma.

Antihypertensives for hypertension in **pregnancy** are β_1-selective adrenoceptor-blockers, methyldopa (p. 96), and dihydralazine (i.v. infusion) for eclampsia (massive rise in blood pressure with CNS symptoms).

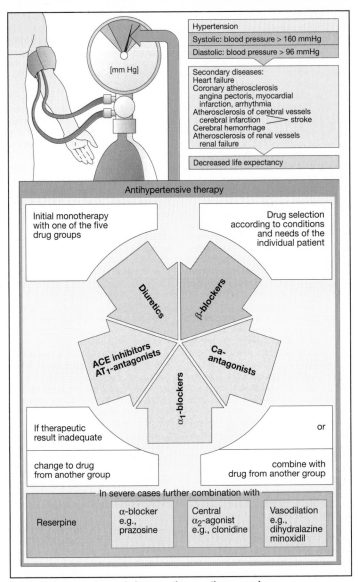

Hypertension
Systolic: blood pressure > 160 mmHg
Diastolic: blood pressure > 96 mmHg

Secondary diseases:
Heart failure
Coronary atherosclerosis
  angina pectoris, myocardial
  infarction, arrhythmia
Atherosclerosis of cerebral vessels
  cerebral infarction ———> stroke
Cerebral hemorrhage
Atherosclerosis of renal vessels
  renal failure

Decreased life expectancy

Antihypertensive therapy

Initial monotherapy
with one of the five
drug groups

Drug selection
according to conditions
and needs of the
individual patient

Diuretics

β-blockers

ACE inhibitors
AT₁-antagonists

Ca-
antagonists

α₁-blockers

If therapeutic
result inadequate

or

change to drug
from another group

combine with
drug from another group

In severe cases further combination with

| Reserpine | α-blocker e.g., prazosine | Central α₂-agonist e.g., clonidine | Vasodilation e.g., dihydralazine minoxidil |

A. Arterial hypertension and pharmacotherapeutic approaches

Hypotension

The venous side of the circulation, excluding the pulmonary circulation, accommodates ~ 60% of the total blood volume; because of the low venous pressure (mean ~ 15 mmHg) it is part of the *low-pressure system*. The arterial vascular beds, representing the *high-pressure system* (mean pressure, ~ 100 mmHg), contain ~ 15%. The arterial pressure generates the driving force for perfusion of tissues and organs. Blood draining from the latter collects in the low-pressure system and is pumped back by the heart into the high-pressure system.

The arterial blood pressure (ABP) depends on: (1) the volume of blood per unit of time that is forced by the heart into the high-pressure system—cardiac output corresponding to the product of stroke volume and heart rate (beats/min), stroke volume being determined *inter alia* by venous filling pressure; (2) the counterforce opposing the flow of blood, i.e., peripheral resistance, which is a function of arteriolar caliber.

Chronic hypotension (systolic BP < 105 mmHg). *Primary idiopathic hypotension* generally has no clinical importance. If symptoms such as lassitude and dizziness occur, a program of physical exercise instead of drugs is advisable.

Secondary hypotension is a sign of an underlying disease that should be treated first. If stroke volume is too low, as in heart failure, a cardiac glycoside can be given to increase myocardial contractility and stroke volume. When stroke volume is decreased due to insufficient blood volume, plasma substitutes will be helpful in treating blood loss, whereas aldosterone deficiency requires administration of a mineralocorticoid (e.g., fludrocortisone). The latter is the drug of choice for orthostatic hypotension due to autonomic failure. A parasympatholytic (or electrical pacemaker) can restore cardiac rate in bradycardia.

Acute hypotension. *Failure of orthostatic regulation.* A change from the recumbent to the erect position (orthostasis) will cause blood within the low-pressure system to sink towards the feet because the veins in body parts below the heart will be distended, despite a reflex venoconstriction, by the weight of the column of blood in the blood vessels. The fall in stroke volume is partly compensated by a rise in heart rate. The remaining reduction of cardiac output can be countered by elevating the peripheral resistance, enabling blood pressure and organ perfusion to be maintained. An orthostatic malfunction is present when counter-regulation fails and cerebral blood flow falls, with resultant symptoms, such as dizziness, "black-out," or even loss of consciousness. In the *sympathotonic form,* sympathetically mediated circulatory reflexes are intensified (more pronounced tachycardia and rise in peripheral resistance, i.e., diastolic pressure); however, there is failure to compensate for the reduction in venous return. Prophylactic treatment with sympathomimetics therefore would hold little promise. Instead, cardiovascular fitness training would appear more important. An increase in venous return may be achieved in two ways. Increasing NaCl intake augments salt and fluid reserves and, hence, blood volume (contraindications: hypertension, heart failure). Constriction of venous capacitance vessels might be produced by dihydroergotamine. Whether this effect could also be achieved by an α-sympathomimetic remains debatable. In the very rare *asympathotonic form,* use of sympathomimetics would certainly be reasonable.

In patients with hypotension due to high thoracic spinal cord transections (resulting in an essentially complete sympathetic denervation), loss of sympathetic vasomotor control can be compensated by administration of sympathomimetics.

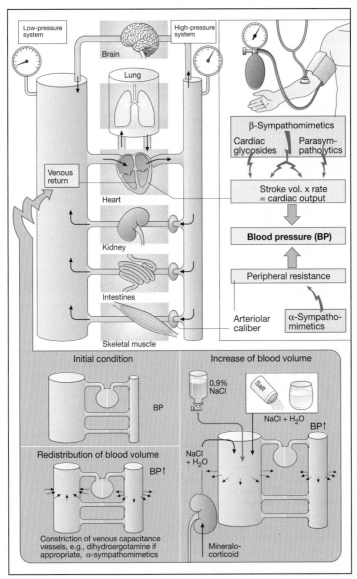

A. Treatment of hypotension

Gout

Gout is an inherited metabolic disease that results from **hyperuricemia,** an elevation in the blood of uric acid, the end-product of purine degradation. The typical **gout attack** consists of a highly painful inflammation of the first metatarsophalangeal joint ("podagra"). Gout attacks are triggered by precipitation of sodium urate crystals in the synovial fluid of joints.

During the early stage of inflammation, urate crystals are phagocytosed by polymorphonuclear leukocytes (1) that engulf the crystals by their ameboid cytoplasmic movements (2). The phagocytic vacuole fuses with a lysosome (3). The lysosomal enzymes are, however, unable to degrade the sodium urate. Further ameboid movement dislodges the crystals and causes rupture of the phagolysosome. Lysosomal enzymes are liberated into the granulocyte, resulting in its destruction by self-digestion and damage to the adjacent tissue. Inflammatory mediators, such as prostaglandins and chemotactic factors, are released (4). More granulocytes are attracted and suffer similar destruction; the inflammation intensifies—the gout attack flares up.

Treatment of the gout attack aims to interrupt the inflammatory response. The drug of choice is *colchicine,* an alkaloid from the autumn crocus *(Colchicum autumnale).* It is known as a "spindle poison" because it arrests mitosis at metaphase by inhibiting contractile spindle proteins. Its antigout activity is due to inhibition of contractile proteins in the neutrophils, whereby ameboid mobility and phagocytotic activity are prevented. The most common *adverse effects* of colchicine are abdominal pain, vomiting, and diarrhea, probably due to inhibition of mitoses in the rapidly dividing gastrointestinal epithelial cells. Colchicine is usually given orally (e.g., 0.5 mg hourly until pain subsides or gastrointestinal disturbances occur; maximal daily dose, 10 mg).

Nonsteroidal anti-inflammatory drugs, such as **indomethacin** and **phenylbutazone,** are also effective. In severe cases, **glucocorticoids** may be indicated.

Effective **prophylaxis of gout attacks** requires urate blood levels to be lowered to less than 6 mg/100 mL.

Diet. Purine (cell nuclei)-rich foods should be avoided, e.g., organ meats. Milk, dairy products, and eggs are low in purines and are recommended. Coffee and tea are permitted since the methylxanthine caffeine does not enter purine metabolism.

Uricostatics decrease urate production. **Allopurinol,** as well as its accumulating metabolite alloxanthine (oxypurinol), inhibit xanthine oxidase, which catalyzes urate formation from hypoxanthine via xanthine. These precursors are readily eliminated via the urine. Allopurinol is given orally (300–800 mg/d). Except for infrequent allergic reactions, it is well tolerated and is the drug of choice for gout prophylaxis. At the start of therapy, gout attacks may occur, but they can be prevented by concurrent administration of colchicine (0.5–1.5 mg/d). **Uricosurics,** such as **probenecid, benzbromarone** (100 mg/d), or **sulfinpyrazone,** promote renal excretion of uric acid. They saturate the organic acid transport system in the proximal renal tubules, making it unavailable for urate reabsorption. When underdosed, they inhibit only the acid secretory system, which has a smaller transport capacity. Urate elimination is then inhibited and a gout attack is possible. In patients with urate stones in the urinary tract, uricosurics are contraindicated.

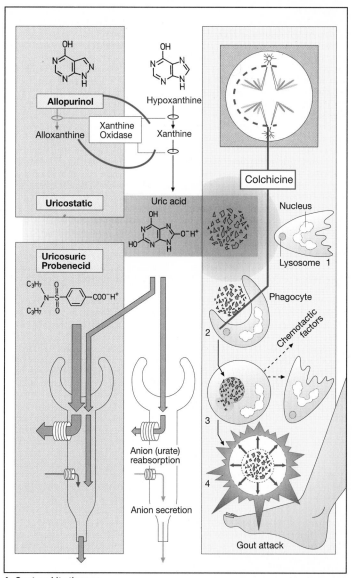

Allopurinol

Hypoxanthine

Alloxanthine

Xanthine Oxidase

Xanthine

Uricostatic

Colchicine

Uric acid

Nucleus

Lysosome 1

Uricosuric Probenecid

C_3H_7

N—SO_2—COO^-H^+

C_3H_7

Phagocyte

2

Chemotactic factors

Anion (urate) reabsorption

3

Anion secretion

4

Gout attack

A. Gout and its therapy

Osteoporosis

Osteoporosis is defined as a generalized decrease in bone mass (osteopenia) that affects bone matrix and mineral content equally, giving rise to fractures of vertebral bodies with bone pain, kyphosis, and shortening of the torso. Fractures of the hip and the distal radius are also common. The underlying process is a disequilibrium between bone formation by osteoblasts and bone resorption by osteoclasts.

Classification: *Idiopathic osteoporosis* type I, occurring in postmenopausal females; type II, occurring in senescent males and females (>70 y). *Secondary osteoporosis:* associated with primary disorders such as Cushing's disease, or induced by drugs, e.g., chronic therapy with glucocorticoids or heparin. In these forms, the cause can be eliminated.

Postmenopausal osteoporosis represents a period of accelerated loss of bone mass. The lower the preexisting bone mass, the earlier the clinical signs become manifest.

Risk factors are: premature menopause, physical inactivity, cigarette smoking, alcohol abuse, low body weight, and calcium-poor diet.

Prophylaxis: Administration of estrogen can protect against postmenopausal loss of bone mass. Frequently, conjugated estrogens are used (p. 254). Because estrogen monotherapy increases the risk of uterine cancer, a gestagen needs to be given concurrently (except after hysterectomy), as e.g., in an oral contraceptive preparation (p. 256). Under this therapy, menses will continue. The risk of thromboembolic disorders is increased and that of myocardial infarction probably lowered. Hormone treatment can be extended for 10 y or longer. Before menopause, daily calcium intake should be kept at 1 g (contained in 1 L of milk), and 1.5 g thereafter.

Therapy. Formation of new bone matrix is induced by **fluoride.** Administered as sodium fluoride, it stimulates osteoblasts. Fluoride is substituted for hydroxyl residues in hydroxyapatite to form fluorapatite, the latter being more resistant to resorption by osteoclasts. To safeguard adequate mineralization of new bone, calcium must be supplied in sufficient amounts. However, simultaneous administration would result in precipitation of nonabsorbable calcium fluoride in the intestines. With *sodium monofluorophosphate* this problem is circumvented. The new bone formed may have increased resistance to compressive, but not torsional, strain and paradoxically bone fragility may increase. Because the conditions under which bone fragility is decreased remain unclear, fluoride therapy is not in routine use.

Calcitonin (p. 264) inhibits osteoclast activity, hence bone resorption. As a peptide it needs to be given by injection (or, alternatively, as a nasal spray). Salmonid is more potent than human calcitonin because of its slower elimination.

Bisphosphonates structurally mimic endogenous pyrophosphate, which inhibits precipitation and dissolution of bone minerals. They retard bone resorption by osteoclasts and, in part, also decrease bone mineralization. Indications include: tumor osteolysis, hypercalcemia, and Paget's disease. Clinical trials with etidronate, administered as an intermittent regimen, have yielded favorable results in osteoporosis. With the newer drugs clodronate, pamidronate, and alendronate, inhibition of osteoclasts predominates; a continuous regimen would thus appear to be feasible.

Bisphosphonates irritate esophageal and gastric mucus membranes; tablets should be swallowed with a reasonable amount of water (250 mL) and the patient should keep in an upright position for 30 min following drug intake.

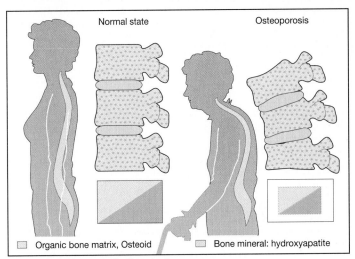

A. Bone: normal state and osteoporosis

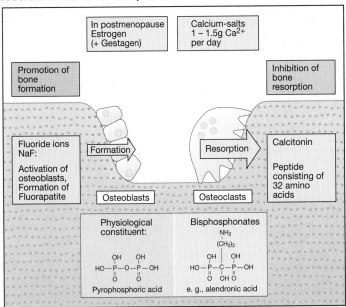

B. Osteoporosis: drugs for prophylaxis and treatment

Rheumatoid Arthritis

Rheumatoid arthritis or **chronic poly-arthritis** is a progressive inflammatory joint disease that intermittently attacks more and more joints, predominantly those of the fingers and toes. The probable cause of rheumatoid arthritis is a pathological reaction of the immune system. This malfunction can be promoted or triggered by various conditions, including genetic disposition, age–related wear and tear, hypothermia, and infection. An initial noxious stimulus elicits an **inflammation of synovial membranes** that, in turn, leads to release of antigens through which the inflammatory process is maintained. Inflammation of the synovial membrane is associated with liberation of inflammatory mediator substances that, among other actions, chemotactically stimulate migration (diapedesis) of phagocytic blood cells (granulocytes, macrophages) into the synovial tissue. The phagocytes produce destructive enzymes that promote tissue damage. Due to the production of prostaglandins and leukotrienes (p. 196) and other factors, the inflammation spreads to the entire joint. As a result, joint cartilage is damaged and the joint is ultimately immobilized or fused.

Pharmacotherapy. Acute relief of inflammatory symptoms can be achieved by **prostaglandin synthase inhibitors; nonsteroidal anti-inflammatory drugs,** or NSAIDs, such as diclofenac, indomethacin, piroxicam, p. 200), and glucocorticoids (p. 248). The inevitably chronic use of NSAIDs is likely to cause *adverse effects.* Neither NSAIDs nor glucocorticoids can halt the progressive destruction of joints.

The use of **disease-modifying agents** may reduce the requirement for NSAIDs. The use of such agents does not mean that intervention in the basic pathogenetic mechanisms (albeit hoped for) is achievable. Rather, disease-modifying therapy permits acutely acting agents to be used as add-ons or as required. The common feature of disease-modifiers is their delayed effect, which develops only after *treatment for several weeks.* Among possible mechanisms of action, inhibition of macrophage activity and inhibition of release or activity of lysosomal enzymes are being discussed. Included in this category are: sulfasalazine (an inhibitor of lipoxygenase and cyclooxygenase, p. 272), chloroquine (lysosomal binding), gold compounds (lysosomal binding; i.m.: aurothioglucose, aurothiomalate; p.o.: auranofin, less effective), as well as D-penicillamine (chelation of metal ions needed for enzyme activity, p. 302). Frequent adverse reactions are: damage to skin and mucous membranes, renal toxicity, and blood dyscrasias. In addition, use is made of cytostatics and immune suppressants such as **methotrexate** (low dose, once weekly) and leflumomid as well as of cytokin antibodies (infliximab) and soluble cytokin receptors (etanercept). Methotrexate exerts an anti-inflammatory effect, apart from its anti-autoimmune action and, next to sulfasalazine, is considered to have the most favorable risk:benefit ratio. In most severe cases cytostatics such as azathioprin and cyclophosphamide will have to be used.

Surgical removal of the inflamed synovial membrane (**synovectomy**) frequently provides long-term relief. If feasible, this approach is preferred because all pharmacotherapeutic measures entail significant adverse effects.

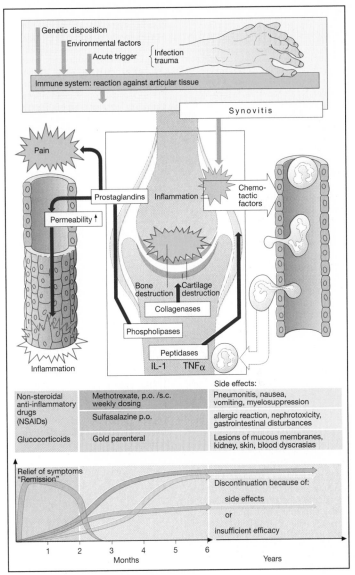

		Side effects:
Non-steroidal anti-inflammatory drugs (NSAIDs)	Methotrexate, p.o. /s.c. weekly dosing	Pneumonitis, nausea, vomiting, myelosuppression
	Sulfasalazine p.o.	allergic reaction, nephrotoxicity, gastrointestinal disturbances
Glucocorticoids	Gold parenteral	Lesions of mucous membranes, kidney, skin, blood dyscrasias

A. Rheumatoid arthritis and its treatment

Migraine

Migraine is a syndrome characterized by recurrent attacks of intense headache and nausea that occur at irregular intervals and last for several hours. In classic migraine, the attack is typically heralded by an "aura" accompanied by spreading homonymous visual field defects with colored sharp edges ("fortification" spectra). In addition, the patient cannot focus on certain objects, has a ravenous appetite for particular foods, and is hypersensitive to odors (hyperosmia) or light (photophobia). The exact cause of these complaints is unknown; however, a disturbance in cranial blood flow is the likely underlying pathogenetic mechanism. In addition to an often inherited predisposition, precipitating factors are required to provoke an attack, e.g., psychic stress, lack of sleep, certain foods. Pharmacotherapy of migraine has two aims: stopping the acute attack and preventing subsequent ones.

Treatment of the attack. For symptomatic relief, headaches are treated with analgesics (acetaminophen, acetylsalicylic acid), and nausea is treated with metoclopramide (p. 330) or domperidone. Since there is delayed gastric emptying during the attack, drug absorption can be markedly retarded, hence effective plasma levels are not obtained. Because metoclopramide stimulates gastric emptying, it promotes absorption of ingested analgesic drugs and thus facilitates pain relief.

If acetylsalicylic acid is administered i.v. as the lysine salt, its bioavailability is complete. Therefore, i.v. injection may be advisable in acute attacks.

Should analgesics prove insufficiently effective, ergotamine or one of the 5-HT$_1$, agonists may help control the acute attack in most cases or prevent an imminent attack. The probable common mechanism of action is a stimulation of serotonin receptors of the 5-HT$_{1D}$ (or perhaps also the 1B and 1F) subtype. Moreover, ergotamine has affinity for dopamine receptors ($\rightarrow$ nausea, emesis), as well as α-adrenoceptors and 5-HT$_2$ receptors ($\uparrow$ vascular tone, $\uparrow$ platelet aggregation). With frequent use, the vascular side effects may give rise to severe peripheral ischemia (ergotism). Overuse (>once per week) of ergotamine may provoke "rebound" headaches, thought to result from persistent vasodilation. Though different in character (tension-type headache), these prompt further consumption of ergotamine. Thus, a vicious circle develops with chronic abuse of ergotamine or other analgesics that may end with irreversible disturbances of peripheral blood flow and impairment of renal function.

Administered orally, ergotamine and sumatriptan, eletriptan, naratriptan, rizatriptan, and zolmitriptan have only limited bioavailability. Dihydroergotamine may be given by i.m. or slow i.v. injection, sumatriptan subcutaneously or by nasal spray.

Prophylaxis. Taken regularly over a longer period, a heterogeneous group of drugs comprising propranolol, nadolol, atenolol, and metoprolol (β-blockers), flunarizine (H$_1$-histamine, dopamine, and calcium antagonist), pizotifen (pizotyline, 5-HT-antagonist), methysergide (partial 5-HT$_{1D}$-agonist and nonselective 5-HT-antagonist, p. 126), NSAIDs (p. 200), and calcitonin (p. 264) may decrease the frequency, intensity, and duration of migraine attacks. Among the β-blockers (p. 90), only those lacking intrinsic sympathomimetic activity are effective.

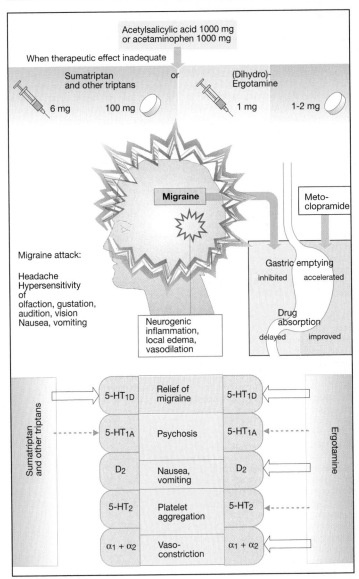

A. Migraine and its treatment

Common Cold

The **common cold**—colloquially the flu, catarrh, or grippe (strictly speaking, the rarer infection with influenza viruses)—is an acute infectious inflammation of the upper respiratory tract. Its symptoms, sneezing, running nose (due to rhinitis), hoarseness (laryngitis), difficulty in swallowing and sore throat (pharyngitis and tonsillitis), cough associated with first serous then mucous sputum (tracheitis, bronchitis), sore muscles, and general malaise can be present individually or concurrently in varying combination or sequence. The term stems from an old popular belief that these complaints are caused by exposure to chilling or dampness. The causative pathogens are different viruses (rhino-, adeno-, parainfluenza v.) that may be transmitted by aerosol droplets produced by coughing and sneezing.

Therapeutic measures. First attempts at a causal treatment consist of zanamavir, an inhibitor of viral neuraminidase, an enzyme necessary for virus adsorption and infection of cells. However, since symptoms of common cold abate spontaneously, there is no compelling need to use drugs. Conventional remedies are intended for symptomatic relief.

Rhinitis. Nasal discharge could be prevented by *parasympatholytics;* however, other atropine–like effects (pp. 104ff) would have to be accepted. Therefore, parasympatholytics are hardly ever used, although a corresponding action is probably exploited in the case of *H₁ antihistamines,* an ingredient of many cold remedies. Locally applied (nasal drops) vasoconstricting α-sympathomimetics (p. 90) decongest the nasal mucosa and dry up secretions, clearing the nasal passage. Long-term use may cause damage to nasal mucous membranes (p. 90).

Sore throat, swallowing problems. Demulcent lozenges containing *surface anesthetics* such as ethylaminobenzoate (benzocaine) or tetracaine (p. 208) may provide relief; however,

the risk of allergic reactions should be borne in mind.

Cough. Since coughing serves to expel excess tracheobronchial secretions, suppression of this physiological reflex is justified only when coughing is dangerous (after surgery) or unproductive because of absent secretions. *Codeine* and *noscapine* (p. 212) suppress cough by a central action.

Mucous airway obstruction. *Mucolytics,* such as acetylcysteine, split disulfide bonds in mucus, hence reduce its viscosity and promote clearing of bronchial mucus. Other expectorants (e.g., hot beverages, potassium iodide, and ipecac) stimulate production of watery mucus. Acetylcysteine is indicated in cystic fibrosis patients and inhaled as an aerosol. Whether mucolytics are indicated in the common cold and whether expectorants like bromohexine or ambroxole effectively lower viscosity of bronchial secretions may be questioned.

Fever. *Antipyretic analgesics* (acetylsalicylic acid, acetaminophen, p. 198) are indicated only when there is high fever. Fever is a natural response and useful in monitoring the clinical course of an infection.

Muscle aches and pains, headache. *Antipyretic analgesics* are effective in relieving these symptoms.

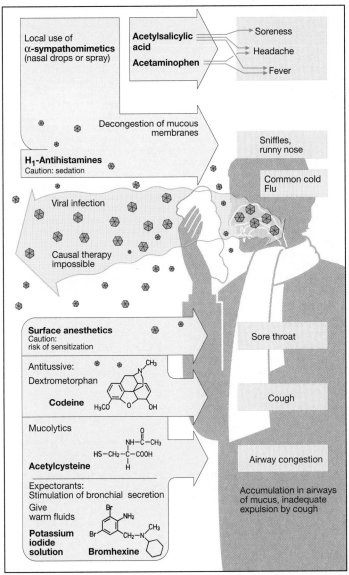

Local use of
α-sympathomimetics
(nasal drops or spray)

Acetylsalicylic acid → Soreness

Acetaminophen → Headache

→ Fever

Decongestion of mucous
membranes

Sniffles,
runny nose

H₁-Antihistamines
Caution: sedation

Common cold
Flu

Viral infection

Causal therapy
impossible

Surface anesthetics
Caution:
risk of sensitization

Sore throat

Antitussive:

Dextrometorphan

Codeine

Cough

Mucolytics

Acetylcysteine

Airway congestion

Expectorants:
Stimulation of bronchial secretion
Give
warm fluids

**Potassium
iodide
solution**

Bromhexine

Accumulation in airways
of mucus, inadequate
expulsion by cough

A. Drugs used in common cold

Allergic Disorders

IgE-mediated allergic reactions (p. 72) involve mast cell release of histamine (p. 114) and production of other mediators (such as leukotrienes, p. 196). Resultant responses include: *relaxation of vascular smooth muscle*, as evidenced locally by vasodilation (e.g., conjunctival congestion) or systemically by hypotension (as in anaphylactic shock); *enhanced capillary permeability* with transudation of fluid into tissues—swelling of conjunctiva and mucous membranes of the upper airways ("hay fever"), cutaneous wheal formation; *contraction of bronchial smooth muscle*—bronchial asthma; *stimulation of intestinal smooth muscle*—diarrhea.

1. Stabilization of mast cells. *Cromolyn* prevents IgE-mediated release of mediators, although only after *chronic treatment.* Moreover, by interfering with the actions of mediator substances on inflammatory cells, it causes a more general inhibition of allergic inflammation. It is applied *locally* to: conjunctiva, nasal mucosa, bronchial tree (inhalation), intestinal mucosa (absorption almost nil with oral intake). Indications: *prophylaxis of hay fever, allergic asthma,* and *food allergies.*

2. Blockade of histamine receptors. Allergic reactions are predominantly mediated by H_1 receptors. *H_1 antihistamines* (p. 114) are mostly used orally. Their therapeutic effect is often disappointing. Indications: allergic rhinitis *(hay fever).*

3. Functional antagonists of mediators of allergy. a) α-Sympathomimetics, such as naphazoline, oxymetazoline, and tetrahydrozoline, are applied topically to the conjunctival and nasal mucosa to produce local vasoconstriction, and decongestion and to dry up secretions (p. 90), e.g., in hay fever. Since they may cause mucosal damage, their use should be short-term.

b) Epinephrine, given i.v., is the *most important drug in the management of anaphylactic shock:* it constricts blood vessels, reduces capillary permeability, and dilates bronchi.

c) β_2-Sympathomimetics, such as terbutaline, fenoterol, and albuterol, are employed in *bronchial asthma,* mostly by inhalation, and parenterally in emergencies. Even after inhalation, effective amounts can reach the systemic circulation and cause side effects (e.g., palpitations, tremulousness, restlessness, hypokalemia). During chronic administration, the sensitivity of bronchial musculature is likely to decline.

d) Theophylline belongs to the methylxanthines. Whereas caffeine (1,3,7-trimethylxanthine) predominantly stimulates the CNS and constricts cerebral blood vessels, theophylline (1,3-dimethylxanthine) possesses additional marked bronchodilator, cardiostimulant, vasorelaxant, and diuretic actions. These effects are attributed to both inhibition of phosphodiesterase ($\rightarrow$ c AMP elevation, p. 66) and antagonism at adenosine receptors. In *bronchial asthma,* theophylline can be given orally for prophylaxis or parenterally to control the attack. Manifestations of overdosage include tonic-clonic seizures and cardiac arrhythmias as early signs.

e) Ipratropium (p. 104) can be inhaled to induce bronchodilation; however, it often lacks sufficient effectiveness in allergic bronchospasm.

f) Glucocorticoids (p. 248) have significant anti-allergic activity and probably interfere with different stages of the allergic response. Indications: *hay fever, bronchial asthma* (preferably local application of analogues with high presystemic elimination, e.g., beclomethasone, budesonide); *anaphylactic shock* (i.v. in high dosage)—a probably nongenomic action of immediate onset.

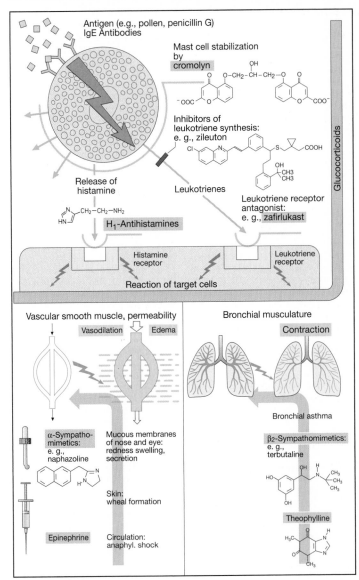

Antigen (e.g., pollen, penicillin G)
IgE Antibodies

Mast cell stabilization by cromolyn

Inhibitors of leukotriene synthesis: e. g., zileuton

Release of histamine

Leukotrienes

Leukotriene receptor antagonist: e. g., zafirlukast

H₁-Antihistamines

Histamine receptor

Leukotriene receptor

Glucocorticoids

Reaction of target cells

Vascular smooth muscle, permeability

Vasodilation   Edema

Bronchial musculature

Contraction

α-Sympatho-mimetics: e. g., naphazoline

Mucous membranes of nose and eye: redness swelling, secretion

Skin: wheal formation

Epinephrine

Circulation: anaphyl. shock

Bronchial asthma

β₂-Sympathomimetics: e. g., terbutaline

Theophylline

A. Anti-allergic therapy

Bronchial Asthma

Definition: a recurrent, episodic shortness of breath caused by bronchoconstriction arising from airway inflammation and hyperreactivity.

Asthma patients tend to underestimate the true severity of their disease. Therefore, self-monitoring by the use of home peak expiratory flow meters is an essential part of the therapeutic program. With proper education, the patient can detect early signs of deterioration and can adjust medication within the framework of a physician-directed therapeutic regimen.

Pathophysiology. One of the main pathogenetic factors is an allergic inflammation of the bronchial mucosa. For instance, leukotrienes that are formed during an IgE-mediated immune response (p. 326) exert a chemotactic effect on inflammatory cells. As the inflammation develops, bronchi become hypersensitive to spasmogenic stimuli. Thus, stimuli other than the original antigen(s) can act as triggers **(A)**; e.g., breathing of cold air is an important trigger in exercise-induced asthma. Cyclooxygenase inhibitors (p. 196) exemplify drugs acting as asthma triggers.

Management. Avoidance of asthma triggers is an important prophylactic measure, though not always feasible. Drugs that inhibit allergic inflammmatory mechanisms or reduce bronchial hyperreactivity, viz., *glucocorticoids,* *"mast-cell stabilizers,"* and *leukotriene antagonists,* attack crucial pathogenetic links. Bronchodilators, such as *β₂-sympathomimetics, theophylline, and ipratropium,* provide symptomatic relief.

The **step scheme (B)** illustrates successive levels of pharmacotherapeutic management at increasing degrees of disease severity.

First treatment of choice for the acute attack are *short-acting, aerosolized β₂-sympathomimetics,* e.g., salbutamol, albuterol, terbutaline, fenoterol, and others. Their action occurs within minutes and lasts for 4 to 6 h.

If β₂-mimetics have to be used more frequently than three times a week, more severe disease is present. At this stage, management includes anti-inflammatory drugs, such as *"mast-cell stabilizers"* (in children or juvenile patients) or else *glucocorticoids.* Inhalational treatment must be administered regularly, improvement being evident only after several weeks. With proper use of glucocorticoids undergoing high presystemic elimination, concern about systemic adverse effects is unwarranted. Possible local adverse effects are: oropharyngeal candidiasis and dysphonia. To minimize the risk of candidiasis, drug administration should occur before morning or evening meals, or be followed by rinsing of the oropharynx. Anti-inflammatory therapy is the more successful the less use is made of as-needed β₂-mimetic medication.

Severe cases may, however, require an *intensified bronchodilator treatment* with *systemic β₂-mimetics* or *theophylline* (systemic use only; low therapeutic index; monitoring of plasma levels needed). *Salmeterol* is a long-acting inhalative β₂-mimetic (duration: 12 h; onset ~20 min) that offers the advantage of a lower systemic exposure. It is used prophylactically at bedtime for nocturnal asthma.

Zafirlukast is a long-acting, selective, and potent leukotriene receptor (LTD₄, LTE₄) antagonist with anti-inflammatory/antiallergic activity and efficacy in the maintenance therapy of chronic asthma. It is given both orally and by inhalation. The onset of action is slow (3 to 14 d). Protective effects against inhaled LTD₄ last up to 12 to 24 h.

Ipratropium may be effective in some patients as an adjunct anti-asthmatic, but has greater utility in preventing bronchospastic episodes in chronic bronchitis.

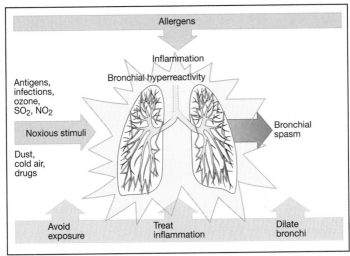

A. Bronchial asthma, pathophysiology and therapeutic approach

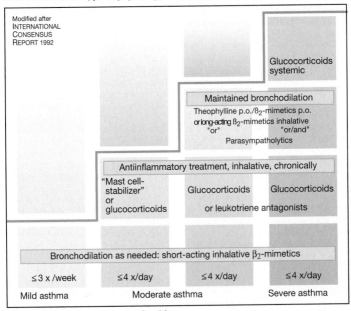

B. Bronchial asthma treatment algorithm

Emesis

In emesis the stomach empties in a retrograde manner. The pyloric sphincter is closed while the cardia and esophagus relax to allow the gastric contents to be propelled orad by a forceful, synchronous contraction of abdominal wall muscles and diaphragm. Closure of the glottis and elevation of the soft palate prevent entry of vomitus into the trachea and nasopharynx. As a rule, there is prodromal salivation or yawning. Coordination between these different stages depends on the **medullary center for emesis,** which can be activated by diverse stimuli. These are conveyed via the **vestibular apparatus, visual, olfactory, and gustatory inputs,** as well as **viscerosensory afferents** from the upper alimentary tract. Furthermore, **psychic experiences** may also activate the emetic center. The mechanisms underlying **motion sickness** (kinetosis, sea sickness) and vomiting during pregnancy are still unclear.

Polar substances cannot reach the emetic center itself because it is protected by the blood-brain barrier. However, they can indirectly excite the center by activating **chemoreceptors** in the **area postrema** or receptors on peripheral vagal nerve endings.

Antiemetic therapy. Vomiting can be a useful reaction enabling the body to eliminate an orally ingested poison. Antiemetic drugs are used to prevent kinetosis, pregnancy vomiting, cytotoxic drug-induced or postoperative vomiting, as well as vomiting due to radiation therapy.

Motion sickness. Effective prophylaxis can be achieved with the parasympatholytic scopolamine (p. 106) and H$_1$ antihistamines (p. 114) of the diphenylmethane type (e.g., diphenhydramine, meclizine). Antiemetic activity is not a property shared by all parasympatholytics or antihistamines. The efficacy of the drugs mentioned depends on the actual situation of the individual (gastric filling, ethanol consumption), environmental conditions (e.g., the behavior of

fellow travellers), and the type of motion experienced. The drugs should be taken 30 min before the start of travel and repeated every 4 to 6 h. Scopolamine applied transdermally through an adhesive patch can provide effective protection for up to 3 d.

Pregnancy vomiting is prone to occur in the first trimester; thus pharmacotherapy would coincide with the period of maximal fetal vulnerability to chemical injury. Accordingly, antiemetics (antihistamines, or neuroleptics if required) should be used only when continuous vomiting threatens to disturb electrolyte and water balance to a degree that places the fetus at risk.

Drug-induced vomiting. To prevent vomiting during anticancer chemotherapy (especially with cisplatin), effective use can be made of 5-HT$_3$-receptor antagonists (e.g., *ondansetron, granisetron,* and *tropisetron*), alone or in combination with glucocorticoids *(methylprednisolone, dexamethasone).* **Anticipatory nausea** and vomiting, resulting from inadequately controlled nausea and emesis in patients undergoing cytotoxic chemotherapy, can be attenuated by a benzodiazepine such as *lorazepam.* Dopamine agonist-induced nausea in parkinsonian patients (p. 188) can be counteracted with D$_2$-receptor antagonists that penetrate poorly into the CNS (e.g., *domperidone, sulpiride). Metoclopramide* is effective in nausea and vomiting of gastrointestinal origin (5-HT$_4$-receptor agonism) and at high dosage also in chemotherapy- and radiation-induced sickness (low potency antagonism at 5-HT$_3$- and D$_2$-receptors). Phenothiazines (e.g., *levomepromazine, trimeprazine, perphenazine*) may suppress nausea/emesis that follows certain types of surgery or is due to opioid analgesics, gastrointestinal irritation, uremia, and diseases accompanied by **elevated intracranial pressure.**

The synthetic cannabinoids *dronabinol* and *nabilone* have antinauseant/antiemetic effects that may benefit AIDS and cancer patients.

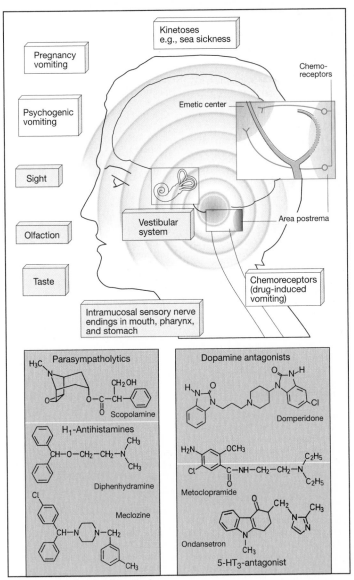

A. Emetic stimuli and antiemetic drugs

Further Reading

A. Foundations and basic principles of pharmacology

Hardman JG, Limbird LE. Goodman & Gilman's. The pharmacological basis of therapeutics. 9th ed. New York: McGraw-Hill; 1996.

Levine RR. Pharmacology: drug actions and reactions. 5th ed. New York: Parthenon Publishing Group; 1996.

Munson PL, Mueller RA, Breese GR. Principles of pharmacology. London: Chapman & Hall; 1995.

Mutschler E, Derendorf H. Drug actions—basic principles and therapeutic aspects. Stuttgart: Medpharm Scientific Pub.; Boca Raton: CRC Press; 1995.

Page CR, Curtis MJ, Sutter MC, Walker MJA, Hoffman BB. Integrated pharmacology. London: Mosby; 1997.

Pratt WB, Taylor P. Principles of drug action—the basis of pharmacology. 3rd ed. New York: Churchill Livingstone; 1990.

Rang HP, Dale MM, Ritter JM, Gardiner P. Pharmacology. 4th ed. New York: Churchill Livingstone; 1999.

B. Clinical pharmacology

Dipiro JT, Talbert RL, Yee GC, Matzke GR, Wells BG, Posey LM. Pharmacotherapy–a pathophysiological approach. 3rd ed. Norwalk, Conn: Appleton & Lange; 1997.

Kuemmerle H, Shibuya T, Tillement JP. Human pharmacology: the basis of clinical pharmacology. Amsterdam: Elsevier; 1991.

Laurence DR, Bennett PN. Clinical pharmacology. 8th ed. Edinburgh: Churchill Livingstone; 1998.

Melmon KL, Morelli HF, Hoffman BB, Nierenberg DW. Clinical Pharmacology—basic principles in therapeutics. 3rd ed. New York: McGraw-Hill; 1992.

The Medical Letter on Drugs and Therapeutics. New Rochelle NY: The Medical Letter Inc.; published bi-weekly.

Clinical Pharmacology—Electronic drug reference. Tampa, Florida: Gold Standard Multimedia Inc.; updated every 4 months.

C. Drug interactions and adverse effects

D'Arcey PF, Griffin JP. Iatrogenic diseases. Oxford: Oxford University Press; 1986.

Davies DM. Textbook of adverse drug reactions. 4th ed. Oxford: Oxford University Press; 1992.

Hansten PD, Horn JR. Drug interactions, analysis and management. Vancouver, WA: Applied Therapeutics Inc.; 1999; updated every 4 months.

D. Drugs in pregnancy and lactation

Briggs GG, Freeman RK, Yaffe SJ. Drugs in pregnancy and lactation: a reference guide to fetal and neonatal risk. 5th ed. Baltimore: Williams & Wilkins; 1998.

Rubin PC. Prescribing in pregnancy. London: British Medical Journal; 1987

E. Pharmacokinetics

Rowland M, Tozer TN. Clinical pharmacokinetics: concepts and applications. 3rd ed. Baltimore: Williams & Wilkins; 1995.

F. Toxicology

Amdur MO, Doull J, Klaassen CD. Casarett and Doull's toxicology: the basic science of poisons. 5th ed. New York: McGraw-Hill; 1995.

Drug Indexes

Nomenclature. The terms *active agent* and *pharmacon* designate substances that are capable of modifying life processes irrespective of whether the effects elicited may benefit or harm the organisms concerned. By this definition, a toxin is also a pharmacon. Taken in a narrower sense, a pharmacon means a substance that is used for therapeutic purposes. An unequivocal term for such a substance is *medicinal drug.*

A drug can be identified by different designations:
– the chemical name
– the generic (nonproprietary) name
– a trade or brand name

The drug diazepam may serve as an illustrative example. Chemically, this compound is called 7-chloro-1,3-dihydro-1-methyl-5-phenyl-2H-1,4-benzodiazepin-2-one, a term too unwieldy for everyday use. A simpler name is diazepam. This is not a legally protected name but a *generic (nonproprietary) name.* An INN (= international nonproprietary name) is a generic name that has been agreed upon by an international commission.

Preparations containing diazepam were first marketed under the *trade name* Valium by its manufacturer, Hoffmann–La Roche, Inc. This name is a registered trademark. After patent protection for the manufacture of diazepam-containing drug preparations expired, other companies were free to produce preparations containing this drug. Each invented a proprietary name for its "own" preparation. As a result, there now exists a plethora of proprietary labels for diazepam preparations (as of 1991, more than 50). Some of these easily reveal the active ingredient, because the company name is simply added to the generic name, e.g., Diazepam- (company's name). Other designations are new creations, as for example, Vivol.

Similarly, some other commercially successful drugs are sold under more than 20 different brand labels. The number of proprietary names, therefore, greatly exceeds the number of available drugs.

For the sake of clarity, only INNs or generic (nonproprietary) names are used in this atlas to designate drugs, such as the name "diazepam" in the above example.

Use of Indexes

The indexes are meant to help the reader:

1. identify a commercial preparation for a given drug. This information is found in the index "Generic Name → Proprietary Name."

2. obtain information about the pharmacological properties of the active ingredient in a commercial preparation. In order to find the generic (nonproprietary) name, the second index "Proprietary Name → Generic Name" can be consulted. Page references pertaining to the drug can then be looked up in the Index. The list of proprietary names given below will necessarily be incomplete due to their multitude. For drugs that are marketed under several brand names, the trade name of the original manufacturer will be listed; in the case of some frequently prescribed generics, some proprietary names of other manufacturers will also be listed. Brand names that clearly reveal the drug's identity have been omitted. Combination preparations have not been included, barring a few exceptions.

Many a brand name is not listed in the index "Proprietary Name → Generic Name." In these cases, it will be useful to consult the packaging information, which should list the generic (nonproprietary) name or INN.

Drug Index

Drug Name	Trade Name
	(* denotes investigational drug status in USA)
A	
Abacavir	Ziagen
Abciximab	ReoPro
Acarbose	Precose
Acebutolol	Monitan, Sectral
Acenocoumarin (= Nicoumalone)	Sintrom
Acetaminophen	see Paracetamol
Acetazolamide	Diamox, Glaupax
Acetylcysteine	Airbron, Fabrol, Mucomyst, Parvolex
Acetyldigoxin	Acylanid
Acetylsalicylic acid	Aspirin, Arthrisin, Asadrine, Ecotrin, Entrophen, Pyronoval, Supasa
Aciclovir	Zovirax
ACTH	Acthar, Cortrophin
Actinomycin D	Cosmegen
Acyclovir	Zovirax
ADH (= Vasopressin)	Pitressin, Presyn
Adrenalin	see epinephrine
Adriamycin	See doxorubicin
Ajmaline	Cardiorhythmino; Gilurytmal
Albuterol	See Salbutamol
Alcuronium	Alloferin
Aldosterone	Aldocorten
Alendronate	Fosamax
Alfentanil	Alfenta
Alfuzosin	Alfoten, Xatral
Allopurinol	Alloprin, Novopurol, Urosin, Zyloprim, Zyloric
Alprazolam	Xanax
Alprenolol	Aprobal, Aptine, Gubernal
Alprostadil (= PGE_1)	Prostin VR, Minprog
Alteplase	Activase
Aluminium hydroxide	Aldrox, Alu-Tab, Amphojel, Fluagel
Amantadine	Solu-Contenton, Virofral, Symmetrel
Ambroxol	Ambril, Bronchopront, Mucosolvan, Surfactal
Amikacin	Amikin, Briclin, Novamin
Amiloride	Arumil, Colectril, Midamor, Nilurid
Amiloride + Hydrochlorothiazide	Moduret
ε-Aminocaproic acid	Amicar, Afibrin, Capramol
ε-Aminocaproic acid + Thromboplastin	Epsilon-Tachostyptan
Aminomethylbenzoic acid	Gumbix, Pamba
5-Aminosalicylic acid	Propasa, Rezipas
Amiodarone	Cordarex, Cordarone
Amitriptyline	Amitril, Elavil, Endep, Enovil, Levate, Mevaril
Amodiaquine	Camoquin, Flavoquine
Amoxicillin	Amoxil, Clamoxyl, Moxacin, Novamoxin

d-Amphetamine	Dexedrine, Synatan
Amphotericin B	Amphozone, Fungilin, Fungizone, Moronal
Ampicillin	Amcill, Omnipen, Penbritin, Polycillin, Principen, Totacillin
Amrinone	Inocor, Wincoram
Ancrod*	Arvin, Arwin, Viprinex
Angiotensin II	Hypertensin
Aprindine	Amidonal, Aspenon, Fibocil
Ardeparin	Normiflo
Articaine	Ultracain, Ubistesin
Astemizole	Hismanal
Atenolol	Prenormine, Tenormin
Atorvastatin	Lipitor
Atracurium	Tracrium
Atropine	Atropisol, Borotropin
Auranofin	Ridaura
Aurothioglucose	Aureotan, Auromyose, Solganal
Azapropazone	Prolixan
Azathioprine	Azanin, Imuran, Imurek
Azidothymidine	Retrovir
Azithromycin	Zithromax
Azlocillin	Azlin, Securopen
Aztreonam	Azactam

B

Bacitracin	Altracin, Baciguent, Topitracin
Baclofen	Lioresal
Basiliximab	Simulect
Beclomethasone	Aldecin, Beclovent, Beconase, Becotide, Propaderm, Vanceril
Benazepril	Lotensin
Benserazide	Madopar (plus Levodopa)
Benzathine-Penicillin G	Bicillin, Megacillin, Tardocillin
Benztropine	Cogentin
Benzbromarone	Desuric, Narcaricin, Normurat, Uricovac
Benzocaine	Anaesthesin, Americaine, Anacaine
Betaxolol	Betoptic, Kerlone
Bezafibrate	Befizal, Bezalip, Bezatol, Cedur
Bifonazole	Amycor, Bedriol, Mycospor, Mycosporan
Biperiden	Akineton, Akinophyl
Bisacodyl	Bicol, Broxalax, Durolax, Dulcolax, Laxanin, Laxbene, Nigalax, Pyrilax, Telemin, Ulcolax
Bismuth subsalicylate	Pepto-Bismol
Bisoprolol	Concor, Detensiel, Emcor, Isoten, Soprol, Zebeta
Bitolterol	Effectin, Tornalate
Bleomycin	Blenoxane
Botulinum Toxin Type A	Oculinum
Bromazepam	Durazanil, Lectopam, Lexotan
Bromhexine	Auxit, Bisolvon, Ophthosol
Bromocriptine	Parlodel, Pravidel, Serono-Bagren
Brotizolam	Lendorm (A), Lendormin
Bucindolol*	Bextra

Budesonide	Pulmicort, Spirocort
Bumetanide	Bumex, Burinex, Fontego, Fordiuran
Bunitrolol	Betriol, Stresson
Bupranolol	Betadran, Betadrenol, Looser, Panimit
Buprenorphine	Buprene, Temgesic
Bupropion	Wellbatrin, Wellbutrin
Buserelin	Sprecur, Suprefact
Buspirone	Buspar
Busulfan	Mielucin, Mitosan, Myleran, Sulfabutin
Butizid	Saltucin
N-Butyl-scopolamine	Buscopan, Hyoscin-N-Butylbromid

C

Calcifediol	Calderol, Dedrogyl, Hidroferol
Calcitonin	Calcimer, Calsynar, Cibacalcin, Karil
Calcitriol	Rocaltrol
Calcium carbonate	Calsan, Caltrate, Nu-Cal
Camazepam	Albego
Canrenone	Kanrenol, Soldactone, Venactone
Candesartan	Atacand
Capreomycin	Capastat, Caprolin
Captopril	Acediur, Acepril, Alopresin, Capoten, Cesplon, Hypertil, Lopirin, Tensobon
Carazolol	Conducton, Suacron
Carbachol	Doryl, Miostat, Lentin
Carbamazepine	Epitol, Mazepine, Sirtal, Tegretol, Timonil
Carbenicillin	Anabactyl (A), Carindapen, Geopen, Pyopen
Carbenoxolone	Biogastrone, Bioplex, Neogel, Sanodin
Carbidopa + Levodopa	Isicom, Nacom, Sinemet
Carbimazole	Neo-Mercazole, Neo-Thyreostat
Carboplatin	Paraplatin
Carteolol	Arteoptic, Caltidren, Carteol, Endak, Ocupress, Tenalin
Carvedilol	Coreg
Cefalexin	Keflex, Keftab
Cefazolin	Ancef, Ketzol
Cefixime	Suprax
Cefmenoxime	Bestcall, Cefmax, Cemix, Tacef
Cefoperazone	Cefobid, Cefobis, Tomabef
Cefotaxime	Claforan
Cefoxitin	Mefoxin
Ceftazidime	Fortaz, Fortum, Tacicef
Ceftriaxone	Acantex, Rocephin
Cefuroxime axetil	Ceftin
Cellulose	Avicel
Cephalexin	Cepexin (A), Ceporex, Keflex, Losporal
Cerivastatin	Baycol
Chenodeoxycholic acid	Chenix
Chloralhydrate	Lorinal, Noctec, Somnos
Chlorambucil	Chloraminophene, Leukeran
Chloramphenicol	Chloromycetin, Chloroptic, Leukomycin, Paraxin, Sopa-mycetin, Spersanicol
Chlorhexidine	Baxedin, Chlor-hex, Hibidil, Hibitane, Plak-out

Chlormadinone acetate	Gestafortin
Chloroquine	Aralen, Avloclor, Quinachlor
Chlorpromazine	Largactil, Hibanil, Megaphen, Thorazine
Chlorpropamide	Diabinese
Chlorprothixene	Taractan, Tarasan, Truxal
Chlorthalidone	Hygroton
Cholecalciferol	D-Tabs, Vigantol, Vigorsan
Clorazepate	Novoclopate, Tranxene
Cilazapril	Inhibace
Cimetidine	Peptol, Tagamet
Ciprofloxacin	Ciprobay, Cipro
Cisapride	Propulsid
Cisplatin	Platinex, Platinol
Citalopram	Celexa
Clarithromycin	Biaxin
Clavulanic Acid + Amoxicillin	Augmentin
Clemastine	Tavist
Clindamycin	Cleocin, Dalacin, Sobelin
Clobazam	Frisium
Clodronate*	Clasteon, Ossiten, Ostac
Clofazimine	Lampren
Clofibrate	Atromid-S, Claripex, Skleromexe
Clomethiazole	Distraneurin, Hemineurin
Clomiphene	Clomid, Dyneric, Omifin, Pergotime, Serophene
Clonazepam	Clonopin, Iktorivil, Rivotril
Clonidine	Catapres, Dixarit
Clopidogrel	Plavix
Clostebol	Macrobin, Steranabol
Clotiazepam	Clozan, Rize, Tienor, Trecalmo, Veratran
Clotrimazole	Canesten, Clotrimaderm, Gyne-Lotrimin, Mycelex, Trimysten
Cloxacillin	Clovapen, Tegopen
Clozapine	Clozaril
Codeine	Codicept, Paveral
Colestipol	Cholestabyl, Cholestid
Colestyramine	Questran, Cuemid
Corticotropin	Acthar, Cortigel, Cortrophin
Cortisol (Hydrocortisone)	Alocort, Cortate, Cortef, Cortenema, Hyderm, Hyocort, Rectocort, Unicort
Cortisone	Cortelan, Cortogen, Cortone
Cotrimoxazole	Bactrim, Novotrimel, Protrin Septra
Cromoglycate (Cromolyn)	Intal, Nalcrom, Opticrom, Rynacrom, Vistacrom
Cyanocobalamin	Anacobin, Bedoz, Rubion, Rubramin
Cyclofenil	Fertodur, Ondogyne, Ondonid, Sanocrisin, Sexovid
Cyclopenthiazide	Navidrix, Salimid
Cyclophosphamide	Cytoxan, Endoxan, Procytox
Cyclosporine	Neoral, Sandimmune, Sang-35
Cyproheptadine	Anarexol, Nuran, Periactin, Peritol, Vimicon
Cyproterone-acetate	Androcur
Cytarabine	Udicil, Cytosar

D

Drug	Trade
Daclizumab	Zenapax
Dactinomycin	See Actinomycin D
Dalteparin	Fragmin
Danaparoid	Orgaran
Dantrolene	Dantrium
Dapsone	Avlosulfone, Eporal, Diphenasone, Udolac
Daunorubicin	Cerubidine, Daunoblastin, Ondena
Deferoxamine	Desferal
Delavirdine	Rescriptor
Desipramine	Pertofran, Norpramin
Desmopressin	DDAVP, Minirin, Stimate
Desogestrel + Ethinylestradiol	Marvelon
Dexamethasone	Decadron, Deronil, Hexadrol, Spersadex
Dexetimide	Tremblex
Dextran	Hyskon
Diazepam	Apaurin, Atensine, Diastat, Dizac, Eridan, Lembrol, Meval, Noan, Tensium, Valium, Vatran, Vivol
Diazoxide	Eudemine, Hyperstat, Mutabase, Proglicem
Diclofenac	Allvoran, Diclophlogont, Rhumalgan, Voltaren, Voltarol
Dicloxacillin	Diclocil, Dynapen, Pathocil
Didanosine (ddl)	Videx
Diethylstilbestrol	Honvol
Digitoxin	Crystodigin, Digicor, Digimerck, Digacin, Lanicor, Lanoxin, Lenoxin, Novodigoxin
Digoxin immune FAB	Digibind
Dihydralazine	Dihyzin, Nepresol, Pressunic
Dihydroergotamine	Angionorm, D.E.H.45, Dihydergot, Divegal, Endophleban
Diltiazem	Cardizem
Dimenhydrinate	Dimetab, Dramamine, Dymenate, Marmine
Dinoprost	Minprostin $F_{2\alpha}$, Prostarmon, Prostin F_2 Alpha
Dinoprostone	Prepidil, Prostin E_2
Diphenhydramine	Allerdryl, Benadryl, Insommal, Nautamine
Diphenoxylate	Diarsed, Lomotil, Retardin
Disopyramide	Norpace, Rythmodan
Dobutamine	Dobutrex
Docetaxel	Taxotere
Dolasetron	Anzemet
Domperidone*	Euciton, Evoxin, Motilium, Nauzelin, Peridon
Dopamine	Dopastat, Intropin
Dorzolamide	Trusopt
Doxacurium	Nuromax
Doxazosin	Cardura, Carduran
Doxepin	Adapin, Sinequan, Triadapin
Doxorubicin	Adriblastin, Adriamycin
Doxycycline	C-Pak, Doxicin, Vibramycin
Doxylamine	Decapryn
Dronabinol	Marinol
Droperidol	Inapsine, Droleptan

E

Econazole	Ecostatin, Gyno-Pevaryl
Ecothiopate	Phospholine Iodide
Enalapril	Vasotec, Xanef
Enflurane	Ethrane
Enoxacin	Bactidan, Comprecin, Enoram
Enoxaparin	Lovenox
Entacapone*	Comtan
Epinephrine	Adrenalin, Bronchaid, Epifin, Epinal, EpiPen, Epitrate, Lyophrin, Simplene, Suprarenin, Vaponefrine
Ephedrine	Bofedrol, Efedron, Va-tro-nol
Eprosartan	Teveten
Eptifibatide	Integriline
Ergocalciferol	Drisdol
Ergometrine (= Ergonovine)	Ergotrate Maleate, Ermalate
Ergonovine	Ergotrate
Ergotamine	Ergomar, Gynergen, Migril
Erythomcyin	E-mycin, Eryc, Erythromid
Erythromycin-estolate	Dowmycin, Ilosone, Novorythro
Erythromycin-ethylsuccinate	EES, Erythrocin, Wyamycin
Erythromycin-propionate	Cimetrin
Erythromycin-stearate	Erymycin, Erythrocin
Erythromycin-succinate	Monomycin
Erythropoietin (= epoetin alfa)	Epogen
Esmolol	Brevibloc
Estradiol	Estrace
Estradiol-benzoate	Progynon B
Estradiol-valerate	Delestrogen, Dioval, Femogex, Progynova
Estratriol = Estriol	Theelol
Etanercept	Enbrel
Ethacrynic acid	Edecrin, Hydromedin, Reomax
Ethambutol	Etibi, Myambutol
Ethinylestradiol	Estinyl, Feminone, Lynoral
Ethionamide	Trecator
Ethopropazine	Parsitan, Parsitol
Ethosuximide	Petinimid, Suxinutin, Zarontin
Etidocaine	Duranest
Etidronate	Calcimux, Diodronel, Diphos
Etilefrine	Apocretin, Effontil, Effortil, Ethyl Adrianol, Circupon, Kertasin, Pulsamin,
Etodolac	Lodine
Etomidate	Amidate
Etoposide	Toposar, VePesid
Etretinate	Tegison, Tigason

F

Famotidine	Pepcid, Pepdul
Felbamate	Felbatol
Felodipine	Plendil
Felypressin	Octapressin
Fenfluramine	Ganal, Ponderal, Pondimin

Fenofibrate	Lipidyl, Tricor
Fenoldopam	Corlopam
Fenoprofen	Nalfon, Nalgesic
Fenoterol	Berotec, Partusisten
Fentanyl	Sublimaze
Fentanyl + Droperidol	Innovar
Finasteride	Propecia, Proscar
Flecainide	Tambocor
Flucloxacillin	Fluclox
Fluconazole	Diflucan
Flucytosine	Alcoban, Ancotil
Fludrocortisone	Alflorone, F-Cortef, Florinef
Flumazenil	Anexate, Romazicon
Flunarizine	Dinaplex, Flugeral, Sibelium
Flunisolide	Aerobid, Bronalide, Nasalide, Rhinalar
Flunitrazepam*	Hypnosedon, Narcozep, Rohypnol
Fluoxetine	Prozac
5-Fluorouracil	Adrucil, Effudex, Effurix
Flupentixol	Depixol, Fluanxol
Fluphenazine	Moditen, Prolixin
Flurazepam*	Dalmane
Flutamide	Drogenil, Eulexin
Fluticasone	Cutivate, Flixonase, Flonase, Flovent
Fluvastatin	Lescol
Fluvoxamine	Floxifral, Faverin, Luvox
Folic acid	Foldine, Folvite, Leucovorin
Foscarnet	Foscavir
Fosinopril	Monopril
Furosemide	Fusid, Lasix, Seguril, Uritol

G

Gabapentin	Neurontin
Gallamine	Flaxedil
Gallopamil	Algocor, Corgal, Procorum, Wingom
Ganciclovir	Cytovene, Vitrasert
Gelatin-colloids	Gelafundin, Haemaccel
Gemfibrozil	Lopid
Gentamicin	Cidomycin, Garamycin, Refobacin, Sulmycin
Glibenclamide (= glyburide)	Daonil, DiaBeta, Euglucon, Glynase, Micronase
Glimepiride	Amaryl
Glipizide	Glucotrol
Glyceryltrinitrate (= nitroglycerin)	Ang-O-Span, Nitrocap, Nitrogard, Nitroglyn, Nitrolingual, Nitrong, Nitrostat
Glycopyrrolate	Robinul
Gonadorelin	Factrel, Kryptocur, Relefact
Goserelin	Zoladex
Gramicidin	Gramoderm
Granisetron	Kytril
Griseofulvin	Fulvicin, Grisovin, Likuden
Guanabenz	Wytensin
Guanethidine	Ismelin, Visutensil
Guanfacine	Tenex

H

Halofantrine	Halfan
Haloperidol	Haldol, Serenace
Halothane	Fluothane, Narkotan
HCG (= chorionic gonadotropin)	Chorex, Choron, Entromone, Follutein, Gonic, Pregnesin, Pregnyl, Profasi
Heparin	Calciparin, Hepalean, Liquemin
Heparin, low molecular	Fragmin, Fraxiparin
Hetastarch (HES)	Hespan
Hexachlorophane	see Lindane
Hexobarbital	Evipal
Hydralazine	Alazine, Apresoline
Hydrochlorothiazide	Aprozide, Diaqua, Diuchlor, Esidrex, Hydromal, Neo-Codema, Oretic
Hydromorphone	Dilaudid, Hymorphan
Hydroxocobalamin	Acti-B_{12}, Alpha-redisol, Sytobex
Hydroxychloroquine	Plaquenil
Hydroxyethyl starch	Hespan
Hydroxyprogesterone caproate	Duralutin, Gesterol L.A., Hylutin, Hyroxon, Pro-Depo
Hyoscyamine sulfate	Cystospaz-M, Levbid, Levsin

I

Ibuprofen	Actiprophen, Advil, Motrin, Nuprin, Trendar
Idoxuridine	Dendrid, Herplex, Kerecid, Stoxil
Ifosfamide	Ifex
Iloprost	Latanaprost
Imipramine	Dynaprin, Impril, Janimine, Melipramin, Tofranil, Typramine
Indapamide	Lozide, Lozol, Natrilix
Indinavir	Crixivan
Indomethacin	Ammuno, Indocid, Indocin, Indome, Metacen
Infliximab	Remicade
Insulin	Humalog, Humulin, Iletin, Novolin, Velosulin
Interferon-α2	Berofor alpha 2
Interferon-α2b	Intron A
Interferon-α2a	Roferon A3
Interferon-β	Fiblaferon 3
Interferon-β-1a	Avonex
Interferon-β-1b	Betaseron
Interferon-γ	Actimmune
Ipratropium	Atrovent, Itrop
Irbesartan	Avapro
Isoconazole	Gyno-Travogen, Travogen
Isoetharine	Arm-a-Med, Bisorine, Bronkosol, Dey-Lute
Isoflurane	Forane
Isoniazid	Armazid, Isotamine, Lamiazid, Nydrazid, Rimifon, Tee-baconin
Isoprenaline (= Isoproterenol)	Aludrin, Isuprel, Neo Epinin, Saventrine
Isosorbide dinitrate	Cedocard, Coradus, Coronex, Isordil, Sorbitrate
5-Isosorbide mononitrate	Coleb, Elantan, Ismo
Isotretinoin	Acutane Roche, Roaccutan

Isoxsuprine	Rolisox, Vasodilan, Vasoprine
Isradipine	DynaCirc
Itroconazole	Sporanox

K

Kanamycin	Anamid, Kantrex, Klebcil
Kaolin + Pectin (= attapulgite)	Kaopectate, Donnagel-MB, Pectokay
Ketamine	Ketalar
Ketoconazol	Nizoral
Ketorolac	Acular, Toradol
Ketotifen	Zaditen

L

Labetalol	Normodyne, Trandate
Lactulose	Cephulac, Chronulac, Duphalac
Lamivudine (3TC)	Epivir
Lamotrigine	Lamictal
Lansoprazole	Prevacid
Leflunomide	Arava
Lepirudin	Refludan
Leuprorelide	Lupron
Levodopa	Larodopa, Dopar, Dopaidan
Levodopa + Benserazide	Madopar, Prolopa
Levodopa + Carbidopa	Sinemet
Levomepromazine	Levoprome, Nozinan
Lidocaine	Dalcaine, Lidopen, Nulicaine, Xylocain, Xylocard
Lincomycin	Albiotic, Cillimycin, Lincocin
Lindane	Hexit, Kwell, Kildane, Scabene
Liothyronine	Cytomel, Triostat
Lisinopril	Prinivil, Zestril
Lispro insulin	Humalog
Lisuride	Cuvalit, Dopergin, Eunal, Lysenyl
Lithium carbonate	Carbolite, Duoralith, Eskalith
Lithium carbonate	Lithane, Lithobid, Lithotabs
Lomustine	CeeNu
Loperamide	Imodium, Kaopectate II
Loratidine	Claritin
Lorazepam	Alzapam, Ativan, Loraz
Lorcainide	Lopantrol, Lorivox, Remivox
Lormetazepam	Ergocalm, Loramet, Noctamid
Losartan	Cozaar
Lovastatin	Mevacor, Mevinacor
Lypressin	Diapid, Vasopressin Sandoz

M

Mannitol	Isotol, Osmitrol
Maprotiline	Ludiomil
Mazindol	Mazonor, Sanorex
Mebendazole	Vermox
Mechlorethamine	Mustargen

Meclizine (meclozine)	Antivert, Antrizine, Bonamine, Whevert
Meclofenamate	Meclomen
Medroxyprogesterone-acetate	Amen, Depo-Provera, Oragest
Mefloquine	Lariam
Melphalan	Alkeran
Menadione	Synkayvit
Meperidine	Demerol
Mepindolol	Betagon, Caridian, Corindolan
Mepivacaine	Carbocaine, Isocaine
6-Mercaptopurine	Purinethol
Mesalamine (Mesalazine)	Asacol, Pentasa, Rowasa
Mesna	Mesnex, Uromitexan
Mesterolone	Androviron, Proviron
Mestranol	Menophase, Norquen, Ovastol
Metamizol (= Dipyrone)	Algocalmin, Bonpyrin, Divarine, Feverall, Metilon, No-valgin, Paralgin, Sulpyrin
Metaproterenol	Alupent, Metaprel
Metformin	Diabex, Glucophage
Methadone	Dolophine, Methadose, Physoseptone
Methamphetamine	Desoxyn, Methampex
Methimazole	Tapazole
Methohexital	Brevital
Methotrexate	Folex, Mexate
Methoxyflurane	Penthrane, Methofane
Methyl-Dopa	Aldomet, Amodopa, Dopamet, Novomedopa, Presinol, Sembrina
Methylcellulose	Celevac, Cellothyl, Citrucel, Cologel, Lacril, Murocel
Methylergometrine (Methylergonovine)	Methergine, Metenarin, Methylergobrevin, Ryegono-vin, Partergin, Spametrin-M
Methylphenidate	Ritalin
Methylprylon	Noludar
Methyltestosterone	Android, Metandren, Testred, Virilon
Methysergide	Sansert
Metipranolol	Optipranolol
Metoclopramide	Clopra, Emex, Maxeran, Maxolan, Reclomide, Reglan
Metoprolol	Betaloc, Lopressor
Metronidazole	Clont, Femazole, Flagyl, Metronid, Protostat, Satric
Mexiletin	Mexitil
Mezlocillin	Mezlin
Mianserin	Bolvidon, Norval
Mibefradil	Posicor
Miconazole	Micatin, Monistat
Midazolam	Versed
Mifepristone	RU 486
Milrinone	Primacor
Minocycline	Minocin, Vectrin
Minoxidil	Loniten, Rogaine
Misoprostol	Cytotec
Mithramycin	Mithracin
Mitoxantrone	Novantrone
Mivacurium	Miracron
Moclobemide	Aurorix
Molsidomine	Corvaton, Duracoron, Molsidolat

Montelukast	Singulair
Morphine hydrochloride	Morphitec
Morphine sulfate	Astramorph, Duramorph, Epimorph, Roxanol, Statex
Muromonab-CD3	Orthoclone OKT3
Mycophenolate Mofetil	CellCept

N

Nabilone	Cesamet
Nadolol	Corgard
Naftifin	Naftin
Nalbuphine	Nubain
Nalidixic acid	Negram, Nogram
Naloxone	Narcan
Naltrexone	Nalorex, Revia, Trexan
Nandrolone	Anabolin, Androlone, Deca-Durabolin, Hybolin Decano-ate, Kabolin
Naphazoline	Albalon, Degest-2, Privine, Vasocon
Naproxen	Aleve, Naprosyn, Naxen
Narcotine (= Noscapine)	Coscopin, Coscotab
Nadroparin*	Fraxiparine
Nedocromil	Tilade
Nelfinavir	Viracept
Neomycin	Mycifradin, Myciguent
Neostigmine	Prostigmin
Netilmicin	Netromycin
Nevirapine	Viramune
Nicardipine	Cardene
Niclosamide	Niclocide, Yomesan
Nifedipine	Adalat, Procardia
Nimodipine	Nimotop
Nisoldipine	Sular
Nitrazepam	Atempol, Mogadon
Nitrendipine	Bayotensin, Baypress
Nitroglycerin	See Glyceryl trinitrate
Nitroprusside sodium	Nipride, Nitropress
Nizatidine	Axid
Nor-Diazepam	Tranxilium N, Vegesan
Noradrenalin (= Norepinephrine)	Arterenol, Levophed
Norethisterone	Micronor
= Norethindrone	Norlutin, Nor-Q D
Norfloxacin	Noroxin
Noscapine (= Narcotine)	Coscopin, Coscotab
Nortriptyline	Pamelor
Nystatin	Korostatin, Mycostatin, Mykinac, Nilstat, Nystex, O-V Statin

O

Octreotide	Sandostatin
Ofloxacin	Tarivid
Olanzapine	Zyprexa
Omeprazole	Losec, Prilosec

Ondansetron	Zofran
Opium Tincture (laudanum)	Paregoric
Orciprenaline (= Metaproterenol)	Alupent
Ornipressin	POR 8
Oxacillin	Bactocill, Prostaphlin
Oxatomide	Tinset
Oxazepam	Oxpam, Serax, Zapex
Oxiconazole	Oxistat
Oxprenolol	Trasicor
Oxymetazoline	Afrin, Allerest, Coricidin, Dristan, Neo-Synephrine, Sinarest
Oxytocin	Pitocin, Syntocinon

P

Paclitaxel	Taxol
Pamidronate	Aminomux
Pancuronium	Pavulon
Pantoprazole*	Pantolac
Papaverine	Cerebid, Cerespan, Delapav, Myobid, Papacon, Pavabid, Pavadur, Vasal
Paracetamol = acetaminophen	Acephen, Anacin-3, Bromo-Seltzer, Datril, Tempra, Tylenol, Valadol, Valorin
Paromomycin	Humatin
Paroxetine	Paxil
Penbutolol	Levatol
Penciclovir	Denavir
D-Penicillamine	Cuprimine, Depen
Penicillin G	Bicillin, Cryspen, Deltapen, Lanacillin, Megacillin, Par-cillin, Pensorb, Pentids, Permapen, Pfizerpin
Pencillin V	Betapen-VK, Bopen-VK, Cocillin-VK, Lanacillin-VK, Le-dercillin VK, Nadopen-V, Novopen-VK, Penapar VK, Penbec-V, Pen-Vee K, Pfizerpen VK, Robicillin-VK, Uti-cillin-VK, V-Cillin K, Veetids
Pentazocine	Fortral, Talwin
Pentobarbital	Butylone, Nembutal, Novarectal, Pentanca
Pentoxifylline	Trental
Pergolide	Permax
Perindopril	Coversum
Permethrin	Elimite, Nix, Permanone
Pethidine = Meperidine	Demerol, Dolantin
Phencyclidine	Sernyl
Pheniramine	Daneral, Inhiston
Phenobarbital	Barbita, Gardenal, Solfoton
Phenolphthalein	Alophen, Correctol, Espotabs, Evac-U-gen, Evac-U-Lax, Ex-Lax, Modane, Prulet
Phenoxybenzamine	Dibenzyline
Phenprocoumon	Liquamar, Marcumar
Phentolamine	Regitin, Rogitin
Phenylbutazone	Algoverine, Azolid, Butagen, Butazolidin, Malgesic
Phenytoin	Dilantin
Physostigmine	Antilirium
Phytomenadione	Konakion

Pilocarpine	Akarpine, Almocarpine, I-Pilopine, Miocarpine, Isopto-Carpine, Pilokair
Pindolol	Visken
Piperacillin	Pipracil
Pipecuronium	Arduan
Pirenzepine	Gastrozepin
Piroxicam	Felden
Pizotifen = Pizotyline	Litec, Mosegor, Sandomigran
Plicamycin	Mithracin
Polidocanol	Thesit
Pranlukast*	Ultair
Pravastatin	Pravachol
Prazepam	Centrax
Praziquantel	Biltricide
Prazosin	Minipress
Prednisolone	Articulose, Codelsol, Cortalone, Delta-Cortef, Deltastab, Econopred, Hydeltrasol, Inflamase, Key-Pred, Metalone, Metreton, Pediapred, Predate, Predcor, Prelone
Prednisone	Meticorten, Orasone, Panasol, Winpred
Prilocaine	Citanest, Xylonest
Primaquine	Primaquine
Primidone	Myidone, Mysoline, Sertan
Probenecid	Benemid, Probalan
Probucol	Lovelco
Procaine	Novocaine
Procainamide	Procan SR, Promine, Pronestyl, Rhythmin
Procarbazine	Natulan
Procyclidine	Kemadrin
Progabide	Gabren(e)
Progesterone	Femotrone, Progestasert
Promethazine	Anergan, Ganphen, Mallergan, Pentazine, Phenazine, Phenergan, Prometh, Prorex, Provigan, Remsed
Propafenone	Rhythmol
Propofol	Diprivan
Propranolol	Detensol, Inderal
Propylthiouracil	Propyl-Thyracil
Pyrantel Pamoate	Antiminth
Pyrazinamide	Aldinamide, Tebrazid
Pyridostigmine	Mestinon, Regonol
Pyridoxine	Bee-six, Hexa-Betalin, Pyroxine
Pyrimethamine	Daraprim
Pyrimethamine + Sulfadoxine	Fansidar

Q

Quazepam	Doral
Quinacrine	Atabrine
Quinapril	Accupril
Quinidine	Cardioqin, Cin-Quin, Quinalan, Quinidex, Quinora
Quinine	Quinaminoph, Quinamm, Quine, Quinite

R

Raloxifene	Evista
Ramipril	Altace
Ranitidine	Zantac
Remifentanil	Ultiva
Repaglinide	Actulin, NovoNorm, Prandin
Reserpine	Sandril, Serpalan, Serpasil, Zepine
Ribavirin	Virazole, Rebetol
Rifabutin	Mycobutin
Rifampin	Rifadin, Rimactan
Ritodrine	Yutopar
Ritonavir	Norvir
Rocuronium	Zemuron
Rolitetracyclin	Reverin, Transcycline, Velacycline
Ropinirole*	ReQuip
Roxithromycin	Rulid

S

Salazosulfapyridine = sulfasalazine	Azaline, Azulfidine, S.A.S.-500, Salazopyrin
Salbutamol (= Albuterol)	Proventil, Novosalmol, Ventolin
Salicylic acid	Acnex, Sebcur, Soluver, Trans-Ver-Sal
Sameterol	Serevent
Saquinavir	Fortovase, Invirase
Scopolamine	Transderm Scop, Triptone
Selegeline	Carbex, Deprenyl, Eldepryl
Senna	Black Draught, Fletcher's Castoria, Genna, Gentle Nature, Nytilax, Senokot, Senolax
Sertindole*	Serlect
Sibutramine	Reductil
Sildenafil	Viagra
Simethicone	Gas.X, Mylicon, Phazyme, Silain
Simvastatin	Zocor
Sitosterol	Sito-Lande
Sotalol	Sotacor
Spectinomycin	Trobicin
Spiramicin	Rovamycin, Selectomycin
Spironolactone	Aldactone
Stavudine (d4T)	Zerit
Streptokinase	Kabikinase, Streptase
Streptomycin	Strepolin, Streptosol
Streptozocin	Zanosar
Succinylcholine	Anectine, Quelicin, Succostrin
Sucralfate	Carafate, Sulcrate
Sufentanil	Sufenta
Sulfacetamide	AK-Sulf Forte, Cetamide, Sulamyd, Sulair, Sulfex, Sulten
Sulfacytine	Renoquid
Sulfadiazine	Microsulfon
Sulfadoxine + Pyrimethamine	Proklar
Sulfamethoxazole	Gamazole, Gantanol, Methanoxazol
Sulfapyridine	Dagenan
Sulfisoxazole	Gantrisin, Gulfasin

Sulfasalazine	Azaline, Azulfidine, Salazopyrin
Sulfinpyrazone	Anturan, Aprazone
Sulprostone	Nalador
Sulthiame	Ospolot
Sumatriptan	Imitrex

T

t-PA (= alteplase)	Activase
Tacrine	Cognex
Tacrolimus	Prograf
Tamoxifen	Nolvadex, Tamofen
Temazepam	Euhypnos, Restoril
Teniposide	Vumon
Terazosin	Hytrin
Terbutalin	Brethine, Bricanyl
Terfenadine	Seldane
Testosterone cypionate	Androcyp, Andronate, Duratest, Testoject
Testosterone enantate	Andro, Delatestryl, Everone, Testone
Testosterone propionate	Testex
Testerone undecanoate	Andriol
Tetracaine	Anethaine, Pontocaine
Tetryzoline (= tetrahydrozoline)	Collyrium, Murine, Tyzine, Visine
Thalidomide	Contergan, Synovir
Theophylline	Aerolate, Bronkodyl, Constant-T, Elixophyllin, Quibron-T, Slo-bid, Somophyllin-T, Sustaire, Theolair, Uniphyl
Thiabendazole	Mintezol
Thiamazole (= Methimazole)	Tapazole, Mercazol
Thiopental	Pentothal, Trapanal
Thio-TEPA	Thiotepa Lederle
Thrombin	Thrombinar, Thrombostat
Thyroxine	Choloxin
Tiagabine	Gabitril
Ticarcillin	Ticar
Ticlopidine	Ticlid
Timolol	Blocadren, Timoptic
Tinidazol	Fasigyn(CH), Simplotan, Sorquetan
Tinzaparin*	Innohep
Tirofiban	Aggrastat
Tizanidine	Zanaflex
Tobramycin	Nebcin, Tobrex
Tocainide	Tonocard
Tolbutamide	Mobenol, Oramide, Orinase
Tolcapone	Tasmar
Tolmetin	Tolectin
Tolnaftate	Pitrex, Tinactin
Tolonium chloride	Klot, Toazul
Tolterodine tartrate	Detrol
Topiramate	Topamex
Tramadol	Tramal
Trandolapril	Mavik
Tranexamic acid	Cyklocapron
Tranylcypromine	Parnate

Trazodone	Desyrel, Trialodine
Triamcinolone	Aristocort, Azmacort, Kenacort, Ledercort(CH), Volon
Triamcinolone acetonide	Adicort, Azmacort, Kenalog, Kenalone, Triam-A
Triamterene	Dyrenium
Triazolam	Halcion
Trichlormethiazide	Metahydrin, Naqua, Trichlorex
Trifluoperazine	Stelazine
Trifluridine	Viroptic
Trihexipheidyl	Aparkane, Artane, Tremin, Trihexane
Triiodothyronine (= Liothyronine)	Cytomel
Trimethaphan	Arfonad
Trimethoprim	Proloprim, Trimpex
Triptorelin	Decapeptyl
Troglitazone	Rezulin
Tropicamide	Mydriacyl, Mydral
Tropisetron	Navoban
d-Tubocurarine	Tubarine
Tyrothricin	Hydrotricin

U

Urokinase	Abbokinase, Ukidan
Ursodeoxycholic acid = ursodiol	Actigall, Destolit, Ursofalk

V

Valacyclovir	Valtrex
Valproic Acid	Depakene
Valsartan	Diovan
Vancomycin	Vancocin, Vancomycin CP Lilly
Vasopressin	Pitressin
Vecuronium	Norcuron
Venlafaxine	Effexor
Verapamil	Calan, Isoptin, Verelan
Vidarabine	Vira-A
Vigabatrin*	Sabril
Vinblastine	Velban, Velbe
Vincamine	Cerebroxine
Vincristine	Oncovin
Viomycine	Celiomycin,Vinactane, Viocin, Vionactane
Vit. B_{12}	Bay-Bee, Berubigen, Betalin 12, Cabadon, Cobex, Cyanoject, Cyomin, Pemavit, Redisol, Rubesol, Sytobex, Vibal
Vit. B_6	Bee Six, Hexa-Betalin, Pyroxine
Vit. D	Calciferol, Drisdol

W

Warfarin	Coumadin, Panwarfin, Sofarin

X

Xanthinol nicotinate	Complamin
Xylometazoline	Chlorohist, Neosynephrine II, Sinutab, Sustaine

Z

Zafirlukast	Accolate
Zalcitabine	Hivid
Zidovudine	Retrovir
Zileuton	Zyflo
Zolpidem	Ambien
Zopiclone	Amoban, Amovane, Imovane, Zimovane

Drug Name	Trade Name	Drug Name	Trade Name
A		Albiotic	Lincomycin
		Alcoban	Flucytosine
Abbokinase	Urokinase	Aldactone	Spironolactone
Acantex	Ceftriaxone	Aldecin	Beclomethasone
Accolate	Zafirlukast	Aldinamide	Pyrazinamide
Accupril	Quinapril	Aldocorten	Aldosterone
Acediur	Captopril	Aldomet	Methyl-Dopa
Acephen	Paracetamol = acetami-nophen	Aldrox	Aluminium hydroxide
		Alfenta	Alfentanil
Acepril	Captopril	Alflorone	Fludrocortisone
Acnex	Salicylic acid	Alfoten	Alfuzosin
Acthar	ACTH	Algocalmin	Metamizol (= Dipyrone)
Acthar	Corticotropin	Algocor	Gallopamil
Acti-B 12	Hydroxocobalamin	Algoverine	Phenylbutazone
Actigall	Ursodeoxycholic acid = ursodiol	Alkeran	Melphalan
		Allerdryl	Diphenhydramine
Actimmune	Interferon-γ	Allerest	Oxymetazoline
Actiprophen	Ibuprofen	Alloferin	Alcuronium
Activase	t-PA (= alteplase)	Alloprin	Allopurinol
Actulin	Repaglinide	Allvoran	Diclofenac
Acular	Ketorolac	Almocarpine	Pilocarpine
Acutane Roche	Isotretinoin	Alocort	Cortisol (Hydrocortiso-ne)
Acylanid	Acetyldigoxin		
Adalat	Nifedipine	Alophen	Phenolphthalein
Adapin	Doxepin	Alopresin	Captopril
Adicort	Triamcinolone aceto-nide	Alpha-redisol	Hydroxocobalamin
		Altace	Ramipril
Adrenalin	Epinephrine	Altracin	Bacitracin
Adriamycin	Doxorubicin	Alu-Tab	Aluminium hydroxide
Adriblastin	Doxorubicin	Aludrin	Isoprenaline (= Isopro-terenol)
Adrucil	5-Fluorouracil		
Advil	Ibuprofen	Alupent	Metaproterenol
Aerobid	Flunisolide	Alzapam	Lorazepam
Aerolate	Theophylline	Amaryl	Glimepiride
Afibrin	ε-Aminocaproic acid	Ambien	Zolpidem
Afrin	Oxymetazoline	Ambril	Ambroxol
Aggrastat	Tirofiban	Amcill	Ampicillin
Airbron	Acetylcysteine	Amen	Medroxyprogesterone-acetate
Akarpine	Pilocarpine		
Akineton	Biperiden	Americaine	Benzocaine
Akinophyl	Biperiden	Amicar	e-Aminocaproic acid
AK-Sulf Forte	Sulfacetamide	Amidate	Etomidate
Alazine	Hydralazine	Amidonal	Aprindine
Albalon	Naphazoline	Amikin	Amikacin
Albego	Camazepam	Aminomux	Pamidronate

Amitril	Amitriptyline	Aristocort	Triamcinolone
Ammuno	Indomethacin	Arm-a-Med	Isoetharine
Amoban	Zopiclone	Armazid	Isoniazid
Amodopa	Methyl-Dopa	Artane	Trihexiphenidyl
Amovane	Zopiclone	Arteoptic	Carteolol
Amoxil	Amoxicillin	Arterenol	Noradrenalin (= Nore-
Amphojel	Aluminium hydroxide		pinephrine)
Amphozone	Amphotericin B	Arthrisin	Acetylsalicylic acid
Amycor	Bifonazole	Articulose	Prednisolone
Anabactyl(A)	Carbenicillin	Arumil	Amiloride
Anabolin	Nandrolone	Arvin	Ancrod
Anacaine	Benzocaine	Arwin	Ancrod
Anacin-3	Paracetamol = acetami-	Asacol	Mesalamine
	nophen	Asadrine	Acetylsalicylic acid
Anacobin	Cyanocobalamin	Aspenon	Aprindine
Anaesthesin	Benzocaine	Aspirin	Acetylsalicylic acid
Anamid	Kanamycin	Astramorph	Moiphine sulfate
Anarexol	Cyproheptadine	Atabrine	Quinacrine
Ancef	Cefazolin	Atacand	Candesartan
Ancotil	Flucytosine	Atempol	Nitrazepam
Andriol	Testerone undecanoate	Atensine	Diazepam
Andro	Testosterone enantate	Ativan	Lorazepam
Androcur	Cyproterone-acetate	Atromid-S	Clofibrate
Androcyp	Testosterone cypionate	Atropisol	Atropine
Android	Methyltestosterone	Atrovent	Ipratropium
Androlone	Nandrolone	Augmentin	Clavulanic Acid + Amo-
Andronate	Testosterone cypionate		xicillin
Androviron	Mesterolone	Aureotan	Aurothioglucose
Anectine	Succinylcholine	Auromyose	Aurothioglucose
Anergan	Promethazine	Aurorix	Moclobemide
Anethaine	Tetracaine	Auxit	Bromhexine
Anexate	Flumazenil	Avapro	Irbesartan
Ang-O-Span	Glyceryltrinitrate (=	Avicel	Cellulose
	nitroglycerin)	Avloclor	Chloroquine
Angionorm	Dihydroergotamine	Avlosulfone	Dapsone
Antilirium	Physostigmine	Axid	Nizatidine
Antiminth	Pyrantel Pamoate	Azactam	Aztreonam
Antivert	Meclizine (meclozine)	Azaline	Salazosulfapyridine =
Antrizine	Meclizine (meclozine)		sulfasalazine
Anturan	Sulfinpyrazone	Azanin	Azathioprine
Anzemet	Dolasetron	Azlin	Azlocillin
Aparkane	Trihexiphenidyl	Azmacort	Triamcinolone
Apaurin	Diazepam	Azmacort	Triamcinolone aceto-
Apocretin	Etilefrine		nide
Aprazone	Sulfinpyrazone	Azolid	Phenylbutazone
Apresoline	Hydralazine	Azulfidine	Salazosulfapyridine =
Aprobal	Alprenolol		sulfasalazine
Aprozide	Hydrochlorothiazide	Azulfdine	Sulfasalazine
Aptine	Alprenolol		
Aralen	Chloroquine	**B**	
Arava	Leflunomide		
Arduan	Pipecuronium	Baciguent	Bacitracin
Arfonad	Trimethaphan	Bactidan	Enoxacin

Bactocill	Oxacillin	Bromo-Seltzer	Paracetamol = acetami-nophen
Bactrim	Cotrimoxazole	Bronalide	Flunisolide
Barbita	Phenobarbital	Bronchaid	Epinephrine
Baxedin	Chlorhexidine	Bronchopront	Ambroxol
Bay-Bee	Vit. B12	Bronkodyl	Theophylline
Baycol	Cerivastatin	Bronkosol	Isoetharine
Bayotensin	Nitrendipine	Broxalax	Bisacodyl
Baypress	Nitrendipine	Bumex	Bumetanide
Beclovent	Beclomethasone	Bunitrolol	Bumetanide
Beconase	Beclomethasone	Buprene	Buprenorphine
Becotide	Beclomethasone	Burinex	Bumetanide
Bedoz	Cyanocobalamine	Buscopan	N-Butyl-scopolamine
Bedriol	Bifonazole	Buspar	Buspirone
Bee Six	Vit. B6 Pyridoxine	Butagen	Phenylbutazone
Befizal	Bezafbrate	Butazolidin	Phenylbutazone
Benadryl	Diphenhydramine	Butylone	Pentobarbital
Benemid	Probenecid		
Berofor alpha 2	Interferon-a2	**C**	
Berotec	Fenoterol		
Berubigen	Vit. B12	C-Pak	Doxycycline
Bestcall	Cefmenoxime	Cabadon	Vit. B12
Betadran	Bupranolol	Calan	Verapamil
Betadrenol	Bupranolol	Calciferol	Vit.D
Betagon	Mepindolol	Calcimer	Calcitonin
Betalin 12	Vit. B12	Calcimux	Etidronate
Betaloc	Metoprolol	Calderol	Calcifediol
Betapen-VK	Pencillin V	Calsan	Calcium carbonate
Betoptic	Betaxolol	Calsynar	Calcitonin
Bextra	Bucindolol*	Caltidren	Carteolol
Bezalip	Bezafibrate	Caltrate	Calcium carbonate
Bezatol	Bezafibrate	Camoquin	Amodiaquine
Biaxin	Clarithromycin	Canesten	Clotrimazole
Bicillin	Benzathine-Penicillin G	Capastat	Capreomycin
Bicol	Bisacodyl	Capoten	Captopril
Biltricide	Praziquantel	Capramol	ε-Aminocaproic acid
Biogastrone	Carbenoxolone	Caprolin	Capreomycin
Bioplex	Carbenoxolone	Carafate	Sucralfate
Bisolvon	Bromhexine	Carbex	Selegeline
Bisorine	Isoetharine	Carbocaine	Mepivacaine
Black Draught	Senna	Carbolite	Lithium carbonate
Blenoxane	Bleomycin	Cardene	Nicardipine
Blocadren	Timolol	Cardioqin	Quinidine
Bofedrol	Ephedrine	Cardiorhythmino	Ajmaline
Bolvidon	Mianserin	Cardizem	Diltiazem
Bonamine	Meclizine (meclozine)	Cardura	Doxazosin
Bonpyrin	Metamizol (= Dipyrone)	Carduran	Doxazosin
Bopen-VK	Pencillin V	Caridian	Mepindolol
Borotropin	Atropine	Carindapen	Carbenicillin
Brethine	Terbutalin	Carteol	Carteolol
Brevibloc	Esmolol	Catapres	Clonidine
Brevital	Methohexital	Cedocard	Isosorbide dinitrate
Bricanyl	Terbutalin	Cedur	Bezafibrate
Briclin	Amikacin		

CeeNu	Lomustine
Cefmax	Cefmenoxime
Cefobis	Cefmenoxime
Cefoperazone	Cefmenoxime
Ceftin	Cefuroxime axetil
Celevac	Methylcellulose
Celiomycin	Viomycine
CellCept	Mycophenolate Mofetil
Cellothyl	Methylcellulose
Cemix	Cefmenoxime
Centrax	Prazepam
Cepexin(A)	Cephalexin
Cephulac	Lactulose
Ceporex	Cephalexin
Cerebid	Papaverine
Cerebroxine	Vincamine
Cerespan	Papaverine
Cerubidine	Daunorubicin
Cesamet	Nabilone
Cesplon	Captopril
Cetamide	Sulfacetamide
Chenix	Chenodeoxycholic acid
Chlor-hex	Chlorhexidine
Chloraminophene	Chlorambucil
Chlorohist	Xylometazoline
Chloromycetin	Chloramphenicol
Chloroptic	Chloramphenicol
Cholestabyl	Colestipol
Cholestid	Colestipol
Choloxin	Thyroxine
Chorex	HCG (= chorionic gona-dotropin)
Choron	HCG (= chorionic gona-dotropin)
Chronulac	Lactulose
Cibacalcin	Calcitonin
Cidomycin	Gentamicin
Cillimycin	Lincomycin
Cimetrin	Erythromycin-propio-nate
Cin-Quin	Quinidine
Cipro	Ciprofloxacin
Ciprobay	Ciprofloxacin
Circupon	Etilefrine
Citanest	Prilocaine
Citrucel	Methylcellulose
Claforan	Cefotaxime
Clamoxyl	Amoxicillin
Claripex	Clofibrate
Claritin	Loratidine
Clasteon	Clodronate*
Cleocin	Clindamycin
Clobazam	Clindamycin

Clomid	Clomiphene
Clonopin	Clonazepam
Clont	Metronidazole
Clopra	Metoclopramide
Clotrimaderm	Clotrimazole
Cloxacillin	Clotrimazole
Clozan	Clotiazepam
Clozaril	Clozapine
Cobex	Vit. B12
Cocillin-VK	Pencillin V
Codelsol	Prednisolone
Codicept	Codeine
Cogentin	Benztropine
Cognex	Tacrine
Coleb	5-Isosorbide mono-nitrate
Colectril	Amiloride
Collyrium	Tetryzoline (= tetrahy-drozoline)
Cologel	Methylcellulose
Complamin	Xanthinol nicotinate
Comprecin	Enoxacin
Comtan	Entacapone*
Concor	Bisoprolol
Conducton	Carazolol
Constant-T	Theophylline
Contergan	Thalidomide
Coradus	Isosorbide dinitrate
Cordarex	Amiodarone
Cordarone	Amiodarone
Coreg	Carvedilol
Corgal	Gallopamil
Corgard	Nadolol
Coricidin	Oxymetazoline
Corindblan	Mepindolol
Corlopam	Fenoldopam
Coronex	Isosorbide dinitrate
Correctol	Phenolphthalein
Cortalone	Prednisolone
Cortate	Cortisol (Hydrocortiso-ne)
Cortef	Cortisol (Hydrocortiso-ne)
Cortelan	Cortisone
Cortenema	Cortisol (Hydrocortiso-ne)
Cortigel	Corticotropin
Cortogen	Cortisone
Cortone	Cortisone
Cortrophin	Corticotropin
Corvaton	Molsidomine
Coscopin	Noscapine (= Narcoti-ne)

Coscotab	Narcotine (= Noscapine)
Coscotab	Noscapine (= Narcotine)
Cosmegen	Actinomycin D
Coumadin	Warfarin
Coversum	Perindopril
Cozaar	Losartan
Crixivan	Indinavir
Cryspen	Penicillin G
Crystodigin	Digitoxin
Cuemid	Colestyramine
Cuprimine	D-Penicillamine
Cutivate	Fluticasone
Cuvalit	Lisuride
Cyanoject	Vit. B 12
Cyklocapron	Tranexamic acid
Cyomin	Vit. B 12
Cystospaz-M	Hyoscyamine sulfate
Cytomel	Triiodothyronine (= Liothyronine)
Cytosar	Cytarabine
Cytotec	Misoprostol
Cytovene	Ganciclovir
Cytoxan	Cyclophosphamide

D

D-Tabs	Cholecalciferol
D.E.H.45	Dihydroergotamine
DDAVP	Desmopressin
Dagenan	Sulfapyridine
Dalacin	Clindamycin
Dalcaine	Lidocaine
Dalmane	Flurazepam
Daneral	Pheniramine
Dantrium	Dantrolene
Daonil	Glibenclamide (= glyburide)
Daraprim	Pyrimethamine
Datril	Paracetamol = acetaminophen
Daunoblastin	Daunorubicin
Deca-Durabolin	Nandrolone
Decadron	Dexamethasone
Decapeptyl	Triptorelin
Decapryn	Doxylamine
Dedrogyl	Calcifediol
Degest-2	Naphazoline
Delapav	Papaverine
Delatestryl	Testosterone enantate
Delestrogen	Estradiol-valerate
Delta-Cortef	Prednisolone

Deltapen	Penicillin G
Deltastab	Prednisoloneduisolme
Demerol	Meperidine
Demerol	Pethidine = Meperidine
Denavir	Penciclovir
Dendrid	Idoxuridine
Depakene	Valproic Acid
Depen	D-Penicillamine
Depixol	Flupentixol
Depo-Provera	Medroxyprogesterone-acetate
Deprenyl	Selegeline
Deronil	Dexamethasone
Desferal	Deferoxamine
Desoxyn	Methamphetamine
Destolit	Ursodeoxycholic acid = ursodiol
Desuric	Benzbromarone
Desyrel	Trazodone
Detensiel	Bisoprolol
Detensol	Propranolol
Detrol	Tolteridine tartrate
Dexedrine	d-Amphetamine
Dey-Lute	Isoetharine
DiaBeta	Glibenclamide (= glyburide)
Diabex	Metformin
Diamox	Acetazolamide
Diapid	Lypressin
Diaqua	Hydrochlorothiazide
Diarsed	Diphenoxylate
Diastat	Diazepam
Dibenzyline	Phenoxybenzamine
Diclocil	Dicloxacillin
Diclophlogont	Diclofenac
Diflucan	Fluconazole
Digacin	Digoxin
Digibind	Digoxin immune FAB
Digicor	Digitoxin
Digimerck	Digitoxin
Digitaline	Digitoxin
Dihydergot	Dihydroergotamine
Dihyzin	Dihydralazine
Dilantin	Phenytoin
Dilaudid	Hydromorphone
Dimetab	Dimenhydrinate
Dinaplex	Flunarizine
Diodronel	Etidronate
Dioval	Estradiol-valerate
Diovan	Valsartan
Diphenasone	Dapsone
Diphos	Etidronate
Diprivan	Propofol

Distraneurin	Clomethiazole
Diuchlor	Hydrochlorothiazide
Divarine	Metamizol (= Dipyrone)
Divegal	Dihydroergotamine
Dixarit	Clonidine
Dizac	Diazepam
Dobutrex	Dobutamine
Dolantin	Pethidine = Meperidine
Dolophine	Methadone
Donnagel-MB	Kaolin + Pectin (= atta-pulgite)
Dopaidan	Levodopa
Dopamet	Methyl-Dopa
Dopar	Levodopa
Dopastat	Dopamine
Dopergin	Lisuride
Doral	Quazepam
Doryl	Carbachol
Dowmycin	Erythromycin-estolate
Doxicin	Doxycycline
Doxylamine	Doxycycline
Dramamine	Dimenhydrinate
Drisdol	Ergocalciferol Vit. D
Dristan	Oxymetazoline
Drogenil	Flutamide
Droleptan	Droperidol
Dulcolax	Bisacodyl
Duoralith	Lithium carbonate
Duphalac	Lactulose
Duracoron	Molsidomine
Duralutin	Hydroxyprogesterone caproate
Duramorph	Morphine sulfate
Duranest	Etidocaine
Duratest	Testosterone cypionate
Durazanil	Bromazepam
Durolax	Bisacodyl
Dymenate	Dimenhydrinate
DynaCirc	Isradipine
Dynapen	Dicloxacillin
Dynaprin	Imipramine
Dyneric	Clomiphene
Dyrenium	Triamterene

E

Econopred	Prednisolone
Enbrel	Etanercept
E-mycin	Erythomcyin
Ecostatin	Econazole
Ecotrin	Acetylsalicylic acid
Edecrin	Ethacrynic acid
Efedron	Ephedrine

Effectin	Bitolterol
Effexor	Venlafaxine
Effontil	Etilefrine
Effortil	Etilefrine
Effudex	5-Fluorouracil
Effurix	5-Fluorouracil
Elantan	5-Isosorbide mono-nitrate
Elavil	Amitriptyline
Eldepryl	Selegeline
Elimite	Permethrin
Elixophyllin	Theophylline
Emcor	Bisoprolol
Emex	Metoclopramide
Endak	Carteolol
Endep	Amitriptyline
Endophleban	Dihydroergotamine
Endoxan	Cyclophosphamide
Enoram	Enoxacin
Enovil	Amitriptyline
Entromone	HCG (= chorionic gona-dotropin)
Entrophen	Acetylsalicylic acid
EpiPen	Epinephrine
Epifin	Epinephrine
Epimorph	Morphine sulfate
Epinal	Epinephrine
Epitol	Carbamazepine
Epitrate	Epinephrine
Epivir	Lamivudine (3TC)
Epogen	Erythropoietin (= epoe-tin alfa)
Eporal	Dapsone
Ergocalm	Lormetazepam
Ergomar	Ergotamine
Ergotrate	Ergonovine
Ergotrate Maleate	Ergometrine (= Ergono-vine)
Eridan	Diazepam
Ermalate	Ergometrine (= Ergono-vine)
Eryc	Erythromcyin
Erymycin	Erythromycin-stearate
Erythrocin	Erythromycin-estolate
Erythromid	Erythomcyin
Esidrex	Hydrochlorothiazide
Eskalith	Lithium carbonate
Espotabs	Phenolphthalein
Estinyl	Ethinylestradiol
Estrace	Estradiol
Ethrane	Enflurane
Ethyl Adrianol	Etilefrine
Etibi	Ethambutol

Euciton	Domperidone*
Eudemine	Diazoxide
Euglucon	Glibenclamide (= glyburide)
Euhypnos	Temazepam
Eulexin	Flutamide
Eunal	Lisuride
Evac-U-Lax	Phenolphthalein
Evac-U-gen	Phenolphthalein
Everone	Testosterone enantate
Evipal	Hexobarbital
Evista	Raloxifene
Evoxin	Domperidone*
Ex-Lax	Phenolphthalein

F

F-Cortef	Fludrocortisone
Fabrol	Acetylcysteine
Factrel	Gonadorelin
Fansidar	Pyrimethamine + Sulfadoxine
Fasigyn(CH)	Tinidazol
Faverin	Fluvoxamine
Felbatol	Felbamate
Felden	Piroxicam
Femazole	Metronidazole
Feminone	Ethinylestradiol
Femogex	Estradiol-valerate
Femotrone	Progesterone
Fertodur	Cyclofenil
Feverall	Metamizol (= Dipyrone)
Fiblaferon 3	Interferon-b
Fibocil	Aprindine
Flagyl	Metronidazole
Flavoquine	Amodiaquine
Flaxedil	Gallamine
Fletcher's Castoria	Senna
Flixonase	Fluticasone
Flonase	Fluticasone
Florinef	Fludrocortisone
Flovent	Fluticasone
Floxifral	Fluvoxamine
Fluagel	Aluminium hydroxide
Fluanxol	Flupentixol
Fluclox	Flucloxacillin
Flugeral	Flunarizine
Fluothane	Halothane
Foldine	Folic acid
Folex	Methotrexate
Follutein	HCG (= chorionic gonadotropin)
Folvite	Folic acid

Fontego	Bumetanide
Forane	Isoflurane
Fordiuran	Bumetanide
Fortaz	Ceftazidime
Fortovase	Saquinavir
Fortral	Pentazocine
Fortum	Ceftazidime
Fosamax	Alendronate
Foscavir	Foscarnet
Fragmin	Dalteparin
Fraxiparine	Nadroparin*
Frisium	Clobazam
Fulvicin	Griseofulvin
Fungilin	Amphotericin B
Fungizone	Amphotericin B
Fusid	Furosemide

G

Gabitril	Tiagabine
Gabren(e)	Progabide
Gamazole	Sulfamethoxazole
Ganal	Fenfluramine
Ganphen	Promethazine
Gantanol	Sulfamethoxazole
Gantrisin	Sulfisoxazole
Garamycin	Gentamicin
Gardenal	Phenobarbital
Gas. X	Simethicone
Gastrozepin	Pirenzepine
Gelafundin	Gelatin-colloids
Genna	Senna
Gentle Nature	Senna
Geopen	Carbenicillin
Gestafortin	Chlormadinone acetate
Gesterol L.A.	Hydroxyprogesterone caproate
Gilurytmal	Ajmaline
Glaupax	Acetazolamide
Glucophage	Metformin
Glucotrol	Glipizide
Gonic	HCG (= chorionic gonadotropin)
Gramoderm	Gramicidin
Grisovin	Griseofulvin
Gubernal	Alprenolol
Gulfasin	Sulfisoxazole
Gumbix	Aminomethylbenzoic acid
Gyne-Lotrimin	Clotrimazole
Gynergen	Ergotamine
Gyno-Pevaryl	Econazole
Gyno-Travogen	Isoconazole

H

Haemaccel	Gelatin-colloids
Halcion	Triazolam
Haldol	Haloperidol
Halfan	Halofantrine
Hemineurin	Clomethiazole
Hepalean	HCG (= chorionic gona-dotropin)
Heparin	HCG (= chorionic gona-dotropin)
Herplex	Idoxuridine
Hespan	Hetastarch Hydroxy-ethyl starch (HES)
Hexa-Betalin	Pyridoxine Vit. B6
Hexadrol	Dexamethasone
Hexit	Chlorhexidine
Hidroferol	Calcifediol
Hismanal	Astemizole
Hivid	Zalcitabine
Honvol	Diethylstilbestrol
Humalog	Insulin
Humatin	Paromomycin
Humulin	Insulin
Hybolin Decanoate	
	Nandrolone
Hydeltrasol	Prednisolone
Hyderm	Cortisol (Hydrocortiso-ne)
Hydromal	Hydrochlorothiazide
Hydromedin	Ethacrynic acid
Hydrotricin	Tyrothricin
Hygroton	Chlorthalidone
Hylutin	Hydroxyprogesterone caproate
Hymorphan	Hydromorphone
Hyocort	Cortisol (Hydrocortiso-ne)
Hyoscin-N-Butyl-bromid	N-Butyl-scopolamine
Hyperstat	Diazoxide
Hypertensin	Angiotensin II
Hypertil	Captopril
Hypnosedon	Flunitrazepam*
Hyroxon	Hydroxyprogesterone caproate
Hyskon	Dextran
Hytrin	Terazosin

I

I-Pilopine	Pilocarpine
Ifex	Ifosfamide
Ifosfamide	Idoxuridine
Iktorivil	Clonazepam
Iletin	Insulin
Ilosone	Erythromycin-estolate
Imitrex	Sumatriptan
Imodium	Loperamide
Imovane	Zopiclone
Impril	Imipramine
Imuran	Azathioprine
Imurek	Azathioprine
Inapsine	Droperidol
Inderal	Propranolol
Indocid	Indomethacin
Indocin	Indomethacin
Indome	Indomethacin
Inflamase	Prednisolonechnisolove
Inhibace	Cilazapril
Inhiston	Pheniramine
Innohep	Tinzaparin*
Innovar	Fentanyl + Droperidol
Inocor	Amrinone
Insommal	Diphenhydramine
Intal	Cromoglycate
Integriline	Eptifibatide
Intron A	Interferon-a2b
Intropin	Dopamine
Invirase	Saquinavir
Isicom	Carbidopa + Levodopa
Ismelin	Guanethidine
Ismo	5-Isosorbide mono-nitrate
Isocaine	Mepivacaine
Isoptin	Verapamil
Isopto-Carpine	Pilocarpine
Isordil	Isosorbide dinitrate
Isotamine	Isoniazid
Isoten	Bisoprolol
Isotol	Mannitol
Isuprel	Isoprenaline (= Isopro-terenol)
Itrop	Ipratropium

J

Janimine	Imipramine

K

Kabikinase	Streptokinase
Kabolin	Nandrolone
Kanrenol	Canrenone
Kantrex	Kanamycin

Kaopectate	Kaolin + Pectin (= attapulgite)	Lescol	Noradrenalin (= Norepinephrine)
Kaopectate II	Loperamide	Levoprome	Levomepromazine
Karil	Calcitonin	Levsin	Hyoscyamine sulfate
Keflex	Cefalexin	Lexotan	Bromazepam
Keflex	Cephalexin	Lidopen	Lidocaine
Keftab	Cefalexin	Likuden	Griseofulvin
Kemadrin	Procyclidine	Lincocin	Lincomycin
Kenacort	Triamcinolone	Lindane	Hexachlorophane
Kenalog	Triamcinolone acetonide	Lioresal	Baclofen
		Lipitor	Atorvastatin
Kenalone	Triamcinolone acetonide	Liquamar	Phenprocoumon
		Liquemin	HCG (= chorionic gonadotropin)
Kerecid	Idoxuridine		
Kerlone	Betaxolol	Litec	Pizotifen = Pizotyline
Kertasin	Etilefrine	Lithane	Lithium carbonate
Ketalar	Ketamine	Lithobid	Lithium carbonate
Ketzol	Cefazolin	Lithotabs	Lithium carbonate
Key-Pred	Prednisolone	Lodine	Etodolac
Kildane	Lindane	Lomotil	Diphenoxylate
Klebcil	Kanamycin	Loniten	Minoxidil
Klot	Tolonium chloride	Looser	Bupranolol
Konakion	Phytomenadione	Lopantrol	Lorcainide
Korostatin	Nystatin	Lopid	Gemfibrozil
Kryptocur	Gonadorelin	Lopirin	Captopril
Kwell	Lindane	Lopressor	Metoprolol
Kytril	Granisetron	Loramet	Lormetazepam
		Loraz	Lorazepam
L		Lorinal	Chloralhydrate
		Lorivox	Lorcainide
Lacril	Methylcellulose	Losec	Omeprazole
Lamiazid	Isoniazid	Losporal	Cephalexin
Lamictal	Lamotrigine	Lotensin	Benazepril
Lampren	Clofazimine	Lovelco	Probucol
Lanacillin	Penicillin G	Lovenox	Enoxaparin
Lanacillin-VK	Penicillin V	Lozide	Indapamide
Lanicor	Digoxin	Lozol	Indapamide
Lanoxin	Digoxin	Ludiomil	Maprotiline
Largactil	Chlorpromazine	Lupron	Leuprorelide
Lariam	Mefloquine	Luvox	Fluvoxamine
Larodopa	Levodopa	Lynoral	Ethinylestradiol
Lasix	Furosemide	Lyophrin	Epinephrine
Laxanin	Bisacodyl	Lysenyl	Lisuride
Laxbene	Bisacodyl		
Lectopam	Bromazepam	**M**	
Ledercillin VK	Pencillin V		
Ledercort(CH)	Triamcinolone	Macrobin	Clostebol
Lembrol	Diazepam	Madopar	Levodopa + Benserazide
Lendorm(A)	Brotizolam		
Lendormin	Brotizolam	Madopar (plus Levodopa)	
Lenoxin	Digoxin		Benserazide
Lentin	Carbachol	Malgesic	Phenylbutazone
		Mallergan	Promethazine

Marcumar	Phenprocoumon
Marinol	Dronabinol
Marmine	Dimenhydrinate
Marvelon	Desogestrel + Ethinyle-stradiol
Mavik	Trandolapril
Maxeran	Metoclopramide
Maxolan	Metoclopramide
Mazepine	Carbamazepine
Mazonor	Mazindol
Meclomen	Meclofenamate
Mefoxin	Cefoxitin
Megacillin	Benzathine-Penicillin G
Megaphen	Chlorpromazine
Melipramin	Imipramine
Menophase	Mestranol
Mercazol	Thiamazole (= Methi-mazole)
Mesnex	Mesna
Mestinon	Pyridostigmine
Metacen	Indomethacin
Metahydrin	Trichlormethiazide
Metalone	Prednisolone
Metandren	Methyltestosterone
Metaprel	Metaproterenol
Metenarin	Methylcellulose
Methadose	Methadone
Methampex	Methamphetamine
Methanoxanol	Sulfamethoxazole
Methofane	Methoxyflurane
Methylergobrevin	Methylcellulose
Methylergometrine	
	Methylcellulose
Meticorten	Prednisone
Metilon	Metamizol (= Dipyrone)
Metreton	Prednisolone
Metronid	Metronidazole
Mevacor	Lovastatin
Meval	Diazepam
Mevaril	Amitriptyline
Mevinacor	Lovastatin
Mexate	Methotrexate
Mexitil	Mexiletin
Mezlin	Mezlocillin
Micatin	Miconazole
Micronase	Glibenclamide (= gly-buride)
Micronor	Norethisterone
Microsulfon	Sulfadiazine
Midamor	Amiloride
Mielucin	Busulfan
Migril	Ergotamine
Minipress	Prazosin

Minirin	Desmopressin
Minocin	Minocycline
Minprog	Alprostadil (= PGE1)
Minprostin F2a	Dinoprost
Mintezol	Thiabendazole
Miocarpine	Pilocarpine
Miostat	Carbachol
Mithracin	Mithramycin, Plicamy-cin
Mitosan	Busulfan
Mobenol	Tolbutamide
Modane	Phenolphthalein
Moditen	Fluphenazine
Moduret	Amilorid + Hydrochlo-rothiazide
Mogadon	Nitrazepam
Molsidolat	Molsidomine
Monistat	Miconazole
Monitan	Acebutolol
Monomycin	Erythromycin-succina-te
Monopril	Fosinopril
Moronal	Amphotericin B
Morphitec	Morphine hydrochlori-de
Mosegor	Pizotifen = Pizotyline
Motilium	Domperidone*
Motrin	Ibuprofen
Moxacin	Amoxicillin
Mucomyst	Acetylcysteine
Mucosolvan	Ambroxol
Murine	Tetryzoline (= tetrahy-drozoline)
Murocel	Methylcellulose
Mustargen	Mechlorethamine
Mutabase	Diazoxide
Myambutol	Ethambutol
Mycelex	Clotrimazole
Mycifradin	Neomycin
Myciguent	Neomycin
Mycobutin	Rifabutin
Mycospor	Bifonazole
Mycosporan	Bifonazole
Mycostatin	Nystatin
Mydral	Tropicamide
Mydriacyl	Tropicamide
Myidone	Primidone
Mykinac	Nystatin
Myleran	Busulfan
Mylicon	Simethicone
Myobid	Papaverine
Mysoline	Primidone

N

Nacom	Carbidopa + Levodopa
Nadopen-V	Pencillin V
Naftin	Naftifin
Nalador	Sulprostone
Nalcrom	Cromoglycate
Nalfon	Fenoprofen
Nalgesic	Fenoprofen
Nalorex	Naltrexone
Naprosyn	Naproxen
Naqua	Trichlormethiazide
Narcan	Naloxone
Narcaricin	Benzbromarone
Narcozep	Flunitrazepam*
Narkotan	Halothane
Nasalide	Flunisolide
Natrilix	Indapamide
Natulan	Procarbazine
Nautamine	Diphenhydramine
Nauzelin	Domperidone*
Navidrix	Cyclopenthiazide
Naxen	Naproxen
Nebcin	Tobramycin
Negram	Nalidixic acid
Nembutal	Pentobarbital
Neo Epinin	Isoprenaline (= Isoproterenol)
Neo-Codema	Hydrochlorothiazide
Neo-Mercazole	Carbimazole
Neo-Synephrine	Oxymetazoline
Neo-Thyreostat	Carbimazole
Neogel	Carbenoxolone
Neoral	Cyclosporine
Neosynephrine II	Xylometazoline
Nepresol	Dihydralazine
Netromycin	Netilmicin
Neurontin	Gabapentin
Niclocide	Niclosamide
Nigalax	Bisacodyl
Nilstat	Nystatin
Nilurid	Amiloride
Nimotop	Nimodipine
Nipride	Nitroprusside sodium
Nitrocap	Glyceryltrinitrate (= nitroglycerin)
Nitrogard	Glyceryltrinitrate (= nitroglycerin)
Nitroglyn	Glyceryltrinitrate (= nitroglycerin)
Nitrolingual	Glyceryltrinitrate (= nitroglycerin)
Nitrong	Glyceryltrinitrate (= nitroglycerin)
Nitropress	Nitroprusside sodium
Nitrostat	Glyceryltrinitrate (= nitroglycerin)
Nix	Permethrin
Nizoral	Ketoconazol
Noan	Diazepam
Noctamid	Lormetazepam
Noctec	Chloralhydrate
Nogram	Nalidixic acid
Noludar	Methylprylon
Nolvadex	Tamoxifen
Nor-Q D	Norethindrone
Norcuron	Vecuronium
Norlutin	Norethindrone
Normiflo	Ardeparin
Normodyne	Labetalol
Normurat	Benzbromarone
Noroxin	Norfloxacin
Norpace	Disopyramide
Norpramin	Desipramine
Norquen	Mestranol
Norval	Mianserin
Norvir	Ritonavir
Novalgin	Metamizol (= Dipyrone)
Novamin	Amikacin
Novamoxin	Amoxicillin
Novantrone	Mitoxantrone
Novarectal	Pentobarbital
NovoNorm	Repaglinide
Novocaine	Procaine
Novoclopate	Clorazepate
Novodigoxin	Digoxin
Novolin	Insulin
Novomedopa	Methyl-Dopa
Novopen-VK	Pencillin V
Novopurol	Allopurinol
Novorythro	Erythromycin-estolate
Novosalmol	Salbutamol (= Albuterol)
Novotrimel	Cotrimoxazole
Nozinan	Levomepromazine
Nu-Cal	Calcium carbonate
Nubain	Nalbuphine
Nulicaine	Lidocaine
Nuprin	Ibuprofen
Nuran	Cyproheptadine
Nuromax	Doxacurium
Nydrazid	Isoniazid
Nystex	Nystatin
Nytilax	Senna

O

O-V Statin	Nystatin
Octapressin	Felypressin
Oculinum	Botulinum Toxin Type A
Ocupress	Carteolol
Omifin	Clomiphene
Omnipen	Amphotericin B
Oncovin	Vincristine
Ondena	Daunorubicin
Ondogyne	Cyclofenil
Ondonid	Cyclofenil
Ophthosol	Bromhexine
Opticrom	Cromoglycate
Optipranolol	Metipranolol
Oragest	Medroxyprogesterone-acetate
Oramide	Tolbutamide
Orasone	Prednisone
Oretic	Hydrochlorothiazide
Organan	Danaparoid
Orinase	Tolbutamide
Orthoclone OKT3	Muromonab-CD3
Osmitrol	Mannitol
Ospolot	Sulthiame
Ossiten	Clodronate*
Ostac	Clodronate*
Ovastol	Mestranol
Oxistat	Oxiconazole
Oxpam	Oxazepam

P

POR 8	Ornipressin
Pamba	Aminomethylbenzoic acid
Pamelor	Nortriptyline
Panasol	Prednisone
Panimit	Bupranolol
Pantolac	Pantoprazole*
Panwarfin	Warfarin
Papacon	Papaverine
Paralgin	Metamizol (= Dipyrone)
Paraplatin	Carboplatin
Paraxin	Chloramphenicol
Parcillin	Penicillin G
Paregoric	Opium Tincture (laudanum)
Parlodel	Bromocriptine
Parnate	Tranylcypromine
Paromomycin	Paracetamol = acetaminophen

Parsitan	Ethopropazine
Parsitol	Ethopropazine
Partergin	Methylcellulose
Partusisten	Fenoterol
Parvolex	Acetylcysteine
Pathocil	Dicloxacillin
Pavabid	Papaverine
Pavadur	Papaverine
Paveral	Codeine
Pavulon	Pancuronium
Paxil	Paroxetine
Pectokay	Kaolin + Pectin (= attapulgite)
Pediapred	Prednisolone
Pemavit	Vit. B12
Penapar VK	Penicillin V
Penbec-V	Penicillin V
Penbritin	Amphotericin B
Pensorb	Penicillin G
Pentanca	Pentobarbital
Pentasa	Mesalamine
Pentazine	Promethazine
Penthrane	Methoxyflurane
Pentids	Penicillin G
Pentothal	Thiopental
Pepcid	Famotidine
Pepdul	Famotidine
Pepto-Bismol	Bismuth subsalicylate
Peptol	Cimetidine
Pergotime	Clomiphene
Periactin	Cyproheptadine
Peridon	Domperidone*
Peritol	Cyproheptadine
Permanone	Permethrin
Permapen	Penicillin G
Permax	Pergolide
Pertofran	Desipramine
Petinimid	Ethosuximide
Pfizerpin	Penicillin G
Phazyme	Simethicone
Phenazine	Promethazine
Phenergan	Promethazine
Phospholine Iodide	
	Ecothiopate
Physoseptone	Methadone
Pilokair	Pilocarpine
Pipracil	Piperacillin
Pitocin	Oxytocin
Pitressin	ADH (= Vasopressin)
Pitrex	Tolnaftate
Plak-out	Chlorhexidine
Plaquenil	Hydroxychloroquine
Platinex	Cisplatin

Platinol	Cisplatin
Plavix	Clopidogrel
Plendil	Felodipine
Polycillin	Amphotericin B
Ponderal	Fenfluramine
Pondimin	Fenfluramine
Pontocaine	Tetracaine
Posicor	Mibefradil
Prandin	Repaglinide
Pravachol	Pravastatin
Pravidel	Bromocriptine
Predate	Prednisolone
Predcor	Prednisolone
Precose	Acarbose
Pregnesin	HCG (= chorionic gonadotropin)
Pregnyl	HCG (= chorionic gonadotropin)
Prelone	Prednisolone
Prenormine	Atenolol
Prepidil	Dinoprostone
Presinol	Methyl-Dopa
Pressunic	Dihydralazine
Presyn	ADH (= Vasopressin)
Prevacid	Lansoprazole
Primacor	Milrinone
Primaquine	Primaquine
Principen	Amphotericin B
Prinivil	Lisinopril
Privine	Naphazoline
Pro-Depo	Hydroxyprogesterone caproate
Probalan	Probenecid
Procan SR	Procainamide
Procardia	Nifedipine
Procorum	Gallopamil
Procytox	Cyclophosphamide
Profasi	HCG (= chorionic gonadotropin)
Progestasert	Progesterone
Proglicem	Diazoxide
Prograf	Tacrolimus
Progynon B	Estradiol-benzoate
Progynova	Estradiol-valerate
Proklar	Sulfamethizole
Prolixan	Azapropazone
Prolixin	Fluphenazine
Prolopa	Levodopa + Benserazide
Proloprim	Trimethoprim
Prometh	Promethazine
Promine	Procainamide
Pronestyl	Procainamide

Propasa	5-Aminosalicylic acid
Propecia	Finasteride
Propulsid	Cisapride
Propyl-Thyracil	Propylthiouracil
Prorex	Promethazine
Proscar	Finasteride
Prostaphlin	Oxacillin
Prostarmon	Dinoprost
Prostigmin	Neostigmine
Prostin E2	Dinoprostone
Prostin F2	Dinoprost
Prostin VR	Alprostadil (= PGE1)
Protostat	Metronidazole
Protrin Septra	Cotrimoxazole
Proventil	Salbutamol (= Albuterol)
Provigan	Promethazine
Proviron	Mesterolone
Prozac	Fluoxetine
Prulet	Phenolphthalein
Pulmicort	Budesonide
Pulsamin	Etilefrine
Purinethol	6-Mercaptopurine
Purodigin	Digitoxin
Pyopen	Carbenicillin
Pyrilax	Bisacodyl
Pyronoval	Acetylsalicylic acid
Pyroxine	Pyridoxine, Vit. B6

Q

Quelicin	Succinylcholine
Questran	Colestyramine
Quibron-T	Theophylline
Quinachlor	Chloroquine
Quinalan	Quinidine
Quinaminoph	Quinine
Quinamm	Quinine
Quine	Quinine
Quinidex	Quinidine
Quinite	Quinine
Quinora	Quinidine

R

RU 486	Mifepristone
ReQuip	Ropinirole*
Rebetol	Ribavirin
Reclomide	Metoclopramide
Rectocort	Cortisol (Hydrocortisone)
Redisol	Vit. B12
Refludan	Lepirudin

Refobacin	Gentamicin
Regitin	Phentolamine
Reglan	Metoclopramide
Regonol	Pyridostigmine
Relefact	Gonadorelin
Remicade	Infliximab
Remivox	Lorcainide
Remsed	Promethazine
Renoquid	Sulfacytine
ReoPro	Abciximab
Reomax	Ethacrynic acid
Rescriptor	Delavirdine
Restoril	Temazepam
Retardin	Diphenoxylate
Retrovir	Azidothymidine, Zido-vudine
Reverin	Rolitetracyclin
Revia	Naltrexone
Rezipas	5-Aminosalicylic acid
Rezulin	Troglitazone
Rhinalar	Flunisolide
Rhumalgan	Diclofenac
Rhythmin	Procainamide
Rhythmol	Propafenone
Ridaura	Auranofin
Rifadin	Rifampin
Rimactan	Rifampin
Rimifon	Isoniazid
Ritalin	Methylphenidate
Rivotril	Clonazepam
Rize	Clotiazepam
Roaccutan	Isotretinoin
Robinul	Glycopyrrolate
Rocaltrol	Calcitriol
Rocephin	Ceftriaxone
Roferon A3	Interferon-a2a
Rogaine	Minoxidil
Rogitin	Phentolamine
Rohypnol	Flunitrazepam*
Rolisox	Isoxsuprine
Romazicon	Flumazenil
Rovamycin	Spiramicin
Rowasa	Mesalamine
Roxanol	Moiphine sulfate
Rubesol	Vit. B12
Rubion	Cyanocobalamin
Rubramin	Cyanocobalamin
Rulid	Roxithromycin
Ryegonovin	Methylcellulose
Rynacrom	Cromoglycate
Rythmodan	Disopyramide

S

S.A.S.-500	Salazosulfapyridine = sulfasalazine
Sabril	Vigabatrin*
Salazopyrin	Salazosulfapyridine = sulfasalazine
Salimid	Cyclopenthiazide
Saltucin	Butizid
Sandimmune	Cyclosporine
Sandomigran	Pizotifen = Pizotyline
Sandostatin	Octreotide
Sandril	Reserpine
Sang-35	Cyclosporine
Sanocrisin	Cyclofenil
Sanodin	Carbenoxolone
Sanorex	Mazindol
Sansert	Methysergide
Satric	Metronidazole
Saventrine	Isoprenaline (= Isopro-terenol)
Scabene	Lindane
Sebcur	Salicylic acid
Sectral	Acebutolol
Securopen	Azlocillin
Seguril	Furosemide
Seldane	Terfenadine
Selectomycin	Spiramicin
Sembrina	Methyl-Dopa
Senokot	Senna
Senolax	Senna
Serax	Oxazepam
Serenace	Haloperidol
Serevent	Sameterol
Serlect	Sertindole*
Sernyl	Phencyclidine
Serono-Bagren	Bromocriptine
Serophene	Clomiphene
Serpalan	Reserpine
Serpasil	Reserpine
Sertan	Primidone
Sexovid	Cyclofenil
Sibelium	Flunarizine
Silain	Simethicone
Simplene	Epinephrine
Simplotan	Tinidazol
Simulect	Basiliximab
Sinarest	Oxymetazoline
Sinemet	Levodopa + Carbidopa
Sinequan	Doxepin
Singulair	Montelukast
Sintrom	Acenocoumarin (= Ni-coumalone)

Sinutab	Xylometazoline
Sirtal	Carbamazepine
Sito-Lande	Sitosterol
Skleromexe	Clofibrate
Slo-bid	Theophylline
Sobelin	Clindamycin
Sofarin	Warfarin
Soldactone	Canrenone
Solfoton	Phenobarbital
Solganal	Aurothioglucose
Solu-Contenton	Amantadine
Soluver	Salicylic acid
Somnos	Chloralhydrate
Somophyllin-T	Theophylline
Sopamycetin	Chloramphenicol
Soprol	Bisoprolol
Sorbitrate	Isosorbide dinitrate
Sorquetan	Tinidazol
Sotacor	Sotalol
Spametrin-M	Methylcellulose
Spersadex	Dexamethasone
Spersanicol	Chloramphenicol
Spirocort	Budesonide
Sporanox	Itroconazole
Sprecur	Buserelin
Statex	Morphine sulfate
Stelazine	Trifluoperazine
Steranabol	Clostebol
Stimate	Desmopressin
Stoxil	Idoxuridine
Strepolin	Streptomycin
Streptase	Streptokinase
Streptosol	Streptomycin
Stresson	Bumetanide
Suacron	Carazolol
Sublimaze	Fentanyl
Succostrin	Succinylcholine
Sufenta	Sufentanil
Sulair	Sulfacetamide
Sulamyd	Sulfacetamide
Sular	Nisoldipine
Sulcrate	Sucralfate
Sulfabutin	Busulfan
Sulfex	Sulfacetamide
Sulmycin	Gentamicin
Sulpyrin	Metamizol (= Dipyrone)
Sulten	Sulfacetamide
Supasa	Acetylsalicylic acid
Suprarenin	Epinephrine
Suprax	Cefixime
Suprefact	Buserelin
Surfactal	Ambroxol
Sustaine	Xylometazoline
Sustaire	Theophylline
Suxinutin	Ethosuximide
Symmetrel	Amantadine
Synatan	d-Amphetamine
Synkayvit	Menadione
Synovir	Thalidomide
Syntocinon	Oxytocin
Sytobex	Hydroxocobalamin
Sytobex	Vit. B12

T

Tacef	Cefmenoxime
Tacicef	Ceftazidime
Tagamet	Cimetidine
Talwin	Pentazocine
Tambocor	Flecainide
Tamofen	Tamoxifen
Tapazole	Methimazole
Tapazole	Thiamazole (= Methimazole)
Taractan	Chlorprothixene
Tarasan	Chlorprothixene
Tardigal	Digitoxin
Tardocillin	Benzathine-Penicillin G
Tarivid	Ofloxacin
Tasmar	Tolcapone
Tavist	Clemastine
Taxol	Paclitaxel
Taxotere	Docetaxel
Tebrazid	Pyrazinamide
Teebaconin	Isoniazid
Tegison	Etretinate
Tegopen	Clotrimazole
Tegretol	Carbamazepine
Telemin	Bisacodyl
Temgesic	Buprenorphine
Tempra	Paracetamol = acetaminophen
Tenalin	Carteolol
Tenex	Guanfacine
Tenormin	Atenolol
Tensium	Diazepam
Tensobon	Captopril
Testex	Testosterone propionate
Testoject	Testosterone cypionate
Testone	Testosterone enantate
Testred	Methyltestosterone
Teveten	Eprosartan
Theelol	Estratriol = Estriol
Theolair	Theophylline
Thesit	Polidocanol

Thiotepa Lederle	Thio-TEPA
Thorazine	Chlorpromazine
Thrombinar	Thrombin
Thrombostat	Thrombin
Ticar	Ticarcillin
Ticlid	Ticlopidine
Tienor	Clotiazepam
Tigason	Etretinate
Tilade	Nedocromil
Timonil	Carbamazepine
Timoptic	Timolol
Tinactin	Tolnaftate
Tinset	Oxatomide
Toazul	Tolonium chloride
Tobrex	Tobramycin
Tofranil	Imipramine
Tolectin	Tolmetin
Tomabef	Cefmenoxime
Tonocard	Tocainide
Topamex	Topiramate
Topitracin	Bacitracin
Toposar	Etoposide
Toradol	Ketorolac
Tornalate	Bitolterol
Totacillin	Amphotericin B
Tracrium	Atracurium
Tramal	Tramadol
Trandate	Labetalol
Trans-Ver-Sal	Salicylic acid
Transcycline	Rolitetracyclin
Transderm Scop	Scopolamine
Tranxene	Clorazepate
Tranxilium N	Nor-Diazepam
Trapanal	Thiopental
Trasicor	Oxprenolol
Travogen	Isoconazole
Trecalmo	Clotiazepam
Trecator	Ethionamide
Tremblex	Dexetimide
Tremin	Trihexiphenidyl
Trendar	Ibuprofen
Trental	Pentoxifylline
Trexan	Naltrexone
Triadapin	Doxepin
Trialodine	Trazodone
Triam-A	Triamcinolone aceto-nide
Triamterene	Triamcinolone aceto-nide
Trichlorex	Trichlormethiazide
Tricor	Fenofibrate*
Trihexane	Trihexiphenidyl
Trimpex	Trimethoprim

Trimysten	Clotrimazole
Triostat	Liothyronine
Triptone	Scopolamine
Trobicin	Spectinomycin
Trusopt	Dorzolamide
Truxal	Chlorprothixene
Tubarine	d-Tubocurarine
Tylenol	Paracetamol = acetaminophen
Typramine	Imipramine
Tyzine	Tetryzoline (= tetrahydrozoline)

U

Udicil	Cytarabine
Udolac	Dapsone
Ukidan	Urokinase
Ulcolax	Bisacodyl
Ultair	Pranlukast*
Ultiva	Remifentanil
Ultracain	Articaine
Unicort	Cortisol (Hydrocortisone)
Uniphyl	Theophylline
Uricovac	Benzbromarone
Uritol	Furosemide
Uromitexan	Mesna
Urosin	Allopurinol
Ursofalk	Ursodeoxycholic acid = ursodiol

V

Va-tro-nol	Ephedrine
Valadol	Paracetamol = acetaminophen
Valium	Diazepam
Valorin	Paracetamol = acetaminophen
Valtrex	Valacyclovir
Vancocin	Vancomycin
Vancomycin CP Lilly	Vancomycin
Vaponefrine	Epinephrine
Vasal	Papaverine
Vasocon	Naphazoline
Vasodilan	Isoxsuprine
Vasopressin Sandoz	Lypressin
Vasoprine	Isoxsuprine
Vasotec	Enalapril
Vatran	Diazepam

VePesid	Etoposide
Vectrin	Minocycline
Vegesan	Nor-Diazepam
Velacycline	Rolitetracyclin
Velban	Vinblastine
Velbe	Vinblastine
Velosulin	Insulin
Venactone	Canrenone
Ventolin	Salbutamol (= Albuterol)
Veratran	Clotiazepam
Verelan	Verapamil
Vermox	Mebendazole
Versed	Midazolam
Viagra	Sildenafil
Vibal	Vit. B12
Vibramycin	Doxycycline
Videx	Didanosine (ddI)
Vigantol	Cholecalciferol
Vigorsan	Cholecalciferol
Vimicon	Cyproheptadine
Vinactane	Viomycine
Viocin	Viomycine
Vionactane	Viomycine
Viprinex	Ancrod
Vira-A	Vidarabine
Viracept	Nelfinavir
Viramune	Nevirapine
Virazole	Ribavirin
Virilon	Methyltestosterone
Virofral	Amantadine
Viroptic	Trifluridine
Visine	Tetryzoline (= tetrahydrozoline)
Visken	Pindolol
Vistacrom	Cromoglycate
Visutensil	Guanethidine
Vitrasert	Ganciclovir
Vivol	Diazepam
Volon	Triamcinolone
Voltaren	Diclofenac
Voltarol	Diclofenac
Vumon	Teniposide

W

Wellbatrin	Bupropion
Wellbutrin	Bupropion
Whevert	Meclizine (meclozine)
Wincoram	Amrinone
Wingom	Gallopamil
Winpred	Prednisone
Wyamycin	Erythromycin-estolate
Wytensin	Guanabenz

X

Xanax	Alprazolam
Xanef	Enalapril
Xatral	Alfuzosin
Xylocain	Lidocaine
Xylocard	Lidocaine
Xylonest	Prilocaine

Y

Yomesan	Niclosamide
Yutopar	Ritodrine

Z

Zaditen	Ketotifen
Zanaflex	Tizanidine
Zanosar	Streptozocin
Zantac	Ranitidine
Zapex	Oxazepam
Zarontin	Ethosuximide
Zebeta	Bisoprolol
Zemuron	Rocuronium
Zenapax	Daclizumab
Zepine	Reserpine
Zerit	Stavudine (d4T)
Zestril	Lisinopril
Ziagen	Abacavir*
Zimovane	Zopiclone
Zithromax	Azithromycin
Zocor	Simvastatin
Zofran	Ondansetron
Zoladex	Goserelin
Zovirax	Aciclovir
Zyflo	Zileuton
Zyloprim	Allopurinol
Zyloric	Allopurinol
Zyprexa	Olanzapine

Index